PRACTICAL LESSONS in PSYCHIATRY

By

JOSEPH L. FETTERMAN, M. D.

Director, The Fetterman Clinic, Cleveland, Ohio; Formerly, Assistant Clinical Professor of Nervous Diseases, Western Reserve University School of Medicine; Executive Officer, School of Military Neuropsychiatry; Ret. Diplomate, American Board of Neurology and Psychiatry

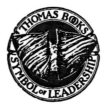

CHARLES C THOMAS • PUBLISHER
Springfield • Illinois

CHARLES C THOMAS · PUBLISHER
Bannerstone House
301-327 East Lawrence Avenue, Springfield, Illinois

Published simultaneously in The British Commonwealth of Nations by
Blackwell Scientific Publications, Ltd., Oxford, England

Published simultaneously in Canada by
The Ryerson Press, Toronto

This book is protected by copyright. No part of it may be duplicated or reproduced in any manner without written permission from the publisher.

Copyright, 1949, by Charles C Thomas · Publisher

FIRST EDITION

Printed in the United States of America

DEDICATION

To my patients who provided the experience which, through the medium of this book, may help other patients.

PREFACE

THIS book aims to present briefly several common neuropsychiatric disorders and the methods by which they are treated. The discussion of these conditions, the lessons which they furnish are based largely upon practical experience with patients. This accounts for the frequent excerpts from clinical case histories which are interspersed throughout the text. It also explains the choice of subject material which has been influenced primarily by personal interest and experience. To this experience the author has added the observations and ideas supplied by a large and extensive literature.

The material here presented in book form is an outgrowth of a series of lectures delivered to the student officers of the School of Military Neuropsychiatry during 1943 and 1944 and of seminars given in Cleveland during 1945 and 1946. I am grateful to my faculty colleagues and to the many student officers who participated in these courses for their contributions. I wish to mention especially Lieutenant Colonel James O'Leary, now Professor of Neurology at Washington University, St. Louis, Missouri.

A book of this kind is the product of combined operations and there are many to whom credit is due. One may start with the authors of textbooks and articles quoted in the references and others whose clinics and lectures have added ideas which are expressed throughout these pages. I have quoted freely from Strecker and Ebaugh's *Practical Clinical Psychiatry*, from Solomon and Yakovlev's *Manual of Military Neuropsychiatry*, from Lennox on epilepsy, from Alexander and French's recent book, *Psychoanalytic Therapy*, and from the writings of Freud.

I wish to thank the members of the staff of The Neuropsychiatric Institute of Cleveland for their contributions during the preparation of the manuscript. Drs. M. D. Friedman, A. A. Weil, Evelyn Katz, and Miss E. J. Wilson have read and offered suggestions to improve the material. These colleagues have supplied case histories for which they are credited in the text.

Several collaborators have been kind enough to review special chapters and to add material to these chapters or advise changes. I would like to express my appreciation to Dr. Foster Kennedy,

Professor of Neurology, Cornell University Medical College, who has checked and written an introductory note to the material on electrocoma therapy; to Dr. Abraham Myerson, Clinical Professor of Psychiatry, Harvard University, who reviewed the chapter on psychopathic personality and made constructive suggestions; to Dr. Claude S. Beck, Professor of Neurosurgery, Western Reserve University, who reviewed the chapter on trauma; to Dr. Frederic A. Gibbs, Associate Professor of Psychiatry, University of Illinois, College of Medicine, for his review of the chapter on epilepsy and the brief section on electroencephalography; to Dr. George W. Binkley, Assistant Clinical Professor of Dermatology and Syphilology, Western Reserve University, who made revisions of the chapter on neurosyphilis; and to Dr. Maurice B. Gordon, Clinical Director, Cleveland State Hospital, who collaborated in the preparation of the material on insulin coma therapy.

In the conversion of an early manuscript to a finished book, my appreciation goes to the publisher, Charles C Thomas, and to his staff for their constructive recommendations and their excellent bookmaking. My gratitude also goes to Miss Phyllis Grothe, who typed the first draft, and to Miss Gertrude E. Craine for the typing of revisions. Mrs. Mary T. Bernstein aided with proofreading and with the bibliography; Dr. Victor M. Victoroff and Virginia Victoroff helped to prepare the index.

The author hopes that this book will help towards a better understanding of these common neuropsychiatric conditions by the general practitioners and by that extensive group of allied workers such as nurses, psychologists, personnel advisers, and social workers who share in the responsibility of guiding those who are mentally ill.

Joseph L. Fetterman, M. D.

Cleveland, Ohio

CONTENTS

Preface vii

Chapter

    I. The Patient and His Personality 3

    II. Psychoneuroses 22

    III. Treatment of Psychoneuroses 58

    IV. Manic-Depressive Psychoses; with Particular Emphasis on Depressions 98

    V. Schizophrenias 127

    VI. Electrocoma Therapy of Psychoses 158

    VII. Psychopathic Personality and Other Abnormalities 204

    VIII. Toxic and Organic Psychoses 243

    IX. Neurosyphilis 258

    X. Epilepsy 280

    XI. The Physical and Mental Sequelae of Head Trauma 301

Index 331

PRACTICAL LESSONS
in
PSYCHIATRY

Chapter I

THE PATIENT AND HIS PERSONALITY

"OF ARMS and the man I sing" is the opening line of Virgil. We may paraphrase this into "of the patient and his sickness I write."

There are innumerable factors in the complex organization that is man. Each plays its role in determining the type of sickness, the symptoms, and the chances of recovery. It is not merely an injury, an infection that constitutes illness, it is also the man himself. What he is, how he reacts to success and failure, his goals, and drives and fears become interwoven in the pattern of symptoms of sickness. Let us therefore begin with a study of the innate factors, both physical and intellectual, and the environmental factors, of home, parents, education, illness and religion which influence personality.

The term personality is used freely to connote the type of the individual in relation to others. Hinsie and Shatzky liken it to a mask worn on the stage and define it as "the habitual patterns of the behavior of the individual in terms of physical and mental activities and attitudes." It is the essence of a man distilled from his energy and intelligence and attitude exhibited in his relations to his fellow men. It has been called a front, a mask, yet it is inseparably tied to his inherent endowments and earlier acquired behavior patterns.

Descriptive terms are also used to single out one feature and label the individual by it - rigid, introvert, extravert, schizoid personality. *A rigid personality* is one who is unusually strict, honest to a fault, overly conscientious, abnormally righteous; *an introvert* is one who is self-concerned, abnormally self-conscious and introspective, meditative, silent; *an extravert* is talkative, friendly, mixes freely, sociable; *a schizoid* possesses introvert traits to a marked degree, becoming seclusive.

Subdivisions of the personality structure, according to Freud, are *the ego* (the conscious self), *the superego* (the conscience, the critical, implanted unconscious voice of parents and teachers, acquired during life), *the id* (the unconscious endowed instincts and acquired patterns). The strength and changing relationships of these forces determine aims and drives of the individual.

Personality, as we will use the term, is the sum total of the complex factors, endowed and acquired, that constitute an individual's makeup. Its basis is constitution, its form shaped by early life experience and later exposures and conflicts.

In the Army I studied two soldiers who can serve as models for our thesis on the importance of the personality in determining the nature and outcome of illness.

P. A. became nervous, shaky and nauseated when he was sent to the rifle range. The sound of gunfire upset him so that he turned pale and limp. For days afterward he could not eat and for nights he could not sleep.

P. A. stated that he was an only son, reared by a devoted overprotective mother. He remembers an illness in childhood, in which his mother stood at his bedside, praying to God, "Don't let my little boy die." This frightened him and made him worse. He said, "When I got older, Mother always warned me to be careful. When I wanted to go swimming, she admonished me, "Please, for my sake, don't go near the water – you might drown, and then I won't have you any more." When I wanted to play football she would not permit me to. She told me about a boy who got a broken leg in football. I was never allowed to play with firecrackers or have a B.B. gun. I was never permitted to go far away, for Mother worried about me. If I had the slightest cold, I was put to bed and kept there until every symptom was gone. I was cautioned about diet, elimination, and warned about diseases." He grew up into an introvert, health conscious to an unhealthy degree and full of fears.

"I had a hard time leaving home to enter the Army. All the time, as we drilled and marched, I could hear Mother's warning, 'Be careful. Don't do that. Don't get hurt – I can't live if anything happens to you.' I was afraid of germs and exposure and always pictured myself getting sick. And so bayonet drill and rifle practice were too much for me. I could see myself being killed and what that would do to my poor mother."

In marked contrast is the case of C. B., who was raised in a family of several children and was allowed to grow up with average restrictions. His parents were poor but industrious and he found his home pleasant, with healthy competition among his brothers, and devoted though seemingly casual supervision by his parents. They loved him but loved each other more. They guided him but did not lead or carry him. They suggested caution but never paralyzing fear. They took care of illness but did not set an example of complaining or magnifying distress. So C. B. swam, played baseball and football with the average amount of scuffling and bruising of his body, but with a joy in living and a certain self-confidence.

C. B. enlisted, went into training wholeheartedly, learned the arts of infantry. Then he reached Sicily and distinguished himself bravely when in battle. "I was scared, sure," he admitted, "yet I hoped for the best. You gotta go sometime, I figured." Crash – something hit him and he fell to the ground. A bullet had fractured his knee cap and injured a nerve in his leg. "Too bad," he said, yet tried to keep going. He fell helpless to the ground. He was flown to North Africa, where the wound was treated and his leg placed in a splint.

I saw C. B. after he was evacuated to the United States. His foot was paralyzed and he was slowly recovering the use of it. He was in bed, but was he moody and depressed? No, he was smiling and cheerful. He vowed he would get a cane and then a lift for his foot and be active again. There was too much to live for. Besides he was in love.

"That's a swell nurse I got," he said. "She's sweet and beautiful. I am going to marry her when the war is over. She gave me her pin. I wear it near my heart instead of the Purple Heart insignia which a general gave me." He was extraverted, confident – more interested in winning the girl than in worrying about illness.

In the book, *The Mind of the Injured Man*, are cited three thumbnail sketches of patients – Tom, Dick, and Harry – who had suffered an identical loss, the amputation of a crushed foot, but whose reactions were totally different. Tom was impatient for the stump to heal, eager for an artificial limb. He practiced on crutches and then without them. He asked to wear a special shoe as soon as possible. Within several months he was back on his strenuous job.

Dick laid awake nights, picturing the horrible deformity: "I'm not the same. I'll be a cripple. I'll have to give up my job. I won't be able to do anything difficult. My wife won't care for me; people will stare at me." He recovered but became self-conscious, brooding and withdrew into himself. "Why did this have to happen to me," he moaned repeatedly. "Why was Tom so careless as to drive that car into a pole? Everyone makes me suffer. I am the unluckiest man in the world – everyone is against me."

Harry was sensitive to pain. He couldn't sleep, couldn't eat. He was relieved only when the nurse held his hand, only when he got a hypodermic of morphine. Even when the stump was healed, he refused to get out of bed. He wanted his leg massaged. He touched it every day and found a sensitive spot. He begged for morphine to ease his pain, begged for an operation to cut out the painful spot (a neuroma). But surgery was tried again and again, morphine again and again, without avail. He has forsaken all struggle and has surrendered as a prisoner to a dependent existence, living only for sympathy, for attention.

Recently I was associated with a large group of amputees. One was minus a foot; another had lost his leg at the middle of the thigh; a third missed his left hand; a fourth had both forearms amputated. The degree of loss was of some significance. A man whose leg was amputated below the knee felt more secure, learned to walk on his prosthesis (artificial leg) more quickly, could go up and down stairs better than the one whose amputation was above the knee. Yet, regardless of the loss, some amputees practiced walking, learned to do crafts with their hands, attended lectures, took up study courses, and made plans for careers. They looked forward toward goals they might attain, even with their obvious handicaps. They were able to strive for self-reliance and independence, *utilizing the intact functions*. But there were many who concentrated attention upon the defect; such self-study added to the discomfort, magnified the disfigurement. Some developed self-pity and depression, thinking and talking of the tragedy: "I can't go back to my home and my family – people will look at me and laugh at me. No one will offer me a job or have anything to do with me." Others were resentful, bitter toward their former officers, displeased with the medical care, hostile toward society – paranoid. Although the Army provided an excellent program of medical care, training and occupational therapy, such soldiers declined to participate and sat on their cots, moping, sighing or cursing. A similar difference in reaction to defect prevails among all persons – in all walks of life. Let us consider certain factors which determine this difference.

Kretschmer subdivided patients into three body types: *the stocky, pyknic; the tall, lean, asthenic;* and *the average or athletic habitus*. On the basis of such types certain psychiatrists built a correlation of distinct mental disease, connecting manic-depressive psychosis with the pyknic type, and schizophrenia with the asthenic build. *This simplification takes into account obvious differences in bodily structure* and can be supported by a few classical illustrations. *It fails to acknowledge the many other and perhaps more influential factors* – drive, dynamic energy, intelligence, family background, education, and especially life's experience. It focuses attention upon the classical instances of illness in characteristic types but tends to overlook the many variations in bodily type, as well as the individual features of the symptoms of every sick man.

More important than body build is the matter of energy, man's physiological processes. His dynamic quotient, his drive is an innate force of importance. Some men are inherently energetic, full of vigor; others are slower, weaker, and fatigue readily. The former are likely to be persons of action, impulsive, extraverted. The latter are more reserved, deliberate, introverted.

Sometimes the very personality and the choice of career are as directly related to the matter of the energy quotient as they are to the intelligence level. Dunbar has shown the distinct difference in the personality profiles of those who have been hospitalized because of accidents and those who have heart trouble. The former are physically well, energetic and impulsive. The latter, perhaps because of physical impairment, are more reserved, more sedentary, fearful. This fundamental difference was well known in ancient times as we may infer from *Deuteronomy 20:17:* "And the officers shall speak further unto the people and they shall say: 'What man is this that is fearful and faint-hearted? Let him go and return unto his house, lest his brother's heart melt as his heart.' "

This connection between personality and physical energy often shows itself quite early in life. Recently, at a bathing beach I watched two youngsters playing. One seemed muscular, healthy and energetic; he was active, running forward to splash in every incoming wave. He seemed to enjoy the spray of the water as each wave struck him. Likewise he greeted strangers with a warm smile and seemed at ease with them. The other child of the same age was pale, thin, and somewhat unsteady in his gait. He was born with a moderate hypotonic weakness of muscles and had acquired some gait defect. He tried to imitate the play of the more vigorous child and ran toward the water, but was thrown down by the waves. A mouthful of salt water seemed to choke him and he began to cry. Thereafter he clung to his mother timidly. He tried again to do tricks in the water but his muscular insecurity once more caused him to falter.

So he gave up and sat down near Mamma, content to play with her. I am sure that he felt jealous of the healthy boy who was being praised by the adults and thus he was embittered even when someone did come to him. A few weeks later I saw these two children again, the vigorous one romping and laughing, the thin child clinging tearfully to his mother. The early pattern of personality was already obvious and the mental reactions seemingly influenced by the physical.

Again and again we see adult patients whose life's story is a continuation of this second child's early experience: physical weakness, easy fatigue, and motor insecurity leading to inaction and feelings of inadequacy. Thus in our approach to patients we must form some estimate of this item of energy, determined as it is by muscular development, metabolism, some quality influenced by the diencephalon. We differ in our dynamic features even more than in our physical structure. This difference in physical status is inherent in every organ: the striped muscles, heart, arteries, and intestines. All of us are acquainted with Herculean men and powerful Katrinkas. We know those who possess the stamina for sustained physical exertion, who can endure the physical collisions of sport and strife with a remarkable capacity to recuperate from exhaustion. Then there are frail and puny persons who, try as they will, do not possess physical vigor.

This physiological quantity of energy, or stamina, has its influence upon traits of personality. Although energy and personality cannot be directly equated, yet it is probable that the vigorous and muscular man is likely to be physically aggressive. Each person elects to do that in which he succeeds and in which he wins the approval of the group. The vigorous is outgoing, extraverted, thus apt to be impulsive, get into accidents. The person with some physical insecurity may withdraw and become the passive, clinging type, developing jealous hostility to others or trying by day-dreams to picture himself as a superman or by strenuous effort to achieve success. The day-dreaming, introverted, seclusive and withdrawn personality may be the echo of physical or organic inferiority.

We recognize, with Alfred Adler, *that symptoms and behavior are not simply the direct expression of such defects or organic inferiority.* The human organization is too complex for such simplicity. Indeed, sometimes the life of an individual seems to be a continuous effort at overcompensation for a defect, either congenital or acquired.

Demosthenes is said to have become a greater orator in his successful effort to overcome a speech handicap; Napoleon a great military leader to rise above the snubs given his slight stature and Corsican origin. Napoleon must have been endowed with an abundance of energy, as may be inferred from his capacity to keep alert and active for long periods of time.

Thus, a weakly child need not directly follow the course of least resistance. Rather, possessing intelligence or talent, he may acquire applause and distinction in such fields as music, writing, the arts, or mechanical invention. A defect need not necessarily extinguish striving. There is need for sensitive poets, for scientists, as well as for wrestlers. It may serve as a challenge, for "sweet are the uses of adversity." Training and ceaseless effort may make it possible to becomes a success in swimming or in golf, if not in sports necessitating bodily collision.

These correlations are mentioned here so that we may better understand *the connection between physical phenomena and the personality traits or even the illness of an individual.* This may be illustrated by the case history of A. C., a youth of seventeen, who was brought to the psychiatrist by his mother because of social maladjustment and nervousness. The history showed that he was a plumpish baby, slow to walk. As he grew, he was clumsy, unsteady and fell often. Later, he clung to his mother's skirts and did not venture out in group play. As he grew older he tried running, baseball, and football, but was always the slowest and most ungainly. His efforts were met with jeers from the superior boys. He withdrew into a shell, reading and listening to the radio. The suggestion that he go out to play induced trembling and sweating. At first his behavior did not arouse much attention, but it became conspicuous when the boy grew up, he avoided sports and dances and refused to date. Any situation which required physical coordination put him in a poor light and he withdrew into the warmer, protected atmosphere of home. The world became a hostile place, to which he reacted as with stage fright.

Along with energy we must consider intelligence. Here again persons are as different as are their statures. We may be pigmies or giants. And not only do we vary in the general level of intelligence but in specific qualities. Some people are more capable in mathematics, others in music, and still others in mechanics. Such intellectual differences help to determine out interests, our *progress,* our professions and our aims in life. The degree to which such intelligence is used, the success that we have, influences our makeup.

The youngster whose I.Q. is low, who cannot grasp theoretical subjects in the classroom, is humiliated by the scolding of the teachers and hurt by the scoffing of his schoolmates. He feels badly too when he fails of promotion and is incensed by the nicknames of "moron" and "dummy" applied to him. Some accept the level of school and job with resignation; others become unhappy and always feel inferior; a few jealous and resentful. Likewise, the intelligent man will be unhappy if he is unable to do the work, get the assignment, or attain the level of achievement which he expects. Attainment of the proper goal will tend to make an individual content and pleased with himself and his fellow men. Failure to obtain the education, the position or the rewards desired may lead to a sense of frustration, attended by depression or resentment. In our evaluation of illness then, we as physicians must reckon with the capacities and intellects of the particular patient and the degree to which effort achieves success or frustration.

The age of the patient is also significant. In the matter of recovery from injury or infection, youth is an advantage, old age a drawback. So too in mental illness, therapy applied early, guidance which directs the patient along the proper road may be more effective in youth than in the later decades. As a rule, youth stands for optimism, a readiness of tissues to heal, a hope for the future, a capacity to look forward. However, the youth of a patient is not always an advantage; cancer in a young individual or hypertension early in life reflects some inherent defect or a more virulent disease process. So too, the occurrence of mental illness in the pre-adolescent or adolescent stage may have sinister meaning. Schizophrenic symptoms occurring before puberty, leading to a withdrawal from normal interests and pursuits and causing the early substitution of a world of fantasy for the concrete though cold world of reality, are usually serious. Indeed, the prognosis is more grave in one who has failed to mature in life's strivings than in an older individual who did attain adult goals and then failed. Although the symptoms be similar, they indicate a deeper and more total defect in the younger person who fails to attain a normal level than in the individual who has once reached a normal state.

Stature and physical appearance are likewise important. We live in a world of comparisons and contrasts. Not only do the dynamic and intelligent persons have advantages, but so also do those of good physique and handsome features. The tiny and the lanky, the painfully thin and those who are too stout, the deformed and disfigured all encounter jibes and rejections and slurs. A young woman consulted me, depressed and disturbed because she was lonesome. She was a painfully thin and extremely tall girl. "All my life I was taller and thinner than most of the girls. From my earliest school days I was always the tallest. It didn't matter so much until high school. Then people called me 'bean pole.' Boys were nice to me but never asked me for a date. And so I've grown up . . . I am an efficient girl and I did well at my work. But now I am thirty-five; my family is gone or dead and I live alone. How I have yearned for companionship, for some man to love me! But fate has been unkind. How I envy the chic and pretty petite girls."

The next patient may be an adolescent boy whose figure is girlish, with large breasts and small genitals (Froelich's syndrome). He complains, "I am so self-conscious. I won't go to gym; I won't have the boys call me names and kid me when they see me under a shower. I'd like to be with others but they won't take me in their games, they say I am too slow. They call me 'fatty' and make fun of me."

Here then are two patients whose symptoms are closely related to deviations in body structure, and our diagnosis and therapy must take this into account. Yet these items alone do not explain illness and personality. *What of the training in childhood, the early life experiences?*

Several important environmental factors seem to modify our later reactions: the examples and attitudes of our parents, the conflicts of our early relations, the illnesses we have sustained. Such early experiences mold the personality out of the basic structure and energy and intelligence with which each man is endowed. As a sword composed of metal must be fashioned by heat and hammering to obtain the finished product, so the human being is not merely the outgrowth of a combination of endowments but is also fashioned by the experiences and impacts of life. Thus the home in which he is raised – its atmosphere, its social position, its members – and later the neighborhood and school all contribute something to the individual's development.

For example, it is recognized that a home affording love and security is more likely to lead to self-assurance than a broken home. So also, children raised in slum areas, in an environment of poverty and filth and alcoholism in the company of those who are lawbreakers, are molded in the direction of anti-social and troublesome individuals.

The parents are the most important influence affecting the personality of the growing child. The example they set is often followed by the child. Indeed, children tend to imitate *the deeds* rather than obey *the "don'ts"* of parents. It is common observation that the fears implanted by parents grow into greater fears and phobias in the child. This was strikingly illustrated by the brief case history of P. A. whose worries about health were but the continuation of his mother's anxieties about him. But even more important than the example of the parents is *the infant's handling of its own attitudes and feelings toward them.* As will be mentioned in greater detail later, the infant finds in its mother the first object that provides warmth, nourishment and satisfaction. In a broad sense, mother is the first love object. How the infant reacts to deprivations of love, to the presence of the father, to the later arrival of another child, how it controls its hostility may determine its later behavior. Neuroses are developed, according to Freud, from such experiences of repressed early hostility, of guilt and frustration.

The earliest years fashion the pattern of our life as to fears, means of attaining attention, attitude toward ourselves, toward sickness, and toward the world in general. The infant who gains a triumph by wailing repeats this technique and may grow into a woman who triumphs with tears. The youngster who, Spartan-like, suffers pain in silence is likely as an adult to endure discomfort without loud complaints. Not so the child who is harassed by inner guilt because of death wishes toward a brother when that brother is ill in the hospital. The child falls and bruises his leg and cries bitterly as he limps painfully along. Mother caresses the injured leg and soothes the crying child. Inwardly the youngster obtains relief – relief for his sense of guilt. Injury has served as an atonement, and also obtained for him the attention he craved from his mother.

A child's illnesses may also affect his later reactions in the pain he suffers, the weakness and disability, and the attitude of his parents. Some insecure parents hover fearfully over the sick bed, express exaggerated concern and show undue anxiety. The child is comforted by such attention, but he too becomes anxious. Perhaps there is some serious condition, he feels. His mother is crying – maybe he is going to die. And he cries too. As he passes through convalescence he demands a continuation of the care and is likely to emphasize such symptoms as pain, dizziness, or a limp. Once a child has profited emotionally from the gains of illness, he is likely to continue such pursuits.

Other forces which help to build personality are *religion and education*. Religion is a particularly potent influence. In religion are hope and fear and sin and punishment. Religion offers comfort to those distressed, guidance to those in doubt. Through prayer man appeals to a power which is reflected back to himself; feels more secure in his actions. Through a feeling of being guided or instructed or watched by a higher authority the individual inhibits acts which might be unsocial. Yet, in one whose superego is unduly strict or whose fear reactions too strong, the influence of religion may be unhealthy. Thus one child may grow into adulthood feeling comforted and secure in the thought of guardianship by an all-seeing God. Another grows up insecure and fearful, hesitant at every step and undecided about every thought. The ideas of sin and guilt and punishment shadow him. It is not rare to meet an adult patient whose sex life is restricted, to whom the sexual act is abhorrent, even when he or she is married. Early ideas of evil and sin have continued into adult life and retain the force to ruin marital happiness. For many, religion is a haven from the cruel realities of life, a compensation for its deprivations.

Education and vocational training impart to some persons a healthy perspective and a sound appreciation. Such training furnishes them with a career which is a means to a livelihood and a source of ego-satisfaction. Unfortunately there are some whose education has been limited and irregular and whose training woefully inadequate. They may succeed in spite of a limited education or they may grow up always unsure, always lacking in confidence, envious of those who are more successful. Some adjust satisfactorily; others are spurred on to effort and win outstanding success; but the less fortunate find sickness a protective screen against failure. A few choose lying or stealing or forging to obtain that which they cannot earn.

The atmosphere of the home and the spirit of the times help to shape the personality pattern. The proud aristocracy of Britain has always inspired its men to bulldog courage on the battlefield. Among the Indians, personal bravery was admired and encouraged. Present-day civilization encourages interest in self and in bodily functions, sometimes to an unhealthy degree.

In the later chapters we will talk of *certain diseases*, some arising from within the individual, as for example endogenous depression, and some occurring from external causes, such as traumatic epilepsy. Yet the symptoms of the disorder, the degree to which it incapacitates, sometimes the very treatment of the illness, depend upon the man, his personality, and his mode of reaction. For each of us enters life with many endowments of color, physique, vigor, intelligence, physiological reaction. Each of us lives in a changing environment with which we must cope. Early in life our basic instincts seek for the goals of food, warmth, security and love, and the elaborated aims of self-importance. These instincts are gratified or refused, attained or frustrated by those in our environment. We respond to such frustration with fear, with anger, with hostility. Some accept difficult situations as they do cold weather, by constructive action; others are allergic to such situations and react with abnormal physiological processes just as they chill, turn blue, or develop rhinitis as a result of cold drafts.

The present reaction thus is an interplay between the person and the situation, modified by the earlier pattern of such reactions. Therefore, a large variety of symptoms is possible and the attitude toward the symptoms will vary greatly. Let us consider *the influence of attitudes and of environment on illness*.

Mental Attitude to Illness and Injury

It is thus obvious that it is not the defect alone, not the anatomic loss that constitutes the disability. Rather it is the relationship of the mental attitude to a particular loss, illness or situation that determines the nature of the symptoms. I have expressed this relationship in a simple algebraic equation:

Defect $\pm$ Mental Attitude = Degree of Disability

In this equation the defect may be fixed – for example, an amputated leg – yet the degree to which this defect incapacitates the individual depends upon the personality, the earlier pattern of reaction, the attitude. Between any situation, illness or injury, and disability is interposed the personality. It may also be likened to a lens which magnifies or contracts. The plus sign in the equation would apply to Harry, who enlarged upon the suffering from his amputation. The minus sign would characterize Tom's mental attitude, his will to ignore his defect and achieve in spite of it.

A mother busily nursing her sick child will be oblivious to a backache, however severe; the star halfback of Notre Dame, limping after a hard tackle, will in the next play run around end, carrying several tacklers with him, and fall over the goal line. He will limp away because of a broken ankle, which had gone unheeded in his sprint for a touchdown. The soldier eager to get revenge against the enemy, to save a buddy, will keep going despite a painful wound. Think of the young French message bearer who hurried to Napoleon with word of victory.

"You're wounded," said Napoleon to the youngster.

"Nay," said the soldier, "I'm killed, Sire," as he fell to the ground – dead.

The spirit that is in a man can ignore or rise above a physical condition, as it can magnify and succumb to it. The degree of disability can thus be made smaller or larger by the mental attitude. If some mature goal be in the foreground – love in the case of C. B. high patriotism in the courier, then disabilities recede into the background. If one gets more security from sickness and dependence, then symptoms occupy the center of attention – as in the case of Harry.

Apropos of this is the case of E. L., an ambitious man of forty, who developed a disease of the arteries of both legs (Buerger's disease). This resulted in gangrene of both feet, necessitating amputations at the middle of the thighs. When the wounds were healed, he procured two artificial limbs and these were strapped to his body by wide leather bands. Then he strove to walk with the aid of crutches. This accomplished, he discarded the crutches for stout canes. Years later, at the age of fifty, he was a successful business man, making sales over the telephone, going out occasionally in a car driven by his wife. He consulted me because of headaches, and not once during the interview did he voluntarily refer to his artificial legs.

A similar attitude was displayed by a man both of whose hands had been amputated. He learned to type and to eat quite efficiently with his artificial appliances. One day we discussed his future and I expected bitterness against the world or self-pity. Instead he remarked, "I sure am getting swell care. I'm learning something new every day. I like the course in salesmanship and I expect to do a lot with sales over the phone. You know, I got a kick out of the fellow who came out here to show what he can do with his two artificial hands. He sure uses them well. He has me beat on tying a tie and buttoning his shirt, but I expect to show him up in one thing. I was an expert shot and I was fond of hunting. So I'm having the gun fixed so that I can fire it—and boy, it'll be good to get out in the woods this fall. This other fellow can't shoot!"

The will to get well and to become useful is an individual attribute. As we look ahead to our problem of rehabilitation of veterans and to the treatment of all patients, we must keep before us two vital points:

(1) The mind of the man is more decisive than the defect.
(2) Rehabilitation is most effective when arising from within man himself.

For the average man illness is hell; for some it is a haven, an escape from the stresses of life. An illness is not a simple episode, a statistical fact in the history of a patient. He reacts to it physically and mentally to a degree influenced by his circumstances and mental attitude. One who is overwhelmed by an inner sense of guilt may accept illness as an opportunity for sacrifice; another considers his suffering as an act of God, a chance to rest and to take inventory. Illness may be a decisive event in the life of one patient, a trivial episode for another.

One patient, absorbed in his work and happy in his home life, is disturbed by the fracture of his leg. "This has interfered with my unfinished work," he complains. "I have a garden to look after; my golf game will be ruined." Another man, crippled by paralysis, accepts his illness with a smile of ecstasy. "God chose me for this. I am the sacrifice for my fellow men. Just as God permitted His Son to be crucified, so He designated me." A third person is miserable at his job, is involved in all kinds of litigation, his home life is wretched. On the way home he wishes for a wreck in the bus, any injury, any illness to escape; an operation would be a relief. Many people welcome a cross to bear.

How an illness or defect fits into the pattern of striving and goals is a fascinating problem of life and medicine.

"There are people," wrote Gorky, "who look upon some disease, either of the body or of the soul, as the best and most precious thing in life. They nurse it all their lives, and only in it do they live at all. Though they suffer by it, yet they live upon it. They complain of it to other people and by means of it attract to themselves the attention of their neighbors. They use it as a means of obtaining sympathy, and without it – they are nothing at all. Take away from them this disease, cure them, and they will be unhappy because they are deprived of the only means of living – then they stand empty."

Such a reaction, interpreted in Freudian language, represents the need for suffering exacted by a relentless sense of guilt, or pleasure in suffering. A physiologist might say that such persons lack the vigor and stamina for competing in the strenuous race for power and approval and become content with a poor substitute and an excuse.

The symptoms of an illness may have unique meaning to the patient. Some symptoms, according to Schilder, affect the periphery of the personality, while others aim at the core. For example, a patient who has a pain in the foot is annoyed by it; the next patient has a pain over the heart and is frightened to death. A soldier who sustained a blow on the back may be annoyed by stiffness; his pal was struck in the head and fears insanity. Certain regions or functions represent the precious, the vital, the indispensable. Symptoms involving the heart or the mind terrify most of us. But the region or the symptoms are not important for their anatomic locations. The meaning of the symptom or illness or the performance of the particular individual is highly significant. A pianist whose index finger was crushed may lose his profession and his very soul. A farmer similarly handicapped may continue to operate his farm successfully.

The unique concern of a patient is shown by the following bedside experience: When I was a senior student in the School of Medicine, Western Reserve University, I approached my first patient, an old negro, who was sitting at the edge of his bed. His abdomen protruded with ascites (fluid), both legs ballooned to bursting, and from the burst skin trickles of serum escaped to drop in pools on the floor. He was struggling, with distended nostrils and open mouth, to catch his breath. My first question was, "Mr. D., what is your *chief* complaint?"

"My chief, complaint?" echoed the patient, panting. "I'm in a bad way. I'm a sick man . . . I've lost my manhood!"

This patient, at the threshold of death because of heart failure, expressed as his tragedy the loss of sex power, his manhood.

Milieu - The Present Situation - Environment

Man does not live in a vacuum; all his thoughts and actions are modified by the setting or environment in which he lives. So also is sickness influenced by the milieu, which includes climate, the social forces, the patient's contacts, his duties. Behavior of man and symptoms of sickness may respond to prevailing customs. Think for a moment of the Spartan, proud to endure hardship, of the Indian woman giving birth to a baby while the tribe is on the march. Picture the fanatical Japanese soldier, surrounded, and choosing (by force of social custom) to pull the pin of a hand grenade which hurls him to his ancestors, rather than surrender. Symptoms are influenced by the examples of others, by the demands of others upon us. Many factors in the social milieu thus determine the intensity of symptoms and their duration. There is a contagiousness of ideas as of germs.

Thus we see styles in nervous manifestations. In the Middle Ages there were epidemics of dancing mania; in Charcot's time dramatic convulsions were a "stylish" form of hysteria. Swooning was popular in Queen Victoria's day, since revived as a form of reaction to a singing star. Colitis was fashionable for a time and is still a common symptom. Patients often imitate other patients' symptoms. The example of one serves as a pattern for others.

In warfare the soldier is in a milieu of hardship, danger and duty. On the one hand is the instinct of self-preservation, which would compel flight for protection. Against this powerful force are arrayed feelings of team partnership, of loyalty to leaders, of patriotism, of a sense of duty, and of fear of disgrace in failing such duty. But when the soldier becomes ill or is wounded, the speed of recovery, the readiness to return to duty will depend not alone upon the wound or the man, but also upon the milieu. If the group spirit has been high, if the company commander has been trustworthy, if the combat be going favorably, then the soldier will be zealous to be back to the front lines. If he be a casual, a man with little outfit loyalty, if he distrust his leaders, if the climate be hot and weakening or muddy and cold, then any injury or illness is likely to lead to a prolonged disability. One recalls the newspaper reports of the high percentage of sickness and the resistance of these patients to returning to duty among soldiers when they felt they had been kept for too long in the jungles. Likewise, our soldiers, stalemated at Anzio and before Cassino - cold, their clothes grimy with mud, buddies wounded, no progress made - were loathe to leave the hospital, once sick or wounded.

Let us consider also *the veteran suffering from some handicap.* If he has an opportunity for work, he may readily relinquish a few residual symptoms (overcompensate for them). But if he be faced with idleness, he may emphasize his troubles and thus be eligible for a pension. This is to say that in a post-war period of industrial depression and unemployment, veterans are likely to remain anxious about themselves, to cling to symptoms and make the most of illness or disability, if idle. On the other hand, these symptoms may recede into the background if the incentive of opportunity attracts the veteran's interest. As a part of effective treatment, the modern medical officer sends a patient out of the milieu of a hospital into the more healthful, more active atmosphere of a health resort or reconditioning center.

The family too has some effect upon the progress of an illness. One man, particularly sharp and unscrupulous in his dealings, was angelic in his overprotectiveness toward his wife. If she had a slight fever or any complaint, he would hover at her bedside, anxiously studying her expression, eager to call specialists or to give medication. His concern seemed to cultivate a neurosis in her. For him it was expiation for his wrongdoing elsewhere. I have also seen a similar devotion of a son for his mother – a son whose career as a gangster was notorious.

This attitude of family may not always be friendly, warm and sympathetic. Some families are cold, critical and particularly unkind to depressed patients. Indeed, the symptoms of a depressed patient are influenced by the helpfulness or hostility of the family.

In our consideration of sickness and symptoms we will try to view *man in relation to his environment*. Even when, for the sake of brevity and accepted usage, we talk of epilepsy and neurosyphilis, it is always the patient with whom we are concerned. To emphasize this point of view I once wrote, "Diseases are fictions; patients are facts." This concept of course applies to the approach of a physician to the sick man, and not to the public health study of leprosy or malaria.

As we approach illnesses, let us always keep before us the man and all that goes into his makeup – his endowments of energy and intelligence and structure, the early life experiences which molded his personality, the present environment, the family of which he is a member, the group or outfit to which he belongs, the job he holds. Each and every one of these factors will modify his reaction to and recovery from the specific illness or injury he has suffered. The personality is like a prism between defect and disability.

The nature of the disease is not negligible, however much we talk of the personality. The soldier who has sustained a head injury resulting in fragments of metal lodged in his brain will exhibit serious disability, regardless of how splendid his personality may have been. Another who has developed encephalitis may show weakness, stiffness, drowsiness and marked alteration of personality. Our respect for disease is not lessened by our consideration of the man who has it.

Man dreams of happiness, reaches for power, craves comfort. Yet everywhere lurk danger, disease, and frustration. During the process of being born, the baby's soft, parchment-like skull must be molded to pass through a narrow space in the bony pelvis of his mother, and some of us bear, throughout life, the damage to our brains when the path of emergence to life is too narrow. During infancy tiny microbes, invisible yet powerful, threaten our right to survival as we come down with measles and colds and infantile paralysis. Later we are exposed to falls from our cribs, to fires, and and to cold. As we grow older, we are subjected to injuries in play and at work, inclement weather, and to changes within ourselves. Although Nature teems with life, in cycles everlasting man occupies but a fragment of time. The very quality of being born and of living, this lease on life furnished by God and Nature, carries with it the changes that lead to death. The instinct for life—the love instinct (Eros) is being challenged as we grow older by the death instinct (Thanatos) (Menninger). Thus we can readily understand the basis for man's fears in the face of such danger—fear which is at the core of neuroses.

REFERENCES

Hinsie, L. E., and Shatzky, J.: *Psychiatric Dictionary.* Oxford University Press, New York, 1940.
Freud, S.: *Psychopathology of Everyday Life.* Benn, London, 1935.
Fetterman, J. L.: *The Mind of the Injured Man.* Industrial Medicine Book Company, Chicago, 1943.
Kretschmer, E.: *Textbook of Medical Psychology.* Tr. from 4th Ger. edition Oxford University Press, New York, 1934.
Dunbar, F.: *Psychosomatic Diagnosis.* Hoeber, New York, 1943.
Adler, A.: *What Life Should Mean to You.* Little, Brown, and Co., Boston, 1931.
Schilder, P.: *Psychotherapy.* Norton, New York, 1938.

Menninger, K. A.: *Man against Himself*. Harcourt Brace, New York, 1938.
Zilboorg, G.: *A History of Medical Psychology*. Norton, New York, 1941.
Cobb, S.: *Foundations of Neuropsychiatry*. Williams & Wilkins, Baltimore, 1941.
Wechsler, D.: *The Measurement of Adult Intelligence*, 3rd edition. Williams & Wilkins, Baltimore, 1944.

Chapter II

PSYCHONEUROSES

A PSYCHONEUROTIC is one whose failure to adjust to life takes the form of physical illness, severe discomfort, or character deviation. He cannot adequately cope with the physical demands and the social stresses imposed upon him. His instinctive drives for love and security and mastery meet with disappointment and he reacts with hostility, usually repressed. Guilt and fear, arising from repressed hostility, dominate his feelings and take hold of his actions. The inner tension, the disappointment, the inadequacy, the fear become translated into bodily symptoms or abnormal behavior. Such symptoms thus represent suffering and yet an escape, an apology; they interfere with successful achievement and place the individual in an infantile dependent position, but one which achieves some protection and security. We may remark that neurotic illness includes both suffering and a solution.

In the development of a psychoneurosis several factors participate – in varying proportions. These are (*1*) inheritance which, though intangible, is highly significant; (*2*) early experiences and exposures which condition the individual; (*3*) reality problems which the person must cope with. Either factor alone may produce a psychoneurosis but it is the combination of all three that is usually responsible. We must reckon first with a particular individual endowed with physique and energy and intelligence, consider how he was modified by childhood training and then what problems he must meet. We may quote Myerson's apt remark: "What happens is important, to whom it happens is equally laden with destiny."

Inheritance

It is difficult among human beings to establish the factor of inheritance in the production of psychoneuroses. Indeed, there are statistical data which make one question its importance. Furthermore, one cannot separate constitutional factors from those of example, identification, and infantile conflicts to which the child is exposed. For the average child derives its nourishment and its early pattern from the same parents who supplied its germ plasm. Granting these doubts, it is my impression that certain individuals are born with the tendency to react "nervously," as they are born with similar, though simpler, physical allergies. I do not mean that an infant is born with a psychoneurosis. Rather, it is my belief that the child may inherit traits such as vigor, intelligence, sensitivity of the autonomic system, and possibly conscience which are so combined as to favor the development of psychoneurotic illness.

Some years ago I treated a patient who complained of precordial pain, shortness of breath, weakness and sleeplessness. Thorough physical examinations had proved negative. The patient described his father as an ambitious, intense person, inclined to sternness. Yet he was often "ailing," calling on doctors and stocking the pantry with enough bottles to honor a pharmacy. His most vivid recollection of his father is that of a sick man and a cruel parent.

For several years the patient himself lived with the constant fear of death. He sought safety in the wards of hospitals and would be relieved in the presence of a physician. Symptoms of this fear began in adolescence, continued through the next two decades, but became pronounced in the early forties when a close friend suddenly died. Under a regime of treatment he showed satisfactory improvement.

Two years later his brother consulted me for almost identical symptoms. He recalled nightmares and fears in childhood, a fear of the dark and of strange people. As he grew older, he acquired self-control, but in his thirties he developed chest pains, dyspnea, giddiness, fear of going out. Again and again he sought the aid of doctors.

These two brothers had lived in different cities, their immediate contacts and situations were entirely dissimilar, yet their physiques and their psychoneurotic symptoms were very similar. One could explain the illness in the two brothers on the basis of their reactions to a stern, cruel father. Yet it was not easy to dismiss the idea of heredity in the face of a similar neurosis in the father and the two sons. History repeats itself in families as in nations.

In my private practice over a period of two decades I have encountered many such examples, or instances like the case of a young woman whose neurotic symptoms and life story were a reproduction of those of her neurotic father. He had been troubled with headaches, insomnia and choking spells for many years. She developed like symptoms and became a psychoneurotic invalid for years. She was preoccupied with bodily functions, feared diseases, and could not enjoy life. She was like her father in intelligence and illness.

Endowment represents constitutional factors of bodily vigor, the presence or absence of energy. It includes physiological reactions in the face of pain or fear or humiliation—possibly inherited patterns. Yet endowment *per se* does not account for psychoneuroses for it usually takes the added factors of childhood training or the later impacts of life to bring out symptoms of illness.

Childhood Experiences and Training

The earlier life experiences stamp the pattern for later reactions. Sickness, example of parents, and especially one's own strivings and failures are highly significant. Freud has pointed out that the infant or child craves attention and affection. Granted this affection, it enjoys pleasure. But life is never a succession of pleasures. There are pains too, even for the young child – the pain of no longer having his mother's breast, of seeing his baby brother or sister take his crib while he is put into a dark and lonely distant room. There is the pain of jealousy when his father claims his mother's affection. Many infants and children accept these disappointments and deprivations without intense reactions. Others react with hate and hostility – a wish to remove the new arrival, to attack and destroy him, or hatred for the father. Such intense feelings bring fear of retaliation and must be forced back out of consciousness and repressed. *However, even though repressed, they exert a dynamic force, influencing the child's behavior.* If the hated rival becomes sick, an overwhelming guilt feeling may develop. Such guilt may even result from the censure of one's own conscience (superego). Fear of retaliation, fear that he will be punished then appears. Such fears, often accompanied by crying, nightmares, and vomiting, provide relief and obtain attention from the parents. The symptoms thus usually bring punishment and also satisfaction.

We may turn back to the case history of P. A. cited in Chapter I, a person who was raised in an environment of anxiety and who was apparently conditioned to react with fear to most situations. An overprotective mother inculcated in him undue caution: "You mustn't go out alone, you may be kidnapped; you'll drown; don't play with the boys after school for I'll be sitting home worrying about you." He complied with his mother's pleading, became overly attached, and was always uneasy lest what he did might be too painful for her. As he grew older, he continued to remain at her side and to do his utmost to win her love and approval. But as he grew older, he developed fears. Indeed, on one occasion he became panicky when his mother left the house and he did not know her whereabouts.

This individual grew into a timid, self-abased person resembling the masochistic type so well described by Horney: "Through a combination of adverse influences, a child's spontaneous assertion of his individual initiative, feelings, wishes, opinions is warped and he feels the world around him to be potentially hostile; under such difficult conditions he must find possibilities of coping with life safely and thus he develops what I have called chronic trends. ... The security offered by any of these ways is real, yet it is precarious because of the never-vanishing fear of being deserted. ... The kind of security that may be achieved by self-belittling is the security of unobtrusiveness. ... The masochistic person tends to be inconspicuous and to cringe in a corner. For instance, if such a person is offered a more favorable position than the one he holds, he becomes alarmed, or a person who in his own mind diminishes his capacities may become frightened when he wishes to assert his opinion in a discussion. He is likely to feel embarrassed and uneasy at any well deserved praise for a job well done. Such persons tend to diminish their value and deprive themselves of the satisfaction to be gained out of achievement.... The resulting feeling toward life can be described as that of a stowaway who has to remain unnoticed and has no rights of his own."

The following excerpt from a case history recounted by Schilder may illustrate: A man, aged 33, complained of an all-pervading anxiety and a fear of death, which hindered him from everything. At four years of age he was afraid of thunderstorms and of God. He felt inferior and weak and was afraid to die. He felt that he would like to poison the bullies who treated him badly. He was afraid to fight. In puberty he had strong sexual wishes concerning his sister, with whom he slept. His present illness began with terrible anxiety.

He wanted to strike the analyst, wanted to use profane language, yet conducted himself politely.

Schilder analyzed this patient and offered these comments: "It seems that he felt weak and helpless, as the youngest child of the family, and unable to express his drives which exceeded the average. In early fantasies and dreams he put all his adversaries and love objects to death. Since he felt tremendously inferior to his love objects, as well as to other boys, his aggressiveness came out against both. He fears retaliation of being dismembered, pulverized, eaten up. This is an individual overpowered by external force. The feeling of weakness and helplessness is supplemented by fear of aggression of others, which is partially patterned according to his own aggressiveness and partially feared as retaliation. This is a type of anxiety which is not merely the fear of losing a love object and of being deserted; it is an anxiety in connection with violent aggressive impulses. His pattern is obviously taken from early situations."

Another interesting case history is presented by Stephen, the analysis of an unmarried woman of thirty-three, who considered herself as Cain, the murderer of Abel. She was suffering from abdominal pain. This pain was so severe that she screamed and said it would drive her mad. She was examined physically and no cause for such symptoms was found. Excerpts from the analysis include these significant data: When she was four years old, her mother had another baby and she, the elder child, was turned out of her cot in the parent's bedroom. The next day she asked to hold the baby but begged the nurse to take it from her because she felt sure she was going to drop it. Several days later the baby died. This did not seem to her a mere coincidence; she appears to have believed that she was in some way responsible. She had wished the new baby might be removed and thus she felt as if the wish had brought this about. She got back her cot.

Four years later another baby came. The patient remembers playing with her doll, getting angry and pushing its eyes in. Then she dropped the doll "accidentally" and it broke into pieces. Later, when she was wheeling the new baby, the carriage overturned and the baby fell into the road.

Stephens describes this patient as timid, soft-spoken and submissive, but considers these traits as overcompensation for her aggressiveness. This meekness was largely the effect of remorse and fear, arising out of her guilt feelings in the death of the first new baby and the intense jealousy toward the second. "We can trace back part of this patient's illness to a repressed murder impulse, the motive for which was jealousy. Deeper analysis offered an explanation for the abdominal pain as due to a fantasy of pregnancy arising from even earlier desires toward the father and replacement of her mother." Stephens remarks, "Those who develop psychogenic illness are those who could not stand disappointment." She neglects to mention the why of this failure – and we must postulate "endowment."

The Freudian concept, correct as it may be, does not sufficiently take into account inherited factors nor the impact of reality and actual life situations of the moment.

The third factor is reality, present life situations, experiences. Rousseau says man was born free and now is in chains. Man was born helpless, dependent, and in no way free from his fellow men. He is born helplessly exposed to the coldness and deprivations of a harsh world. He must compete with his fellow men and with other living things for nourishment and warmth and the opportunity to grow, to reproduce, to live. He craves security and pleasure–he needs protection and satisfaction, yet life teems with denials and dangers, from the apparent harsh act of the mother who withdraws the breast which gave nourishment and warmth and sleep, to the later violent crash of bombs. So it is that man, surrounded by trouble, develops fears. Some dangers are real, obvious, acute; others are slow, insidious, thwarting effort, frustrating hope, causing keen disappointment. All lead to lesser, perhaps diluted forms of fear – self-doubt, uneasiness, worry. Physical illness, disappointments in love, the heat and hazards of a disliked job, cruelties of social and situational impacts, the deprivations and dangers of warfare can upset emotional equilibrium and initiate nervous illness.

A consideration of psychoneuroses then must face these situations, present as well as past. Let us take for example the student who fails to pass his tests and is dismissed from college, or the patriotic youth who is rejected at the Induction Station as a 4-F, or the father of a large family who loses his job. Humiliation, disappointment, insecurity – all disturb bodily functions and may initiate bodily illness. Perhaps we may appreciate the impact of actual experience by a brief clinical sketch:

Mrs. J. H. was referred to me by her physician because of serious nervousness. She had consulted him for a combination of symptoms, including frequency of urination and headaches. He performed a spinal puncture, among other diagnostic procedures. Her headaches became worse. She was brought to my office, moaning and crying, and had to be carried into my consultation room. Her complaint was, "I am afraid I have some incurable disease, maybe meningitis." She appeared pale and weak and frightened. A detailed neurological examination showed normal reflexes and no sensory disturbances. The patient was asked to describe her headaches and how they developed. In telling her story, she sighed and wept, "I remember now, the headaches began several months ago. I was in a family way and I was afraid that my husband, John, would be drafted. I loved him so, that I wanted to be with him in whatever camp he might be stationed. If I were to go on and have my baby, it would be impossible for me to move wherever he would be transferred. I was afraid to have the baby alone while he was away. You know, he means so much to me. I couldn't stand the thought of having to be left behind with a new baby while he was elsewhere. So there was nothing else for me to do but to have it done away with. John and I talked it over, and he agreed that now in wartime we shouldn't have another baby, and so I went to a doctor and had it done.

"But when the abortion was over, I didn't feel relieved; almost that very day I had a terrible burning pressure in my head. At night, when I tried to fall asleep, the pressure was with me, like a heavy fog. In the morning, when I awoke, that terrible feeling came over me. It really wasn't the fog, it wasn't the pressure. I could almost hear the words—'You did wrong. It was a horrible sin. You're a murderer, that's what you are!' Day after day this feeling came over me and I couldn't shake it loose. I was afraid to go to a priest because I was sure I would never be forgiven.

"One day, when I heard of a neighbor who had headaches and then was taken ill with meningitis, I wondered if I might not have the same thing; and thus the fear of meningitis grew on me. When I saw the first doctor, I couldn't bring myself to tell the story of the abortion. It was too awful to bring such words across my lips."

After Mrs. J. H. had unfolded her story, and after she was reassured that she did not have meningitis, she was relieved. She was relieved particularly when she was told that her act was the result of a decision made in the interests of love. Although one could not approve of that decision, yet her confession deserved absolution. She was advised to go to her priest and make a full confession. She walked out of my office, a smile on her face, as though a load had been lifted from her shoulders. I am told that she gradually regained her usual poise and became well again. She had come from out of town so that I have not seen her again. I regret that I did not have the opportunity to learn more about her past. However, the remarkable response to this consultation shows the importance of reality situations.

Mrs. J. H.'s case shows how feelings can produce profound physical distress. The haunting words of accusation, like a tight band of a persecutor, caused her to be troubled by the intense, vise-like pressure. Perhaps she had an ordinary headache, such as we frequently have. The sense of guilt may have attached itself to this discomfort, enlarged upon it, and made it more terrifying. Yet it protects the individual since it conceals the true cause and thus shields one from the accusing finger of guilt. If the headache were due to some physical malady, that sickness is accepted as a concrete, tangible phenomenon which can be cured. To face this concrete fact somehow helps a person to avoid the vague, haunting horror of accusation. Thus, fear of meningitis took over in place of the thought, "I'm a murderer." This fear and the knowledge that a patient so afflicted might become numb, weak and paralyzed, then led to that weak, helpless, faltering gait. Such a pathetic condition might bring some pity to the sufferer. So one situation led to another, until Mrs. J. H. was beside herself with suffering. One might wish to know what infantile experiences made the sense of guilt so overwhelming and why the symptoms took on the form of meningitis. Yet even without such knowledge, the practical approach proved helpful. The event of the abortion coupled with an intense guilt reaction was dominant, however much earlier patterns (Catholic religious training) influenced the development of such a reaction.

Even more striking evidence of the significance of reality situations are the war neuroses. These may be subdivided into those occurring in the pre-combat period and those which occur in combat. The soldier in combat is exposed to a succession of hardships which endanger his life and add up to exhaustion. The psychological hardships of noise, of buddies killed, of danger, and the physical hardships of loss of sleep, deficiencies and fatigue, when taken together, shatter against a man's wall of self-control. Each day of toil and hardship weakens his protection. Finally some men give way.

It has been said that every man has his breaking point but, what is more important, *the direction of the break and the degree of damage vary*. As a glass beaker exposed to excessive pressure may split in a linear direction, may break in several lines or splinter into many pieces, so one soldier weeps, the other cries; one sinks into a stupor, the other runs wildly about; one remains stiff, the other shakes violently. But the analogy of a human being to a fragile glass vessel is not entirely accurate, for it fails to take into account the healing quality in nature, the recoverability of man. Although it is true that every man may have his breaking point, it is equally true that the speed and degree of recovery is different for each person. The more it takes to cause an illness, the more quickly will that person regain his well-being. The resistance to illness means resiliency to rebound in recovery. This leads us to a discussion of exhaustion and neuroses.

Farrell and Appel have stressed "the role of combat as a cause of neuropsychiatric casualties, especially neuroses . . . . The percentage rises in direct proportion to the length of active combat duty. Difficulty in sleeping under shellfire, in open foxholes, extremes of temperature, wetness and mud, cold food, and the constant demands for physical exertion, all produce a state of physical and mental fatigue and induce neuroses, even in otherwise normal soldiers." Let us review the brief case histories of two soldiers who have been hospitalized for psychoneuroses.

Private F. S. was inducted into the Army and assigned to the ground crew of the Air Forces. He was a man of thirty-four, married and fairly successful as a mechanic. His health had been fairly good except for periods of nervousness. In his childhood he was shy, timid, and always avoided strenuous games. He had not been a good sleeper and was frequently awakened by nightmares. In school he trembled and flushed and even stammered when he was called on. He was sensitive to noises and darkness and when the least bit frightened, he would turn pale, "everything seemed to jump inside," and he would stay scared for a long time.

He grew up, found mechanics interesting and enjoyed working in a garage. Several times he took sick – "nervous stomach," the doctors called it. Otherwise he was lucky to escape injury and serious illness. He was saved from guilt and venereal disease by fear. He was devoted to his mother and rarely left his home until, at the age of thirty, he was married.

As a trainee he tried hard to make good, for he knew why we were fighting and had a high sense of duty. But, oh, lonesome nights away from home; oh, the loud voice of the sergeant, and how that food upset his digestion! But he applied himself to his basic training, learned the correct manner of saluting, marched well, and especially enjoyed taking care of planes. Later he was assigned to an airfield and, as usual, found the change difficult. Any change frightened him. Finally he was sent overseas. With all his self-control he restrained a tendency to jitters, fighting hard to keep hopeful and cheerful.

In the theater of operations there were no planes for him to repair, no work except guard duty. Night after night, standing on watch or pacing back and forth in the silent darkness, all the fears of darkness and danger engulfed him. Especially when some noise had frightened him during the day, he could not sleep; he could think only of the terror of the coming night; he could not eat because his stomach seemed jumpy. And again the night vigil. He could not endure the silence, the lonesomeness; all the fears that had been hidden since infancy became intense and alarming "I must desert, I can't take it," he would think to himself. Then, "No, I could never do that. The shame of it would kill my mother. I can't quit. I'd be better off dead, and so why not shoot myself? But I'm a coward, even if no one found out and blamed the enemy."

Thus, frightened, jumpy and sleepless, Private F. S. reported for sick call. He was hospitalized and sent back to the United States. He was invalided, a case of anxiety neurosis. On the ward he spent most of the time in bed. "I am too weak to get out," he explained. He ate little, returning his tray practically untouched. He complained of headache, sleeplessness, palpitation, and a nervous stomach.

Corporal D. J. was a healthy lad, cheerful, active, and not too responsible. He left high school at sixteen and did odd jobs. He was seldom ill and was not troubled by many worries. True, he was always carrying antiseptics with him —"sort of as a precaution." Not being satisfied with his job and being imbued with patriotism, he enlisted in the Army.

After eighteen months of training and with a promotion to corporal, he was sent overseas. He was a member of a medical detachment, driving an ambulance. In North Africa his regiment was exposed to much strafing by enemy planes. Then his outfit took part in many battles: Kasserine, Mateur, El Guitar. Many were the wounded that he helped into litters and into his ambulance. After a cautious journey back to the Battalion Aid Station, the use of plasma, and careful treatment of the wound, another American soldier would be saved. But not always were his efforts thus rewarded. Sometimes he reached a wounded soldier who was ghastly pale, with bubbles of froth coming from his lips, and as he helped the soldier on his litter, Death would enter the scene.

The horror and the groans of the wounded upset him, but he was able to dismiss them as he joined his buddies during the days of rest between battles.

Then came several days and nights of incessant action; trip after trip to the front, during which his ambulance was bombed by strafing enemy planes. He became tired and tense, especially incensed by the bombing of his clearly marked ambulance. One day as his ambulance was carrying several wounded, there came a warning of an approaching plane. He stopped his ambulance and made a dash for the nearest hole. Too late. Minutes later he found himself on the road with blood streaming from his leg and his nearby ambulance demolished. Now he was himself being carried by first-aid men, his leg stiff, sore, and motionless.

When seen at the First Aid Station, he was told that his swollen and deformed leg was fractured. X-rays taken at a hospital in the rear, however, showed only fragments of metal; the bone was not broken. The wounds in the leg healed well, but the corporal became uneasy.

"Will I ever walk again?," he began wondering. "Can I stand going back to combat?"

He became nervous and jittery. When he was permitted up on crutches, he was so weak and his leg seemed so stiff and painful. When allowed to discard the crutches, he found he could not walk straight; his leg had become stiff at the knee. In this condition, he was sent back to the United States.

When examined, he complained of pain and weakness as well as of nervousness. He walked slowly, he arched his back, his right leg seemed short and stiff. Thus his gait showed a pronounced limp. Although he seemed to be deformed, there was no actual damage to bone, nerves, or muscles—nothing except several well-healed scars and three tiny fragments of metal imbedded in the tissues. Neither these scars nor the metal were responsible for the deformity and the limp. It was the corporal's mental attitude, as we shall see later (Chapter III) when his restoration to duty through psychotherapy is described. His illness was a psychoneurosis known as conversion hysteria.

From these case histories and the brief discussion it is apparent that psychoneuroses result from the interplay of endowment, childhood reaction patterns, and actual reality situations. Any one of these alone, if sufficiently powerful, may determine neurotic illness. As we appraise the treatment and the pension problems of veterans we must reckon with this interplay. A veteran whose obvious nervous difficulties appeared in the first days after induction and which have persisted even after his discharge belongs to the group in whom endowment and childhood patterns are fundamental causes. The veteran whose neurosis developed in combat is likely to be well when he returns home. For his illness is largely upon a situational (reality) basis.

Symptoms of Psychoneuroses

GENERAL SYMPTOMS: *Each individual patient manifests specific symptoms which differ more from one person to another than fingerprints. Some are of a general type,* vague, diffuse; *others are referable to a single organ or a specific function,* the skin, the heart, the mind. There are patients in whom one complaint stands out like a bright star, but usually there is a grouping of symptoms like a constellation, shifting, changing, sometimes bright and then dim. We shall describe a few of the common general symptoms and then take up a list of the difficulties which are related to some specific organ of the body.

Weakness is a common symptom, the patient complaining of loss of energy, tiredness, undue fatigue. Such a symptom is prominent in that type of psychoneurosis known as neurasthenia. The patient is too tired to work, too "all in" to participate in any recreational pursuit.

More common than weakness is anxiety, a sense of uneasiness, the dread that something terrible may happen. This anxiety sometimes mounts to the degree of panic in which the patient is almost overcome by fear of impending catastrophe. Again and again patients will say: "I'm afraid, I'm afraid I'm going to lose my mind and do something awful. I'm afraid I'll die." These fears are accompanied by all manner of visceral distress. Along with anxiety is the complaint of tension. "I'm uncomfortable, tense, taut – I'm tied up in a knot; I can't relax." Anxiety and tension are expressed also by specific symptoms as will be mentioned later.

Another symptom group is that of the phobias and compulsions. Patients are afraid of going up in an elevator, of crowds, of dirt. As a defense mechanism, such individuals restrict their activities, wash again and again because of fear of germs. One patient, for instance, would spend an hour bathing herself with utmost thoroughness. Then, upon leaving the bathroom, she would touch a door knob and cry out: "I'll have to wash my hands again because there may be some germs on the knob."

In many patients the symptoms are combined and such obsessional features are attended by physical complaints. This may be illustrated by the case history of N. D. "I must do things three times or I'm afraid something may happen. I must turn off the radio three times, must caress my child three times before I fall asleep. I must turn the pages of a book or newspaper three times."

In addition to the compulsion of the number 3, patient stated: "I can't sleep well; I get nightmares with dreams of falling. I worry a great deal, and when I do, I get pains in my stomach. It all goes back to when I was a child. My mother died when I was very young and my stepmother and stepbrothers were cruel to me. They always made me feel as though I were a bad boy, as though I didn't belong with the family, and I had a sense of loneliness which has been with me. I worry about not being able to talk to anyone. I'm always scared, scared of the future. When I am nervous, I have pains in my stomach and get nauseated."

This patient's symptoms have varied over a period of years, mild and silent at times and then again so severe as to be incapacitating.

MENTAL SYMPTOMS: Many a neurotic is worried about his mind. "I can't concentrate. I can't remember. I am in a fog, I seem so confused. Could it be that I am losing my mind?" It is partially true that many neurotics cannot concentrate – upon outside events. How could they, when so much mental energy and interest are attached to the palpitation of the heart or the paralyzed arm? Neurotic distress so absorbs attention that little capacity remains for other experiences. Likewise the neurotic is partially correct about his failing memory, for among the most common complaints of even healthy persons are not enough money and not enough memory. That's why notebook and memo pads are so popular. Then too, memory is impaired when attention to outside subjects is deficient because of introspection. It is significant that the same patients fail to remember national events, yet give a minute chronological account of every ache, of the disagreeable taste of every medicine and of the exact pulse rate at a specific time of the night. Such retention is a complement to attention to inner processes.

The feeling of being in a fog may result from this same lack of attention and from the widening gap between the patient's self-concern and reality. The growing feeling of weakness leads to self-doubt, a sense of inadequacy.

Of particular interest are the states of amnesia which have been reported. A soldier wanders away from his outfit and is found miles away, "dazed" and blank. He cannot recall his name, his outfit or where he is. "Who am I," he asks. "Where have I been? How did I get here?" The memory of the last day or of a lifetime seems blotted out. For example, a paratrooper was found wandering aimlessly. He could not tell who he was or where he had been. He remained in this state for several weeks and then "came to." In the popular movie film, "Random Harvest," the hero is a British officer of the last war who has been placed in a hospital because he knows nothing of his origin or of his actions. Falling in love and a return to familiar surroundings helped him to revive his forgotten past. The movie portrays a case of hysterical amnesia.

Quite commonly neurotic patients emphasize self-doubt –"I don't amount to anything. I am afraid I'll lose my health and my home." Some depressed features are also present, although not as deep or as prolonged as in true depressions. Patients stress a general sense of discomfort –"I feel tense, quivery, uneasy. I feel all tied up, can't relax, I seem to be afraid."

DISORDERS OF SPECIAL SENSES: Our special senses, like reconnaissance planes and the Signal Corps, bring in reports of the outside world. Good vision, keen hearing, normal taste and smell are helpful to enjoyment of life, and in war may be essential to efficient soldiering. Quite commonly the function of the special senses is disturbed. Sometimes vision seems sharper and everything is painfully bright and dazzling. In another patient, all is dark. Again, a patient may see only a part of an object, one half or one sector only. In a study of hysterical disturbance of vision, cases were reported of trainees suffering from all manner of visual difficulty. Quite common was a narrowing of the field of vision, known as tubular vision. The authors stressed the fact that the soldiers were nervous and inadequate, aside from the impairment of vision.

Hearing troubles are common too, such as fogginess, partial deafness, total deafness, ringing noises in the head. Then there are examples of oversensitivity to sounds. Such difficulties appeared among soldiers who were out on the rifle range or were exposed to artillery fire. The alarming and loudly reverberating noises of gunfire re-echo in the trainee's ears. Even the play of children, traffic sounds, the noise of machinery will become painfully loud to one who is tense, uneasy, and sensitive. Fear adds to the discomfort – the sound, magnified by fear, startles him. All sounds seem so much louder and become painfully annoying. I recall a patient who could not stand the sound of an elevator; the rumbling of the luncheon counter was painful; even a footstep had become jarring. Another form of neurotic reaction may be deafness – a complete exclusion of sound stimuli as a form of hysterical defense.

HEAD SYMPTOMS: The head encases the brain, lodges the special senses. The face is the front which greets and communicates with the world; it expresses joy and sorrow; its muscles denote tenseness or relaxation; its color reveals fear and shame. Emotions may evoke a similar change in circulation within the skull, comparable to pallor and blushing in the skin.

Thus it is that anxiety and fear and tenseness cause uncomfortable sensations in the head. Headache, pressure, tightness, throbbing – these are common nervous complaints. I used to caution my students thus: "Before considering the diagnosis of brain tumor, *remember that life itself is the commonest cause of headaches.*"

The following case history illustrates this point: A woman of forty-two was admitted to the hospital complaining of headaches and fearing that she had a brain tumor. As all diagnostic studies for physical disease were negative, I was asked to see this patient. After a preliminary interview, she broke down and wept: "I am afraid to tell you this because my husband threatened me if I would do so. My headache began a year ago when he stopped coming home on time and I learned that he had a sweetheart. He neglected me, insulted me, stopped supporting me. How my head throbbed! It burned, it seemed to swell – I cried and it made my head worse – I wished I were dead – now it's all settled in my head."

The man who feels the pressure of unsolved problems, the woman troubled by domestic worry, the girl unloved – all may have headache as a result. Some nervous headaches are expressed in this wise: "My headache is violent. There is terrible pounding. I feel such a squeezing, tight band; the pressure is so tight that I am getting narrow-minded. My head feels as though it is divided into two parts." Said one soldier, "I always got a headache when I was scolded by teachers or parents. Now it's worse. When my sergeant yells at me or my C. O. speaks sharply, I get a beating all through my body; my head pounds; I can't stand the pressure."

The patient with a nervous headache not only mentions his discomfort but he fears the worst: "Doctor, I am afraid I am going to have a brain tumor." The suggestible tendency of neurotics and the intensity of this fear accounted for a wave of brain tumor complaints some years ago when the movie, "Dark Victory," was shown. In this picture, Bette Davis portrays the role of the heroine who starts with headaches, develops stumbling, and finally loses her vision because of a brain tumor. When this film was shown in Cleveland, many were the patients who came to doctors sobbing, "I too have headaches and I had some dark spots before my eyes. You don't have to tell me – I can make my own diagnosis – a brain tumor is awful. How long before I'll go blind?"

The intensity of nervous headaches, their appearance during emotional stress and the fear of serious trouble are all common features.

A frequent complaint is dizziness. Patients mention feeling lightheaded, unsteady, a sense of swaying. "I feel unsteady on my feet as though the room were moving." A pianist recently had complained of pain in the chest and the fear of collapsing on the platform. The cardiac symptoms cleared up but he later mentioned dizziness: "I am afraid I will fall; when I play the piano, it seems to wave and move." This patient was troubled by a conflict between love for a beautiful torch singer and his duty towards his plain wife. He could not come to a decision, instinct and inhibition struggled for mastery in his mind, and he became emotionally insecure. The insecurity or imbalance emotionally was translated into the spatial insecurity or dizziness.

Heart and Circulatory Symptoms: The scientist had developed evidence that deep centers at the base of the brain are the seat of the emotions, but the poet has asserted for a long time that this privilege belongs to the heart. Poet and patient record the facts of everyday living, even though behind these facts are involved nerve pathways which link the diencephalon with the rate and vigor of the heartbeat, the caliber of blood vessels, and the changes in blood flow. The poet describes the feelings of man, using language which is packed with physiologic wisdom. Such phrases as "My heart aches for you," "sweetheart," "courage" describe emotions, not heart illness. So a soldier, unhappy during his training, may go to sick call complaining of "pain in my heart, heaviness and weakness." Another in combat exercises remarkable control in the presence of danger, but his rapid heartbeats and faintness betray the inadequate control. The neurotic in a state of anxiety becomes aware of his pulse, conscious of heartbeat, fearful of heart disease. He may count his pulse, again and again. He may scrutinize the color of his nails, even lie awake watching the beating of his heart. Says the patient, "My heart pains me; it skips a beat; it jumps and throbs in my neck. I am short of breath. It is worse when I exert myself. I can't march and I'll keel over if I go on a hike. I am afraid I'll die of it."

A neurotic is aware of his heart and it is this awareness that makes him distressed by its action. In heart disease, the doctor hears the murmur; in a cardiac neurosis the patient does the listening – and taking the pulse.

Sometimes neurotic anxiety is added to actual heart disease. But it is the anxiety which may be the major cause of disability. For instance, P. V. had once contracted rheumatic fever which left her with a valvular heart defect. At the age of fifteen she had a fainting spell and was examined by a physician. When his stethoscope was placed over her heart he must have heard an unusual murmur, for his brow was contracted and his expression anxious. He listened long and attentively. Then he spoke ominously, "Young woman, you have HEART DISEASE. You have a bad murmur. You had better be careful, for you might die of this." *Such utterance is the warning of a man who foresees an autopsy, not one who has feeling for the mental reaction of a living patient.* The young lady was impressed and frightened; her attention was directed to her heart. Thereafter, anxiety about the heart occupied the foreground of consciousness. She lived in constant fear and gave up all activities.

Two years later she was still in bed. She remained awake nights.

She said, "I feel very weak. I am afraid to walk. I stay awake nights for fear my heart may stop." To counteract the unfavorable suggestion and to loosen the fear, this patient was strongly reassured, encouraged to walk. Fortunately she responded as readily to encouragement as she had to unfavorable orders. She has for several years been going out, working, and enjoying life. She still has a murmur, but it is relegated to the valves of the heart and the stethoscope of the physician and is no longer the major concern of the patient.

Closely allied are the respiratory difficulties, shortness of breath, heaviness, panting, choking. It is common for neurotic patients to mention heaviness in breathing, inability to obtain enough air (air hunger), or to exhibit struggling respiration of one kind or another. Even asthmatic breathing has been caused by emotional tension.

DIGESTIVE DISORDERS: Along with circulatory changes, disorders in the gastro-intestinal tract reflect emotional states. "I can't stomach it" reflects the gastric protest to an unpleasant situation. "He hasn't the guts" is an equivalent to "he is yellow." ... One is an intestinal, the other a skin manifestation of fear. Fright affects the bowels–even more violently than does a physic. Emotional states, especially fear, influence the flow of saliva and thus affect taste and appetite; disturb the secretion of gastric juice and change gastric motility leading to "gas, distention, heartburn, pain;" derange intestinal peristalsis, causing diarrhea. From one end to the other, the function of the digestive apparatus registers emotions or, as James put it, "The abdomen is the sounding board of emotions."

Disorders of digestion, such as hyperacidity, intestinal spasm and diarrhea, are examples of psychosomatic disorders. Even duodenal ulcer, according to Alexander, is correlated with personality type. The individual is of the conscientious, industrious type, inclined to worry, gaunt, like Cassius, "who hath a lean and hungry look."

Patients in a gastro-intestinal clinic need not only x-rays of the gastro-intestinal system, but they need a study of their mental processes. During the depression of 1929-32 I saw many patients with gastro-intestinal upsets, whose symptoms were connected with their losses. Indeed, this relationship was so striking that it seemed as though the increase in the use of baking soda reflected the decrease in the quotation of the stock market. Among soldiers, digestive upsets might come from food or from infection, but unpleasant situations or tense danger constitute a more common cause.

A sergeant in the Air Corps, a waist gunner in a bomber crew, had been a splendid soldier. He was fond of his ship and was close to his buddies. They had gone on several missions, long and dangerous ones. Once or twice they were attacked by Messerschmitts en route to and from their target; at their target incessant flak greeted them. On the third mission the plane was badly damaged and one of the crew was wounded. On the next mission our patient himself sustained a small leg wound, which healed promptly. In the hospital, this sergeant spoke cheerfully and insisted upon a return to his plane. But he developed abdominal pain and diarrhea. Careful studies showed no organic cause of his intestinal symptoms. As he was determined to rejoin his outfit, he was permitted to go up again, but when the plane took off he again developed pain, nausea and weakness. His words reflected courage but his intestinal viscera betrayed his fear. He was grounded and his symptoms later cleared up.

MUSCULAR DISORDERS: The soldier uses his muscles even more strenuously than the civilian. A twenty-mile hike is followed by tired, painful legs. Heavy lifting brings lumbago. Bruises, falls and other injuries add up to pain, stiffness, and weakness. Such local pain and injury draw attention in the anxious, neurotic patient. Around this core of pain from muscular exertion there is woven with the endless yarn of man's anxious imagination a larger pattern of disability. To the original pain are added stiffness, weakness and limping. One soldier who is seen limping to sick call has a fractured ankle; the next is an unhappy neurotic. I have seen soldiers shuffling slowly down a hospital corridor, faces drawn in pathetic grimaces, each foot sliding along the floor as though it were glued, and one would think of how badly crippled the poor soldiers might be. *Yet the clinical record may show unmistakably that there is no injured muscle or broken bone or damaged nerve to explain this peculiar gait.* This manner of walking is a pantomime, a dramatic portrayal, which, more eloquently than words, says, "I am helpless. Pity me. I can't drill or march or fight." No wonder such walking has been facetiously labelled the C. D. D. (Certificate for discharge on disability) shuffle. Such a gait disorder "shuffles" a soldier out of the service.

Not only disorders of posture and gait, but all kinds of involuntary movements develop, especially among soldiers in combat. Some twitch, others have tremors, and there are those who shake violently. I recall one such soldier who had "the jitters" in Sicily but was fairly quiet in our hospital in the United States. At the approach of a plane he shook violently and leaped under the bed.

For a period of years I studied a group of patients who presented symptoms of disabling back disorders. As a class, they complained of pain, weakness, inability to lift, and they often walked in a stiff or even awkwardly stooped manner. For the most part they were industrial cases, persons carrying "a heavy burden of physical labor," and an emotional load – resentment against employers. These symptoms were looked upon as vertebral neuroses, caused by, and sometimes relieved by, psychogenic factors. As a rule, the cause was situational, such as a sense of bitterness and resentment or fear building up to a point where a minor fall, a blow, a heavy load induced pain and deformity. The subjective complaint of pain and the objective evidence of deformity and suffering seemed to free the patient from his toil and to provide some revenge against the alleged cruelty of the employer.

Two case histories of vertebral neuroses may be briefly given here:

> M. M., a woman of thirty-two, was referred for study by Dr. McCurdy of the Industrial Commission of Ohio. She had a job as a waitress but found the pay small, the hours long, and the insults many. One day, she slipped and fell down the stairs, sustaining a bruise in the lower back region. She gradually developed pain, stiffness and weakness. In the course of time, there was a visible scoliosis which caused her to walk in a position of pes equinus. This marked postural deformity had already been present for years at the time when she was referred to me.
>
> This patient was sent to the Lakeside Hospital for a thorough study. A routine physical examination, x-rays of the pelvis, and a lumbar puncture all proved negative. Because of the severe postural deformity, Dr. M. Harbin was called in consultation. After many orthopedic tests, Dr. Harbin concurred in the diagnosis of hysteria. The patient was then studied from a psychiatric standpoint

and it was learned that the symptoms were serving as an escape from a home life which was unhappy and a job which was most unpleasant. After our patient's confidence had been gained, it was decided to try a local measure with a psychotherapeutic purpose. She was given an injection of novocain into the area of the painful muscles, with the firm assurance that this would help her. Within an hour after this treatment, the patient could stand erect; the scoliosis had disappeared. In the course of a day or two, her gait had improved remarkably. She was seen several months later, at which time there was no deformity and practically normal posture.

At a later date another troubling experience brought about a return of her symptoms to a slight degree.

A. B., a girl of twenty-two, was seen in the Neuropsychiatric Dispensary at the Lakeside Hospital. She was self-conscious and unhappy. She stated that her home life had been one of uneasiness and insecurity; her father and mother had quarreled a great deal and he had threatened desertion. The patient herself was a bright though obese girl who did well scholastically, but who was poorly adjusted socially. After graduation from high school, she was unable to find employment, her home situation was distressing, and she spent much of her time daydreaming and writing poetry. One day she slipped and struck the end of of her spine. Almost immediately her attention became centered on this region. She palpated the lower end of the spine and would cry out with pain. She went to a clinic, where the x-rays revealed a bent coccyx. On the basis of the x-rays, this bone was removed. However, the pain was not relieved. Indeed, it became stronger than ever. She went back for further surgery, but at this time the psychic aspects were suspected.

A fairly extensive study of this girl showed that the pain in the coccyx was but a focusing point for an introspective, unhappy mental attitude. Over and over again she spoke of the tragedy of living and would write poems such as this:

"Perhaps in later years time shall have passed
Her healing hand across my heart to bring
Blessed relief from this soul-twisting pain;
I may have peace and be content again."

Under a regime of psychotherapy, she showed marked improvement, including a relief of symptoms and a more courageous attitude. This patient states that she has now learned to live with her troubles rather than to flee from them.

GENITO-URINARY COMPLAINTS: Frequency of urination is extremely common; so also are pain and burning. Many emotional experiences are attended by an urge to void. Sometimes there is an inability to empty the bladder. This is particularly common when a male is about to empty his bladder and others are present. Frequency of urination was a distressing symptom in the case of Mrs. J. H. In fact, so marked was the urinary difficulty that a cystoscopic examination had been performed.

SEXUAL SYMPTOMS: Lack of enjoyment of the sexual act is a frequent symptom in neuroses. Some female patients complain of a complete aversion to the approach of their husbands. "I abhor the thought of it. I try to fall asleep or fake sleep so that my husband will let me alone." Others state that they are completely neutral or passive throughout the performance. Then there are those who are physically aroused – to a crescendo of physical warmth, but they fail to reach the climax of an orgasm – and pleasurable relaxation. "The sex act upsets me very much – it excites me but when my partner is finished and falls asleep, I remain stimulated and wakeful."

So also, the male patient who is neurotic may emphasize impairment in the sphere of sex. This may range from marked lack of desire to embarrassing impotence: "I have a tremendous desire, but when I attempt intercourse, I lose my erection – and I am humiliated. I am afraid my wife is going to leave me." Other patients are troubled by premature ejaculation – which is almost equally frustrating to their sexual partners.

Aside from these defects in normal sex acts, there are many perversions and deviations which occur in certain patients. The most common, homosexuality, will be mentioned in a subsequent chapter under the heading of sexual psychopathy.

A recent example of sexual symptoms is the case of a man referred to me because of impotence following head trauma. This patient was a thirty-eight-year-old, vigorous, colored truck driver. About eighteen months prior to my examination he was injured in an explosion, sustaining a laceration of the scalp and a moderate concussion. He complained of headaches and dizziness, but showed no focal cerebral symptoms. He returned to work in two weeks. He did well at work, except that any sudden change of position caused a sense of toppling, a symptom which has but slowly subsided. However, when this patient attempted intercourse, he experienced trouble. "When I was with my girl and came to the point of unloading (orgasm), my head felt like it was going to burst. I tried it again but had to give it up because my head stayed hot and full and all muddled for several days." The patient was asked to discuss his personal life.

"I am the oldest son and I am the chief support of my mother. I have a girl whom I love but I am afraid to get married because I don't want to put anyone ahead of my mother. I like my girl and I enjoy intercourse, but I am afraid that my girl may get pregnant and I would have to marry her."

One may offer this brief interpretation of this so-called impotence. This patient had been confronted with the conflict between duty (toward his mother) and pleasure (with his girl friend). Fear attended every indulgence. Following the head trauma, intercourse was both pleasurable and painful (congestion in the head). This local symptom has been magnified and prolonged and serves as a reason for the renunciation of sex and fulfillment of duty.

MISCELLANEOUS SYMPTOMS: Psychoneurotic patients present many common and also many individual symptoms, the number and types of which are almost endless. We could go on to itemize a much longer list of individual symptoms. We may mention in passing the frequency of disturbed sleep such as restlessness, fatigue upon awakening, nightmares, and sleep walking. Such patients do not get the usual refreshing benefit of normal sleep.

Skin symptoms are frequent, as any dermatologist well knows. Patients complain of flushing or coldness, of itching and burning and crawling. Added to the initial discomfort is the tendency to pinch or scratch, resulting thus in secondary thickening or excoriations of the skin. I recall a patient who, when distressed, was troubled by a burning sensation in the palms and fingers. Indeed, he would hold his hands in front of him in a pathetic, almost pleading manner. His hands revealed suffering which served to allay an inner sense of guilt.

There are all manner of internal discomforts in addition to those already described, but space does not permit further detailed consideration of them.

Choice of Symptoms in Neuroses

Many factors enter into the type of symptomatology of neuroses. Recently Alexander explained hysterical conversion symptoms as a translation of a psychological process into a bodily symptom, the symptom being a symbolic substitute for an unbearable emotion. The vegetative symptoms occurring in the autonomic system are not the substitutes but the accompaniments of emotional states. Alexander believes there is a specific relationship between emotional factors and vegetative expression, stating that patients with gastric neuroses suffer from a constant need to be loved, a persistent wish to be fed.

In the group of neuroses which develop in industrial cases featured by back disabilities of psychic origin, I stressed the importance of local organic pathology as the core of neurotic symptoms. Pain and stiffness resulting from trauma tend to direct attention and to draw anxiety and preoccupation toward the affected region.

As one observes neurotic symptoms, it is apparent that there are many individual factors that guide or determine the type of neurotic symptoms. Some of these are:

1. A Continuation of Unpleasant Physiologic Reactions. Crashing bombs, whistling bullets, lurking danger cause fear. Fear has its physical counterparts: frozen muscles, speechlessness, faintness, and marked trembling. The trembling begun as a physiological reaction continues on and on. Thus many of the soldiers who manifested nervous reactions following the Sicilian invasion were called "jitterers" because of the marked tremors and violent shaking. Thus the form of the neurosis was but the persistence of the initial physiological reaction.

2. Trauma: Prolongation of the Symptoms caused by Trauma. A paratrooper makes a faulty landing and strikes his head. He develops headaches though there has been no serious intracranial injury. The occurrence of the injury becomes a critical event which decided the inner conflict between duty and "disability." The symptom of headache has continued on and on, even though this paratrooper was evacuated to the Zone of the Interior.

We may recall the corporal in the medical detachment who had passed through several harrowing experiences, and was able to exercise self-control over his anxiety. One day he was injured by a bomb explosion, sustaining several shrapnel wounds in the thigh. The wounds healed well, without serious damage to nerves or muscle. However, he developed a marked limp and a peculiar slow gait, keeping his right knee flexed. The hysterical nature of this gait disorder was fully established when the symptom was entirely cleared up by suggestion. The pain, swelling and limitation of motion resulting from injury decided the specific development. The mechanism was a continuation of the original organic lesion, the limping prolonged by autosuggestion, prolonged also because it solved inner problems.

A similar mechanism explains the vertebral neuroses of industry. Neurotic symptoms represent a continuation of distress initiated by trauma. The worker has continued his labors in a state of relative equilibrium, inwardly resentful and unhappy. Then he is knocked down by a vehicle or suffers pain and stiffness after lifting. He becomes disabled by injury – and then the neurotic phase extends the disability.

3. IDENTIFICATION. Frequently the symptoms represent an imitation of, a copy of the symptoms suffered by some person with whom the patient was emotionally linked. We are all familiar with patients who develop hysterical hemiplegias similar to father's stroke. Imitation of fellow patients, adopting the type of sickness prevailing at the time may explain the forms of expression of the neurosis. The occurrence of a dramatic exhibition such as a convulsion may be followed by other like "attacks." Identification means contagion of ideas.

M. C. had complained of anginal pain and palpitation. When asked to tell what scene of his childhood life impressed him most, he replied: "My father used to have pain in his chest – he often rubbed his clothes so hard they got worn there – I was afraid he would die of it."

4. EFFECTIVENESS OF THE SYMPTOMS IN SERVICE OF THE EGO. In civilian practice there are many cases of impotence; in military experience there are few cases with such complaints but an unusual number of postural and gait disabilities of functional origin. Such symptoms become an embodiment of an idea, expressing more eloquently than words, "I cannot march, cannot shoot, I am no longer useful as a soldier." Grinker and Spiegel observed that pilots rarely developed back or leg symptoms, but often complained of visual disturbances which rendered them incapable of combat flying. It is remarkable that once the neuromuscular disability has developed, the patient may appear otherwise content and state verbally, "I'd like to serve my country as a fighting man – if only my paralysis cleared up." Such symptoms do not express anxiety, but an escape from unbearable fear (Goldstein).

As was expressed by Alexander, certain pent-up emotions may be accompanied by visceral manifestation (hypertension) or represent a conversion of inner repressed material. At times viscera betray fear, even though the patient consciously wishes to conceal it. There was the waist gunner in a bomber, deeply attached to the other members of the crew and very fond of his ship. After he had gone through many missions successfully, he was injured slightly. So eager was he to continue with his buddies that he asked quickly to resume his place as soon as the wound healed. On the next mission he developed gastro-intestinal symptoms and the distress grew worse as the bomber was struck by flak and its wing damaged by fighter bullets. Again he insisted on being part of the crew; consciously he wanted to continue, but there was a visceral betrayal of inner anxiety by anorexia and nausea. His gastro-intestinal symptoms led to his being grounded.

5. VULNERABILITY OF CERTAIN REGIONS. Clinical experience shows that certain areas or functions are more sensitive to upset than others. Fatigue causes backaches in one person, insomnia in another, and faintness in a third. The Achilles heel is in a different site or function in different individuals.

Who is Neurotic?

Every human being can develop nervous symptoms. When one is trembly, hot and cold, flushed and perspiring, when he awaits a call from the chairman to address an audience, such "stage fright" causes nervousness. The woman whose son is overseas is tense and trembly at the approach of the postman, hoping, wondering and fearing. Shocking news that her son has been captured leaves her pale and limp and sighing. For days she cannot work because she keeps wondering how her own tender boy is being treated; she cannot sleep for her thoughts travel to distant lands to be with him. There run through her mind the lines he was fond of reciting: "Mother of mine, oh mother of mine, if I were up on the highest hill I know whose love would be with me still." She can't eat or smile for several days. Then gradually she gains self-control, resolves to keep busy, and comforts herself with the hope that her son is well.

A nervous upset or even a nervous illness can affect any of us when we are faced with fright or failure, when those near us are ill. Fortunately the symptoms do not last long, we do not remain overly concerned about our health, we recognize the event that brought about our distress. *But the neurotic has such symptoms without obvious external cause.* The symptoms are but surface bubbles from deeper emotional processes. True, the symptoms are not constant but the tendency remains. This tendency is in part inborn and in part shaped by infancy patterns. The symptoms, however, may be controlled or kept in check by effort, by precautions. Much of the outward appearance of diligence and devotion represents striving against the inner tension. The overcautious, conservative accountant, scrupulous to the minutest fraction, may be overcompensating for the intense fear of doing wrong. The minister in *Rain,* who preached constantly to Sadie Thompson against her life of sin, appeared to be a spokesman for righteousness. His conduct in the last act and his suicide told the truth about his own sex drives. But our concern is not with those who work and struggle and often succeed against their tendency; *it is rather with those who have symptoms.*

Neurotic illness differs from those sicknesses due to external causes, *largely because a neurotic and his neurosis are one.* A soldier may become invalided when he has been shot or his leg broken, confined to a hospital by malarial fever implanted in him by a mosquito. These are organic illnesses. A neurosis is not caused by injury, is not the result of a microbic invasion, is not the result of injury or infection. *It is inextricably connected with the personality of the patient.* This personality, like a tree, grows out of several main roots, in inherited tendency, in early environment of fear and insecurity, and in unsolved conflicts charged with fear and guilt embedded in the past experience. For like a tree which owes its start to the seed and roots, yet the growth of which is modified by environment, so it is the individual's own handling of conflicts, influenced, it is true, by endowment and exposure, which fashions the neurotic features.

Neurotic symptoms fluctuate depending upon the situation. The woebegone look of one neurotic may disappear when the examiner leaves. If the mind of another becomes absorbed in some outside pursuit, the symptoms lessen. The demands and dangers may add to or remove symptoms. For example, a soldier in the invasion of Africa became acutely nervous and trembled so violently that he shook the bed; in fact, he even fell from it. When this same soldier was evacuated to the United States, he remained nervous but his shaking stopped. He merely told how upset he felt. The muscle movement abated; words took over. Even more significant was the striking improvement in many nervous soldiers in the last war after the Armistice was signed.

Not only do neurotic symptoms fluctuate, but they vary strikingly from one patient to the other. One patient tosses in bed, gasping and groaning and pleading for attention. Another lies calmly in bed, yet when asked how he feels, he will describe minutely and picturesquely the rumblings in his intestines, the burning, squeezing and beating of his heart. So vivid is the "organ recital" that I once referred to a neurotic patient as a "poet in the world of his viscera (organs), a poet who hearkens to the splashes of his splanchnic waves (intestines), whose ears are attuned to the tom-tom beat of his heart." Other patients do not act excited or say much but seem unable to carry on their duties. A soldier walks stiffly and limpingly. When you ask him how he feels, he replies, "I'm fine, all but my leg – it's paralyzed. If you get it well, I'll go right back to the front lines." Then too, there are some patients who are busy repeatedly washing their hands, so completely preoccupied are they by their fears of dirt and disease (obsession neuroses).

However variable the symptoms, we find that fear is commonly at the core of neuroses. Sometimes the danger which the patient fears is real and obvious. What could be more real than a bayonet in the hands of a Jap or the sound of a German 88, splashing death? Again the cause is deep within, an anxiety developed because of fear of punishment or guilt linked with some past (repressed) experience. Whether the fear be internal or obvious, or the two combined, such emotion affects the entire body. In the economy of life, fears serve to warn and to protect the individual against dangers. The preparedness for life-saving action involves the nervous system, the endocrines, the blood chemistry and circulation, the muscles. As the outward action of such mobilized preparedness cannot be fulfilled, tensions and tremors and disturbed functions result. When the cause of the fear is deep within, repressed yet emotionally dynamic, the patient exhibits all the signs of anxiety without being able to understand or remove the cause.

Fear is an important factor in the symptoms of war neuroses. Indeed, the pallor and tremors and rapid pulse which are accompaniments of fear may persist as the cardinal symptoms of the neurosis.

Such physical changes of fear are at first a necessary part of the body's preparedness, but later become "fixed" to serve the personality. As a nation prepared for war may be kept militarized, alerted, fearing yet warning others, merely at the instance of the government, even though no real danger is present, so the neurotic personality may maintain bodily preparedness because of inner danger.

There are other factors which determine the type and time of development of nervous symptoms. Injury is one of them. A soldier who falls in the obstacle course or who is injured in a jeep or who is shot in battle suffers pain and weakness, for which he is hospitalized. The pain and suffering became a magnet for drawing attention, interest and anxiety to this region. This painful area may continue to be the source of weakness and pain long after the wound has been healed, because of the worry and attention paid to it and because inner anxiety (free floating) needed an objective attachment. For, this pain and the inability to move an arm or leg occurring accidentally solves an inner conflict and serves the ego. The soldier may have been struggling between the private impulse to escape and the moral duty to fight. The occurrence of the bullet wound settled the issue in favor of an honorable protection of the ego. This service to the ego, called the secondary gain by Freud, may be of prime importance.

We may mention in passing several other features of neurotic symptoms. Frequently they are tenacious – the patient clings to them as though in secret league with them. Likewise there appears a need for some suffering because the removal of a symptom may not bring positive and prolonged relief. Like the two-headed hydra which defied Hercules, another symptom may grow in the place of the one removed.

Let us briefly glance at the observations of fear states as described by an excellent observer, the chief psychiatrist to the Spanish Loyalists. Mira, in discussing fear reactions among Spanish soldiers, lists six stages:

The first is the stage of prudence and self-restraint. The person limits his aims and ambitions and renounces all those pleasures which entail risk or exposure. The caution reflects an inhibitory influence of fear.

The second stage is that of concentration and caution. Actions are no longer spontaneous; they are slow, meticulous, with a waste of energy to review and guard. Subjectively, the person is worried and preoccupied. However calm and confident he pretends to be to the outside world, inwardly there is doubt.

In the third stage, the person is troubled by apprehension and alarm; he is objectively frightened. Attention is restricted and a sense of helplessness and confusion develops. Movements are made hesitantly and there are sudden tremors.

In the next stage, there is anxiety or anguish. Judgment is lost; behavior loses purpose of unity; suffering reaches a marked degree. A visceral storm from a discharge of uncontrolled centers leads to odd movements and trembling and spasms.

The fifth stage is panic. The subject is directed from the thalamic centers. Movements may be of the utmost violence and cannot be restrained either consciously by the victim or externally by change of situation or reassuring measures. In this stage of panic on the battlefield, some soldiers can perform deeds described as heroic. In fact, when "escaping ahead" in a twilight state, soldiers may conquer positions and rouse the courage of their comrades who are unaware of the basis of such actions. However, the performance is usually a source of upset for all who witness it and the subject himself experiences the distress of a nightmare.

In the sixth and final stage of helpless terror, even the automatic actions stop. The patient may lie or stand motionless, as though petrified. His pallor and lack of expression reveal complete exhaustion of psychic life.

A neurotic's symptoms may run the entire gamut of human misery or may be restricted to one part of the body. The clinical description of the neurotic reactions is thus a passing parade of every type of psychological and psychosomatic symptom and unadaptive behavior (Grinker). *They may be of short duration, though more often they run on and on, even though with periods of improvement.*

General Comment

There are many types of psychoneuroses and certainly many classifications of them. Freud made a fundamental subdivision into several groups, the division based upon the life stage at which the stream of libido was "fixated" or dammed. It was Freud's teaching that the instinct of love, expressed also as the stream of energy referred to as the libido, passed through a series of stages much as a stream winds its way through many countries. *In the life of the normal person the stream flows unobstructed from its source to its destination.* Should this instinct be held back by an over-attachment, or frozen by fear, such a cessation may lead to abnormalities in the form of mental illness. Thus the most serious disturbance in the stream of libido, leading to abnormal self-love or narcissism, is supposed to be the basis of schizophrenia. The hysterical and anxiety neuroses are believed to occur in those whose libido disturbances developed later.

There are several distinct types of psychoneuroses, each with specific features. Neurasthenia is a type which occurs in young adults, the chief symptoms of which are undue fatigue, profound weakness. It is attributed to adolescent sex practices failing to attain a normal expression.

Anxiety neurosis is a more common type whose symptoms are fear and panic, with their visceral accompaniments. This malady is explained as due to fear of recurrence of childhood deprivation of love, traced to earlier fears of losing the protection and security of parents.

Hysterical neurosis is characterized by symptoms which may be restricted to the apparent loss of one function (vision, speaking, walking). The inner complex problem has been converted – translated into a paralysis of a limb or loss of vision. The patient may be otherwise comfortable. Such conversion hysterias may be traced back to psychosexual experiences in childhood, though some recent experience reactivates it.

Obsessional neurosis is characterized by undue fears (of going into crowds, of entering an elevator and of going up high, of germs or dirt); by repetitive acts such as counting numbers, or incessant washing. These neuroses are deep-set, have their origin early in childhood, and are difficult to eradicate.

In life these subdivisions are not fixed or constant as in books –patients may have symptoms of several types or the symptoms vary from time to time. Mixed types are most common.

A superficial classification is based upon the major symptom. Thus one encounters in the literature reference to cardiac neuroses or gastric neuroses. Such terms are brief, focus attention upon the obvious symptom, but one should realize that the neurotic state goes far beyond any focal area or one organ disturbance.

Psychoneuroses have been divided according to the circumstances under which they occur. Such terms as combat neurosis emphasize the relationship between the exigencies of fighting and the occurrence of nervous symptoms. War neuroses, menopause neuroses and like terms call attention to such correlation.

A simple distinction as to type is one which I have used in my practice. I divide the psychoneuroses into two major groups: *the situational and the chronic or constitutional.*

The situational neuroses are those which develop largely as the result of a setting, an occasion which is distressing, exhausting or frightening. An individual, upon the occasion of a death in his family, a serious financial loss, an unhappy love affair, or the stress and strain of unpleasant circumstances at work, or during the exhaustion of warfare, develops neurotic symptoms.

Such an individual is of a different type than the *constitutional psychoneurotic,* in whom the factors of endowment and early conditioning are tremendously significant. This latter type has a life story of nervousness. During the infantile period there is sleeplessness, disturbed digestion, ready startle reaction and crying. In early childhood there are fears, nightmares, many complaints, and failure to adjust in play. In adolescence, there may be shyness to an abnormal degree, trembling, palpitation, flushing and sweating, an undue fear and avoidance of physical bodily sports. Then, as this person goes on through life, there may be a succession of symptoms and illnesses for which there is no adequate physical basis. The symptoms fluctuate, although the tendency remains more or less the same. In a normal, untroubled environment, screened from sins by religion, elevated by a gratifying pursuit, the individual may be symptom-free. Confronted by some challenging impacts of life, such as entrance into service, active symptoms appear.

This distinction is important in estimating the capacity of the individual to meet stresses and strains and also in evaluating the effectiveness of therapy. The patient who is more or less normal, but who develops nervous symptoms in a specific setting can be promptly relieved as a rule by appropriate treatment (as will be reviewed in the next chapter).

The constitutional psychoneurotic, however, may continue to have symptoms, even though life runs on quite smoothly and even though treatment be given. This psychoneurotic, however, during his periods of well-being or in an effort to escape his distress, may be an intelligent, charming person of great gifts. He may write well, compose beautiful music or evolve theories of far-reaching significance. The psychoneurotic is frequently sensitive, spurred by fear to create and sometimes to work, and will, if he is endowed with talent, contribute his share to the world's progress. It is well known, for example, that Charles Darwin suffered from nervousness during a great part of his life. He was troubled by digestive symptoms of a definite nervous type. He always had a pathological degree of stage fright. Yet his drive to learn, to achieve honor, his brilliant mind, led him to outstanding discoveries. Indeed, an author recently suggested that the unrest in Darwin, which might have been removed by psychoanalysis, was a great thing for the world.

I do not subscribe to the title of a recently popular book, BE GLAD YOU ARE NEUROTIC. Nevertheless, as we talk about psychoneuroses, we must not look upon such persons with contempt but as average people, and must realize that every living being can develop nervous symptoms for a shorter or longer period. I believe it was Wechsler who remarked, "There is a good deal of the normal in every neurotic and every normal has potential neurotic symptoms."

Psychosomatic Disease

The term, *psychosomatic disease*, has become popular recently as though it were an entirely new concept. Yet the history of medicine shows that *the oneness of psyche and soma is part of life* and that *the tendency to separate the two is incorrect*. Plato some twenty-five hundred years ago criticized the doctors of his day with the remark: "The fault of medicine of our time is the tendency to separate the soul (psyche) from the body (soma)." Plato could have been more outspoken had he witnessed the tendency in the latter part of the nineteenth and early twentieth centuries.

Medicine, under the spell of progress in physical examination and intoxicated by the ability to see lesions, became objective, organic, even mechanical in its concepts. Mental and emotional factors retreated shyly into the background as brilliant clinicians, expert in physical diagnosis and searching for pathological changes, stressed the structural, the microbic causes of illness. That patient was respected whose symptoms could be explained by an infection which might be curable, by a tumor which a surgeon could remove; or if the disease was incurable, the diagnosis could be confirmed at autopsy. Other patients were sometimes dismissed with the then disdainful label of neurotic.

Recognition again of the importance of mental factors came as a refreshing and significant medical truth. *It was the understanding of psychoneuroses that led to a more sincere appreciation of the role of the mind in all illness.* Experiences during the war revealed how vital was the mental attitude of the fighting man in development of psychoneuroses and in all forms of sickness.

Sometimes there were actual structural diseases which had developed as a result of emotional disorders. A group of maladies such as *essential hypertension, peptic ulcer, asthma, dermatitis* could be better understood and more effectively treated when the role of the psyche was recognized. *The term psychosomatic was applied to maladies in which the manifestations were physical but in the cause of which mental factors were extremely important.* This group lies between the psychoneuroses and the so-called organic diseases.

Finesinger and Cobb state: "Psychosomatic disturbances are like the psychoneuroses insofar as they are often part disturbances of the personality and, in the early stages, are reversible. They differ from the neuroses in that (1) they have different symptoms; (2) as a rule they are of much longer duration; (3) they have in most instances a known and demonstrable pathologic basis;(4) the treatment has of necessity been more directly concerned with the symptom itself and hence heretofore it has been directed by different groups of specialists. The patient with anxiety neurosis continues to have symptoms for years without cardiac hypertrophy or any sustained increase in blood pressure, in contrast to the patient with essential hypertension."

The psychosomatic diseases are allied to the psychoneuroses and yet the symptoms and structural changes are those of organic disease. They are believed to arise from emotional tension and drive which cannot attain outward expression. As such emotions produce endocrine and autonomic nerve stimulation, the effect of such stimulation, if persistent and not expressed, eventually results first in altered function and then in pathologic tissue change. It was Alexander and his group at the Psychoanalytical Institute of Chicago who showed how repeated unexpressed hostility may lead to hypertension and how the incessant striving of an overconscientious person to be loved may lead to gastro-intestinal disturbance.

Grinker and Spiegel state: "Since anxiety is part of a preparation for an interpreted danger or a reaction to it, which stimulates the body for action by alerting almost every organ, the resulting energy, if not adequately discharged, accumulates and then its manifestations take the form of symptoms of illness . . . . When we speak of psychosomatic disturbances it is usually with reference to conditions in which persistent and recurring emotion is recognized through those physical activities that normally accompany that emotion, consciousness of that emotion in the form of subjective feeling being absent. It is a state of affairs in which nervous energy is in part or wholly expressed through the vegetative nervous system, because some psychological barrier prevents the person from expressing the feeling at the conscious or behavioral level. The emotion is repressed and only the lower level visceral concomitants are expressed . . . ."

The symptoms of the waist gunner who developed abdominal pain and diarrhea could be classified as psychosomatic. The symptoms were the direct result of overstimulation of the vagus because of fear. The persistent fear of danger could not be expressed verbally because of the man's feeling of camaraderie for his group and because of his high morale. The gunner did not talk about his fear, could not acknowledge it to himself, but his gastro-intestinal symptoms spoke for him. The voice of the vagus expressed the psychosomatic symptoms.

A typical case is that of A. J., a contractor of fifty, a man who was always industrious and conscientious. He was married and had three children. Unusually zealous in his work, aggressive towards his competitors and often unkind to his employees, he overcompensated with kindness to his wife and a display of affection, purchasing jewels and furs for her. Underneath this attitude and display of security was a fear of failure. He craved affection and wanted admiration. He recalled that in his childhood he was obsessed by the fear of poverty and had resolved that he would acquire wealth and security. His entire life's career represented an incessant drive to achieve this security. Even when he was well-to-do, he continued to struggle because he feared he might lose his wealth or his reputation. He was hostile towards any person who might represent an obstacle to the attainment of his goal.

At about fifty, he developed heartburn, eructation, and abdominal pain. Examination showed a peptic ulcer. He received little benefit from diet and the use of antacids. However, several psychiatric interviews and the suggestion that he accept his average level of economic security proved remarkably helpful in the relief of his symptoms. He has remained symptom-free for several years. It has been possible for him to enjoy recreation and to accept others in a social sense as well as to give up acquiring and displaying material evidence of wealth.

Giving Freud credit for the basic idea of psychosomatic disease, Dunbar states that "conflicts excluded from consciousness create a permanent tension which may occasion persistent or recurrent disturbances of organic function." The studies which have followed Freud's ideas, show that emotional conflicts, inadequately expressed, disturb the equilibrium of the organism and thus result in physiological changes which in time may become physical and pathological disturbances.

REFERENCES

Freud, S.: *A General Introduction to Psychoanalysis*. Liveright, New York, 1935.

Stephen, K.: *Psycho-analysis and Medicine, a Study of the Wish To Fall Ill*. University Press, Cambridge, England, 1933.

Schilder, P.: *Introduction to a Psychoanalytic Psychiatry*. Nervous and Mental Disease Pub. Co., New York, 1928.

Farrell, M. J., and Appel, J. W.: Current Trends in Military Neuropsychiatry. *Am. J. Psychiat.*, 101:12, 1944.

Alexander, F.: Fundamental Concepts of Psychosomatic Research, Psychogenesis, Conversion, Specificity. *Psychosomatic Med.*, 5:205, 1943.

Fetterman, J. L.: Back Disorders of Psychic Origin. *Ohio State M. J.*, 33:777, 1937.

Grinker, R. R., and Spiegel, J. P.: Brief Psychotherapy in War Neuroses. *Psychosomatic Med.*, 6:123, 1944.

Goldstein, K.: On So-Called War Neuroses. *Psychosomatic Med.*, 5:376, 1943.

Mira, E.: *Psychiatry in War*. W. W. Norton & Co., New York, 1943.

Wechsler, I.: *A Textbook of Clinical Neurology*, 4th edition. Saunders, Phila., 1939.

Dunbar, F.: *Psychosomatic Diagnosis*. Hoeber, New York, 1943.

Weiss, E., and English, O. S.: *Psychosomatic Medicine*. Saunders, Phila., 1943.

Finesinger, J. E., and Cobb, S.: Psychoneurosis and Psychosomatic Disorders. *Manual of Military Neuropsychiatry*. Saunders, Phila., 1941.

Chapter III

TREATMENT OF PSYCHONEUROSES

THE aims of treatment are to remove symptoms, to promote well-being, and to help the patient get the most out of life. Sometimes these aims can be achieved rapidly, again they may require long effort, or they may never be fully attained. The results will depend upon how deep-set the neurosis is and upon the effectiveness of the treatment.

As the physician views the problems of the patient, certain questions come to his mind. "What do I hope to accomplish?" To answer this question, he should appraise the assets and liabilities of the personality, the meaning of the illness to the individual in the light of his past behavior and present situation. *Schilder points out that the physician should not attempt to remake the patient into a person like himself.* There is too much difference in people. What are the urgent physical needs and what are the emotional conflicts? Are they situational or inherent? What are the most effective remedial steps to be taken?

Treatment may be conducted along one line or along several, all having the same goal. My personal experience consists of using several methods together, each supplementing the other – for mental attitude and physical status are mutually related. We may refer to these methods as improving the patient's point of view (*psychotherapy*), building up his well-being (*physical and medicinal therapy*), and adjusting him more satisfactorily to his environment (*social therapy*). These and other specific procedures, which may draw upon all realms of human endeavor – music, art, recreation, religion and work – serve to benefit the patient. The choice of method and the emphasis used will depend upon the type of symptoms, the make-up of the patient, and the experience of the physician.

Psychotherapy

Psychotherapy is defined as the art of treating mental disorders (Hinsie and Shatzky). Psychotherapy is not one specific method, for every pill a doctor gives, every prescription which he writes, every gesture he makes, every idea which he imparts, all influence the mind of the patient. Yet psychotherapy goes beyond these simple contacts, to relieve the patient's disturbing ideas and feelings, to provide some guidance in resolving the confusion and conflicts of life, to furnish insight into what is going on within himself in relation to others (inter-personal relations). The sum total of these efforts at healing is psychotherapy.

The first essential in psychotherapy is the doctor. He should be sympathetic and possess an understanding both of medicine, mental mechanisms, and of the forces of life. He needs both knowledge and experience. His approach requires a friendly interest and considerable time, for when we say time is a great healer we mean also the time the physician spends with his patients. Rarely is scolding (confrontation therapy) effective. An appeal to will power—"Do as I am doing"—sounds good from the lecturer's platform but in a doctor's office is more effective in building the doctor's ego than in helping the patient's welfare.

The sick man is perplexed, anxious, and absorbed in his one or many symptoms. He is troubled by pain, weakness, sleeplessness, fear. His mental processes are wrapped up in his own distressing sensations and disturbed functions. It is well to obtain a detailed description of such symptoms, how they first appeared, what changes developed. After sufficient history has been taken, a complete physical examination is made. Assuming that this or previous examinations have excluded organic disease and that we look upon the symptoms as psychoneurotic, we must then go further.

We proceed to learn the make-up of the patient, the nature of his illness and the goals of his personality. Whether we label this exploration or analysis, our first step, along with a physical examination, is to encourage the patient to tell his story. At first he will talk only of immediate symptoms and his ideas of their causes, but later he will go back into his earlier life, tying up his present difficulties with a succession of life's experiences, people, work, love, finances, fears. Such telling is encouraged, for not only is it mental catharsis but it permits the patient to gain faith in the physician who acts the role of a father substitute. Most patients are eager to tell their troubles. Like a weary traveler eager to unload the heavy pack from his shoulders, so the neurotic wants to unload thoughts and worries from his harried and overburdened mind. He may continue to talk freely, but if he does not, he is guided to tell of his childhood, of school-day mishaps, of ambitions frustrated, of family discord, of social and economic setbacks. He is encouraged to tell of his sexual impulses and how he has succeeded or failed in his love adjustment. He may relate stories of childhood sexual experiences, of masturbation, of illicit love, which have filled him with a sense of guilt, or of impulses forbidden and thus inhibited by conscience. He may reveal the subjugation of his ego to a strict, scolding superego. This and much more the physician must learn, in one or many visits.

Thus, the patient is urged to talk freely. He will usually discuss his present (surface) difficulties; his work is tense and unpleasant; it is unappreciated. He expected a raise or a promotion and was passed by. His home life is unhappy. His wife drinks or gambles, or is cold and quarrelsome. Sometimes a discussion of such simple, everyday situations related to family or work may uncover disturbing elements which have caused or contributed to the trouble.

Case of Combat Neurosis Relieved by Brief Psychotherapy

An example of symptoms which were situational and which were promptly relieved is provided by the clinical history of N. E., a young man of 21. From his past history it was learned that he had been an intelligent, fairly healthy individual who had gotten along satisfactorily in a happy home environment. He did well at school and showed fairly normal traits. He mentions, however, a tendency to overconscientiousness: "I used to punish myself a great deal more than anyone else could punish me."

N. E. was inducted into service and went through his basic and advanced training efficiently. He became a member of an infantry outfit and went overseas. When his division went into action, he was assigned to a patrol which was to go forward against the enemy. He describes his experiences as follows:

"The lieutenant told us we were going into a difficult patrol between the lines and that this was heavily mined. I remember, as we were going quietly along very close to the German lines, suddenly I saw a big flash of light and then it seemed dark. I opened my eyes and there was dirt all around us. ... In a tree near by was a helmet and I looked around some more to see where everyone else was. On the other side of the road I saw my buddy still twitching and moving. There was a hole in his back. I yelled for medics and the litter bearers came. They looked at his body and said he was dead. ... I became awfully scared. The bottom dropped out of everything. From then on I tried to keep my neck out of danger. ... I said to myself, 'Keep out of the way because I don't want to get hurt.' In the next attack about fifty per cent of our division was wiped out and I often felt, 'Why didn't something happen to me?' "

This soldier maintained his esprit de corps and continued on active duty until V-E Day – struggling with the inner tendency to give up. Then, as he began to rest, he became fearful, sleepless, and was troubled by vivid, tragic dreams. When he was seen at my office, he complained of nervousness: "I am jumpy; I can't concentrate; I feel all mixed up; I am losing weight; I feel sad. The chief trouble is I keep dreaming of my buddy all the time."

The initial physical and neurological studies were negative. During the first psychiatric interview the patient unfolded the following significant material: "The main trouble is that I keep reliving the event of my chum's tragedy. I remember now that we had an argument the night before he died. Some days previously I had a hard time waking him up. I called him a gold brick. He got mad and said, 'What are you going to do about it?' After he was killed I remembered this argument. I remember now that even as we started on the patrol, we were angry at each other. I feel darn sorry that he died when I was mad at him. *When you are mad, you wish someone dead.* I hate to see someone dead because of me. I feel somehow responsible ... I wished him dead and he died. ... I am guilty."

During the subsequent two psychiatric interviews the patient continued to relate the material dealing with his buddy's death and his own sense of responsibility for this tragedy. The intense emotional ordeal of combat surcharged with the sense of guilt arising from the inner belief that his wishes had caused death, were responsible for the recurring dreams and for troublesome somatic sensations. This was a crucial event, the memory of which shadowed him relentlessly because of the terrific emotional content.

In three successive interviews of an hour each he was able to relate the details of his combat experience and of the emotional strain which preceded combat. As he described the events preceding the death of his buddy and the tragedy itself, he gained insight into the nature of his symptoms. There was obvious relief as a result of this opportunity of discussing and confessing before someone who is a representative of society, of someone in authority. He was relieved also by the assurance and explanation of the therapist that the death of his buddy was accidental.

At the third visit the patient himself volunteered: "I suppose that my wishes were like anyone's wishes when he is mad. I am quite sure that I felt that way about other people before and nothing ever happened. You know, I am feeling a great deal better since I have had these talks. During the last few days I can think of other things. In fact I am making plans to go to college next semester and to continue with the education which I dropped when I entered service."

The prompt and remarkable improvement which occurred in this instance is an example of successful brief psychotherapy. It seemed as though the patient's freedom in response to the words of the therapist could be compared with a convict's reaction to a governor's pardon. The scolding voice of the patient's conscience was silenced and his ego strengthened by his own confession, the authority of the therapist, and the convincing force of logic.

Usually it is necessary to explore more deeply and to learn of past problems and former modes of reaction, particularly in the family group. The patient may tell of an insecure childhood, of sickness, of jealousy, of being seduced, or more commonly of masturbation. During such an interview the patient may become hesitant and silent or may begin to cry, as did the woman who related the following: "It happened when I was six years old. We had a boarder who lived on the third floor. He used to invite me up and give me candy. Then one day he put his finger near my vagina and did something. It frightened me, but he made me promise I wouldn't tell my mother. The next day I went up again. I know it's wrong - I shouldn't have done it, but something made me. And he did it again. Ever since then I considered myself a bad girl. I have always been afraid of men and ashamed. Now I am married. I've never told my husband. When he attempts intercourse, I am horrified; I think of the wicked boarder and of my own badness; I am afraid my husband will find out how awful I am. I love my husband but I am afraid I will lose him."

The patient who related this episode cried and trembled, but was relieved to learn that such incidents are common and that no irreparable physical damage was done. She was advised to mention this experience casually to her husband, who was a well informed person. The patient was much relieved after this discussion.

Enough needs to be learned by the physician to understand the deeper problems and the patient needs to tell enough so that he may understand himself. In this preliminary approach, let us keep in mind that as a tool of psychotherapy, listening is more effective than lecturing.

A Clinical Example of Brief Psychotherapy

M. C., a man of 32, had developed nervousness while he was a captain in the Marines. The condition reached such a degree that he was discharged from service because of his symptoms. "I was an expert in codes. I worked very hard. I even drank to get some release from the tension I was under. I developed weak spells and could hardly stand up. One day it was rumored that information had leaked and several of us were suspected. I found out later who was the guilty party, but yet I myself felt guilty, I don't know why. My heart began to race, my blood pressure went up, and I became weak.

"For several years since my discharge from the Marines, I haven't been well; I'm worried about my heart; I'm afraid I may die."

The patient was an intelligent, well developed, healthy-appearing adult whose physical examination was negative except for an increase in blood pressure. At the initial visit the patient stated: "I am anxious, not depressed. The trouble didn't really begin when I was in the service. It must have started when I was seven. I was always nervous and highstrung.

"I was the youngest child and my mother was very close to me. She would teach me things. And even when I went to school, I would hurry home to her.

"One day I went to school and when I returned, Mother was not at home. She was in the hospital, I didn't know why. But two weeks later she came home with a new baby. Almost abruptly my mother seemed to neglect me. She paid no more attention to me. I felt lonesome, unhappy. I wouldn't go in to see the new baby. I would ask my mother if I belonged, if I was adopted. The baby's coming seemed to separate me from Mother.

"I didn't get along well with my father. He was very stern and would scold and strike me. I was always uneasy in his presence. He himself was a very nervous person who was always afraid of dying of heart trouble. My clearest recollection of him is that of his holding the left side of his chest and then rubbing it. On many occasions he cried out that he was dying. It frightened me and yet I wished he would die because the only time I felt happy was when he was away from home. *It's funny, but now that I talk about it, the pains I have in my chest are just like those my father used to complain of.*"

"When I was a child, I often thought of death and was afraid that I would die and go to hell. My mother used to teach me the Ten Commandments. I learned from her and in Sunday School that I must honor my father, but I couldn't honor him and that is why I was afraid that I would be punished and sent to hell.

"I didn't care for my sister. I remember once that she was eating zwieback and choked; she turned blue. Mother cried that she was dying. I was only eight years old then, but I didn't care if she died. In fact I didn't want her around.

"All my life I have felt somewhat insecure but I seemed to get along quite well. My sickness really began in the Marines."

This is an example of anxiety neurosis in which the symptoms in adult life were a reproduction of something the patient had witnessed as a child and were related to a sense of guilt. As Kubie puts it, "The patient's present life is seen to be the screen on which the past continuously throws its shadows."

In several visits M. C. unfolded this history of his past rivalry with his sister and hostility towards his father. The telling of this material, an explanation of his symptoms, as well as sedative therapy have brought about a considerable improvement so that the patient was much more comfortable and was able to resume work. For the first time he was able to be in his father's presence with calmness rather than uneasiness.

The basic features of psychotherapy consist first of permitting the patient to unburden himself and secondly of gaining insight into his problems. Thus relieved of pent-up emotions, seeing himself more accurately in the light of his description, he is ready to go forward, guided by the explanation, reassurance and counsel of his physician.

Education, Reasoning, Persuasion

The very process of the interview, the chance to "confess," the hope of obtaining counsel and comforting guidance from the father figure helps many patients. The patient sees his own symptoms more clearly in the light of his own recital; acts and thoughts lose their shame and horror as the listener calmly accepts them without expression of disgust. The sense of guilt is diminished by the confession and fear is lessened by the implied help of the therapist. Until he came to the physician he looked at himself through the distorted mirror of his own emotions; after his interview he can look outwardly at a true mirror installed by his medical man. This relationship of patient and good physician is of itself beneficial in some cases. However, as a rule more needs to be done. The patient must work his own way out of his troubles, guided by his doctor.

ACTIVE COUNSEL; DISCUSSION AND EXPLANATION: A discussion of symptoms is appropriate only after history-taking and examination. The patient is more conscious of palpitation than of guilt, more troubled by abdominal pain than by his fear. It is true that symptoms are often but surface bubbles which he sees and hears, not the deep unseen chemical changes going on below. His interest is focused upon the apparent reality of the physical distress of his body. The symptoms are painful, objective, immediate, and they exact attention. Hence, a careful physical study is in line with the logic of the patient and the negative findings become a positive fact in reassurance. The physician, too, is reassured by his findings as to the functional nature of the symptoms and better equipped to prescribe for the physical needs of the patient. For it goes without saying that physical disease may coexist with psychoneurosis, either resulting from it (psychosomatic), independent of it, or somewhat responsible for it. There is a continuous fluctuating correlation of psychic and somatic in every patient.

This examination provides a basis for a convincing explanation of the symptoms. Sometimes a brief, clear exposition may prove helpful. In such a discussion I employ a diagram, modified from my article on "Correlation of Psychic and Somatic Disorders."

The symptoms are pronounced and attract attention; hence the anxiety about head and lungs, heart and stomach. It is explained that any thought reaches from the cortex to centers deep in the brain, from which pathways extend to nerves which control breathing and heart rate and digestion. Through the medium of such nerves, as well as through chemical messages, the various organs work differently. Yet the source of the trouble is maladjustment or fear or guilt. I often use such other analogies as the following: "In your own home a bell may ring in the kitchen. You go to the *front* door to greet your caller and not to the room where the sound is made. The button is pressed at the front door;

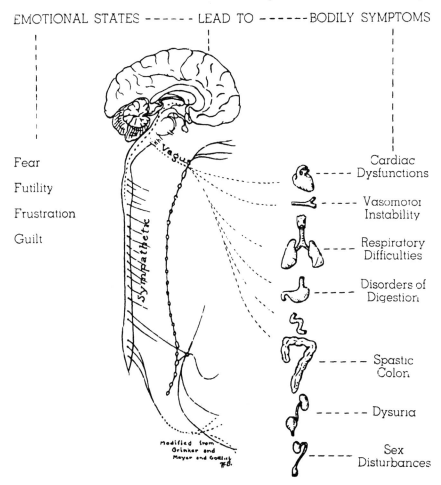

One mechanism explaining how somatic
symptoms arise from psychic causes

the current passes by wires and rings the bell in another part of the house. Or again, you are at a movie and see the action on the screen. When you stop to analyze the source of the action, you know at once that there is a film in the projecting box which provides the image cast on the screen." So it is impressed upon the patient that he is to face the issue squarely, that his trouble is felt as palpitation but does not arise in the heart; rather it comes from fear. He is to look for the cause of the fear, not merely the result.

Such discussion may take the form of education, reassurance or explanation. It is an appeal to reason, and it may work – sometimes. The patient is usually skeptical and will make some inquiry and express some doubt. His questions should be answered as fully as possible.

Such a talk with the patient tends to remove the fears which have magnified the symptoms, to lessen the sense of guilt, and thus re-establish some self-confidence.

A combination of history-taking, physical examination and explanation was effective in the case of J. H. (See Chapter II, page 28.) On the basis of such study, I was able to make the positive statement, "You do not have meningitis." There was an outpouring of ideas laden with a sense of guilt accompanied by evident emotional release. The patient gained relief by the cathartic process of confession, by the self-punishment of having to tell the entire story before a "judge." Her self-confidence was restored, her ego was strengthened by the assurance of the therapist that her "misdeed" was motivated by love and an effort to do good rather than by base, shameful purposes. This patient, who was carried into my examining room, walked out of the office, benefitted by one corrective emotional experience.

Therapy is not usually so quickly successful. In this instance, the thoroughness of the physical examination and the authoritative manner of the physician were convincingly reassuring. More than this was the patient's outpouring of her self-accusatory ideas. The doctor's sincere interest unsealed her lips and her flow of words, mixed with tears, was like the rush of water released when flood gates are opened. She then awaited censure. But the reprimand was gentle, softened by the explanation that the deed was not criminal in intent but inspired by a wish to be with her husband. Thus faith in the physician, reassurance based upon medical knowledge, the emotional release from giving public utterance, the friendly interpretation providing insight which bolstered the ego, all combined to provide definite and prompt improvement. This patient lived out of town and was not seen again, but reports from the referring physician indicated continued well-being.

Explanation and reasoning are not always effective. Additional measures are often necessary. Yet in an intelligent patient, especially if the symptoms be recent and due to some remediable situation, considerable good can be accomplished. The physician depends not alone upon logic and reason; he fortifies these with the authority of his knowledge and experience. He takes the role of a knowing father, leading the timid, dependent child, instructing and reassuring. Such authority, reinforced by the facts of medical study, presented logically, can be remarkably effective. To a patient who is lost in a maze of fears, who has lost all confidence in himself and who is frightened by the terror of the unknown, the physician is like a guide who points to the right road, who inspires renewed energy and confidence. How often has a physician seen a fearful and anxious patient coming frantically to him for help, and if the physician patiently listens to the problems and offers correct counsel, the patient may gain lasting benefit. Wrongly guided or mishandled, the patient's fears mount and his illness persists. Even adolescent problems of masturbation can be helped in adult life as well as in the adolescent by a few interviews – so-called brief psychotherapy.

Therapeutic efforts in the direction of aiding the individuals attitude include the following:

1. Provide an understanding of the symptoms and insight into the illness.
2. Reduce the sense of guilt; lessen the need for self-punishment.
3. Relieve the fear.
4. Provide reassurance and restore confidence (building the ego).
5. Direct thoughts and interest from introspection to outside, constructive activities.

One may be skeptical of the effectiveness of brief psychotherapy. Yet my experience leaves no doubt of its value in many instances and I was impressed by Alexander and French's endorsement of brief procedures. Alexander cites the story of Jean Valjean as an example of the value of one corrective emotional experience in changing the attitude and behavior of a person:

"Every reader is familiar with the classic example of a corrective emotional experience in Victor Hugo's *Les Miserables*. In his account of Jean Valjean's conversion, Hugo anticipated the fundamental principle of every psychotherapy which aims to establish a profound change in the patient's personality. It will be recalled that Jean Valjean, the ex-convict, underwent a dramatic change in his personality because of the overwhelming and unexpected kindness of the bishop whom he had tried to rob. While he was still stunned by being treated for the first time in his life better than he deserved, Valjean met little Gervais playing a hurdy-gurdy on the road. When the little boy's two-franc piece fell to the ground, the ex-convict put his foot on the coin and refused to give it back. Although the little boy cried and pleaded desperately, Valjean remained adamant. In a paralyzed and utterly confused state of mind he was unable to remove his foot from the coin. Only after Gervais left in despair did Valjean awake from his stupor. He ran after the boy in a frantic effort to make good his evil act, but could not find him. This was the beginning of his conversion."

We might question that one favorable experience could undo the cumulative effects of lifelong maltreatment. We are justified, however, in assuming that Valjean, although a hardened criminal, had a conscience which was rendered ineffective only by the hardships of his emotional development. He had to emphasize to himself his adverse fate in order to feel free to act destructively. This equilibrium was disturbed by the bishop's unexpected and extraordinary kindness.

Valjean's conversion took place within a few hours; it is a model of brief psychotherapy. This masterpiece of psychodynamic analysis was written in 1862, about sixty years before Freud introduced his concept of the superego and its compelling influence upon human behavior.

That Hugo's story is no mere creation of fantasy has been proved by many clinical examples. The author has also observed the tremendous effect upon young delinquents of the mere fact that the therapist's attitude was not critical and moralistic but that of a benevolent and helpful friend. In some patients, the pronounced contrast between the patient's own self-critical superego reactions and the analyst's permissive attitude alone may produce profound results."

For an acute neurosis such as those which occurred in warfare, one may combine physical measures, medicinal therapy, and brief analysis. As regards brief analysis, Kubie writes: "Most emotionally disturbed patients try to hide their feelings .... When this effort fails, one sees all degrees of anxiety, with shaking, shivering, chattering, starting, dashing away to hide, sweating, vomiting, urinating and voiding of feces ... there may be a rapid circling through the whole gamut of emotions. Either in the midst of emotional outbursts or in quieter interludes, there may be an uncontrollable need to talk obsessively and endlessly about home and family, about recent experiences, about the men who have been killed, about the conduct of officers, etc. Since human beings like to blame their troubles on superiors or on subordinates, pet hates and resentments will be heard frequently. Such a patient should never, under any circumstances, be shamed, reproved, intimidated or bullied ... he should be freed of the fantastic feeling of guilt that haunts many survivors of terrifying experiences. The feeling that he has survived at the expense of those that were lost, that he is a murderer of his comrades ... is particularly striking among survivors of catastrophies at sea. Here again the patient's feeling of guilt must be heard with respect. During this phase of treatment the physician is an attentive, sympathetic presence who helps the patient to 'discharge his pent-up anguish.' "

Healthful Activities

In addition to and as an aid to a more healthful point of view, the patient should be instructed as to a useful program of activities. Herzberg speaks of "Tasks" which he assigns – a positive program of attitudes and denials to offset or oppose the weakening symptoms of the neurosis. Levine mentions development of hobbies, diversion and entertainment, bibliotherapy and like programs to elevate the ego, remove thoughts from introspection and anxiety. Certainly an absorbing pursuit, be it occupational therapy, a hobby of collecting or creating, or a useful job, is valuable to recovery. For such pursuits remove worry, direct attention to creative goals, provide companionship, and restore confidence in self (ego). The psychoneurotic should be encouraged to leave his passive, dependent, symptom-cultivating manner and take on constructive aims.

Recreations of all kinds should be advised, the type and amount graduated to the needs of the patient. A woman whose goals and dreams placed her in a Versailles salon surrounded by artists and poets, actually lived with a husband completely absorbed in business and with a problem daughter. Thus hemmed in by fate, she developed a series of nervous symptoms, chiefly gastrointestinal. For years she visited doctors and clinics because of "colitis." Then she was invited to attend a garden club and was impressed by its members and by a cultured speaker who was a leading florist. Zealously she took up gardening, raising prize blooms outdoors and exotic flowers indoors. Her garden is a show place which fills her with self-confidence in place of self-pity. The planning and cultivating, the task of watching the growth from seed to fragrant flowers are distracting joys. Proudly she exhibits her work and Nature's, to the praise of her admiring friends. "This is mine; I have grown it," she says to herself – and there is a displacement of affect from family to flowers. She no longer cultivates colitis.

The simple expedient of prescribing a pet helped toward the recovery of a single woman, age 35, lonesome and unhappy. She had developed a neurosis, feeling insecure, shaking and sleepless. After a discussion of symptoms, it was suggested that she get a dog. She followed this advice by studying breeds and visiting kennels and then purchased a cocker spaniel. How tenderly she looked after its needs, got it a warm sweater for outdoors and a soft bed indoors. Her anxiety was transferred from herself to her little puppy. As it grew and she would go walking with it, she would be engaged in conversation by passersby who stopped to admire her dog. Expecially those who also walked with dogs would exchange greetings native to the world of dog lovers. She met and made friends with those who had common interests. Gradually she lost her anxiety about herself and improved remarkably.

I recall also the experience of a nervous man who had been troubled by insomnia. One night, as he wandered about his home, angry with himself, he struck a piece of metal several blows with a hammer. He was attracted by the resemblance to a man he knew. He hammered it more carefully – the resemblance was clearer. The next night, when he couldn't sleep, he went directly to the metal and hammered it carefully and gently. Yes, it became a visible figure. Night after night he worked at it. His skill improved and so did his sleep. This became a hobby which he then pursued diligently. He showed his work to friends, who admired it, so that he was urged to exhibit it in craftsmen's shows. He won prizes. His ego was raised and his self-confidence regained. This hobby, accidentally hit upon, had revealed a hidden talent and aided his mental health.

Another man, who is short in stature, with irregular features, was possessed by a drive for professional success. He had an unhappy childhood; he was envious of the richer and more handsome boys. He developed marked aggressiveness and hostility, which appeared in his tendency to criticize and humiliate any competitor. He developed nervous symptoms – insomnia, abdominal pain, tremors. One day he saw a display of wood carvings and decided to try this himself. He went into it with a vengeance, whittling and cutting into the wood – a socially acceptable substitute for his hostility – and turned out beautiful work. His symptoms decreased as his achievements grew.

Card games too are a miniature substitute for the competitive strife of living. Gardening and golfing, collecting and creating, all such absorbing recreations are a therapeutic tool for psychoneuroses as they are a tonic for all of mankind.

Work

Work removes worry – or action absorbs anxiety. The more a neurotic can utilize his mental energy, the less likely he will be to complain. One major idea can traverse the pathways of the brain, just as one crack train has priority over a railroad track. Hence the counsel to play, to build, to create, is good therapy. In such creating, the patient builds more than an article; he builds his ego. He whittles wood, digs in his garden, plays golf – all outlets for energy and for aggressive impulses. Levine points out the need for such outlets for aggression, which might otherwise be turned against one's self or turned to unhealthy goals.

A satisfactory job has many therapeutic benefits and is strongly urged for veterans with war neuroses. How does this come about and what are some of the factors in the work situation which are helpful in reducing disability?

Work involves not alone muscular effort, and its influence extends beyond the material gains. There is the element of socialization. There is the relationship to fellow employees and to superiors; there is pride in learning and advancing, and in many instances the satisfaction of a job well done. We must also recognize that a job poorly rewarded and work under hazardous conditions in an atmosphere of stress and strain, and particularly labor of a monotonous nature create unhappiness, irritability, and dissatisfaction.

Consider certain individual items in the work situation:

The material reward: If certain features are the poetry of work, the material aspect is its prose. To cope with problems of nature, work is necessary for life. The farmer must till his soil and raise his crop or else face starvation. The miner must dig coal, the tailor sew garments to provide warmth, houses must be built, fuel furnished and food prepared so that man may survive. Life is maintained through painful muscles, toil and sweat. Yet there is a feeling of satisfaction when man has performed his duty and satisfied his needs.

The social aspects of work: Most jobs involve teamwork and supply man with one of his important needs – contact with fellow men. We must share our joys, we need sympathy during periods of sorrow, there must be some rivalry and competition, there is even an instinctive tendency to show our superiority by claim or performance. The relationship of employee and chief, instincts of loyalty, the need for approval and advancement, are all expressed in the work situation. Thus we find that many a person is happier when busy with his fellow workmen than when alone with himself. Of course it is a tragedy all too frequent when a workman receives few rewards and little recognition, and when he is the butt of jokes and pranks and the victim of the condemnation and superiority feelings of others. Under such circumstances, the job is no incentive. It is a painful ordeal to be endured because of necessity and from which the person will remain away as long as possible when sickness and injury afford the opportunity for honorable and compensated escape.

While working and during the rest periods, the employee has a feeling of communal spirit, a sense of belonging to the organization. He participates in discussions, he exchanges views, there is a sense of refreshment in being away from home. The housewife who allows the dinner to burn while she is discussing events and personalities over the back fence demonstrates the importance of the social needs of people.

The interest in work: Our jobs and the products we create are an extension of our personalities. They represent the expression of our dreams, the concrete fulfillment of our manual dexterity and our imaginations. They afford us the opportunity to create, to impress, to achieve. Think for a moment of the writer working on his novel, the sculptor modeling his statue, the master craftsman building his machine. Picture the planning, the labor of love, the anticipation of success, the joy in the work well done.

It would be ideal if all work were creative, safe, and interesting. Most jobs fall far short of this ideal. When the work is unsafe and dangers abound, when the daily routine is monotonous, then there is little stimulus for personality development. Even in such instances the pride in the product of the whole organization, the effort to improve or to better the record, may supply some incentive.

On the positive side, work furnishes substance, socialization, and an interest in the product. There is often the sense of well-being which comes with muscular activity. Furthermore, work absorbs our thoughts and draws them away from introspection or unhappy reflection. It helps to raise the level of the ego.

The need for work is especially prominent in the psychoneurotic. All therapy should attempt to keep the neurotic busy, doing and creating to the extent of his capabilities. There are certain symptoms and periods which render the psychoneurotic disabled. But these are usually temporary. Hence I would discourage weekly insurance payments or pensions for psychoneuroses beyond an initial period for diagnosis and treatment. These subsidize the illness, make a patient more introspective. He strives to earn his pension by retaining his symptoms. We should not remove any incentive to return to work, which is a valuable ally in recovery.

Changing the Environment

Sometimes the point of view cannot be altered by exploration and by discussion, for the individual is reacting unfavorably to his environment, reacting like an allergic patient to an atmosphere laden with pollens to which he is sensitive. One must "purify" the environment and remove the patient from it.

Modifying the environment may mean changing the attitude of those in contact with the patient. His family may be so anxious and overprotective as to cultivate symptoms. A husband may be so unfaithful, so indifferent or cruel that his wife's symptoms are obviously a means of punishing him or of trying to keep him near her. Treatment requires a neutral atmosphere in the first instance and a warmer, more attentive interest in the next. The members of each family must be instructed as to their role in the neurosis and what they can do to help toward recovery.

Modifying the environment may mean a change in the patient's job. There are those whose jobs are too laborious, too unpleasant, who are faced with heat or dust or people who upset them. Going to work is distasteful and each day's endurance adds to nervous tension. So a change of employment is desirable. Previously I recounted the case history of a man who had been persuaded by his wife, or perhaps compelled, to work in a factory, much against his inclination. He told how longingly he looked out from the steamy, dusty furnace room into the green, sunny pastures outside. He craved air and sunshine and freedom from noise. One day he sustained an injury to his foot, a slight fracture of one toe. The fracture healed in six weeks but this man did not return to work then – nor in six months. He continued to complain of pain and weakness and limped pitifully – without organic reason. The condition was diagnosed as an hysterical weakness of his foot - serving as revenge against his domineering wife and as an escape from the factory to the country which he loved.

In another instance a patient had developed marked nervous symptoms when his expected promotion did not come through and when the new superior was a younger man of the "bossy" type. The patient developed loss of appetite, sighing, sleeplessness. He was aware of hostile impulses toward his new superior, whom he hated. Discussion and medication proved of little benefit; a vacation and transfer to another department brought about an improvement. Such a change serves as therapy, in conjunction with the benefits from other procedures – the discussion of symptoms and reassurance by the physician, the chance to unload the pent-up emotions and the practical counsel of the doctor as to medicine, rest, and his recommendation for change of environment. The neurotic symptoms were recently acquired, situational, and thus remedied by a change in the situation.

A change of environment may mean a complete rest, a period away from home, or hospitalization. A period in a hospital is remarkably beneficial to certain patients with anxiety neuroses. It breaks the monotony of the previous weeks and months. It removes the patient from those persons whose attitudes of love and hate may have contributed to the symptoms. It makes possible a neutral environment, as well as examinations and tests which are reassuring. Likewise, the fearful patient knows that a trained nurse and a capable physician are available day and night, in case of an attack. Panicky fears are allayed by the security thus afforded by the findings and the staff ready at hand at all times. Of course, a stay in the hospital is of itself not the complete therapy. Some effort should be made during the hospital period to study the interpersonal problems and the internal conflicts. The opportunity to relieve inner tensions, the insight gained, plus the stay in the hospital, are all three correlated in their influence for improvement.

The tremendous therapeutic value of changing the environment was obvious in dealing with neuroses of war. Certain inductees developed neuroses because of separation from home, deprivation of their accustomed props, inability to adjust to the surroundings of Army life and fear of the dangers ahead. When treatment in the Army setting failed, such soldiers were discharged. The change in environment, namely a return home, resulted in "cures" quite frequently. So too, periods of rest for the pilot or the man in combat, rest with the promise of a change in assignment was sometimes more effective than analysis.

Two case histories are cited showing the injurious effect of an unhealthy (psychological) environment due to improper classification. In the first instance a change of assignment resulted in a striking improvement in well-being and efficiency. In the second case, discharge from the Army and the opportunity to work quietly by himself helped greatly.

Picture the plight of a psychologist, thin, sensitive, shortsighted, and learning bayonet practice in the infantry. Marching fatigued him, his muscles just couldn't take it. He was clumsy in bayonet practice, slow in physical combat, and in running. A sense of exhaustion and futility overcame him. He was on the verge of losing his poise and reporting sick with nervousness when a former colleague, a major in the medical corps, spied him. Six months later this same psychologist was in a Station Hospital, working happily until late into the night, giving mental tests. He was one of the most useful men in the hospital and no amount of work was too hard for him. He loved his job and was adept at it. Prestige and a sense of accomplishment were tonics; a remarkable sense of well-being flowed from this renewed feeling of efficiency and service.

Less fortunate was a clothing fitter assigned to the infantry. Thirty-seven years of age, skilled in needle craft, accustomed to a sedentary life, he exerted himself to do his part as a fighting man. Driven on by a high sense of duty, he drilled and marched and bivouaced and fought with the "enemy" on maneuvers – but he was always behind the others, always exhausted, too tired to relax, too worn out for recreation. Then his outfit went to England and here the training was even more rigid. Others were promoted and he, intelligent and successful in civilian life, never got a rating because he was too slow, too exhausted. Then his company, each man with a full pack, was ordered on a long march. The day was hot and the ex-clothing fitter was fatigued, but he must keep going. Try as he would, he fell behind and then, as the company was given the order to do double time, he started to run and fell flat on his face. All the pride and all the self-control of a year's effort were broken when he fell. Emotion swept through him. He cried openly for the first time in his life, sobbing like a child. A sense of quitting, of failure came over him. He was hospitalized and new symptoms developed.

In the hospital he had many complaints of indigestion, weakness, pain, trembling, weight loss, all of which rendered him unfit for duty. Hospital treatment was of slight benefit. Discharge from the Army, the sympathetic care of his family, living away from fear and exhaustion in an environment which was pleasant for him changed the entire picture.

Such changes may not be permanent "cures" – the personality remains the same. Yet from the standpoint of the individual and society, an unhappy, suffering individual was converted into a comfortable person, working constructively. This may not be total psychotherapy, but it does help considerably. F. R. was a neurotic failure in an artillery outfit but after discharge he was remarkably well doing art work.

Physical measures are also a supplement to therapy. Man is a muscular machine as well as a personality. Well-being that comes from exercise radiates into the mental functions. Thus walking and calisthenics, swimming and bowling and golf should be encouraged. Hydrotherapy has its uses – a warm tub bath in the evening to relax tension and to help sleep; a cool shower for stimulation; swimming for exercise. Sunshine and the scent and breeze of the outdoors are tonics to many. Then too, specific symptoms such as pain, can be eased by heat, massage, passive motion. Diathermy, electric pads and hot packs may furnish relief of pain even if it arises from psychic sources.

Medicinal Measures

As a supplement to other methods, medicines have their place. For the psychoneurotic patient has physical symptoms from his neurosis, or independent of it, which may require relief. The physician of today is the heir of the accumulated wisdom of the ages, entitled to share the treasures stored in the pharmacopeia. Even the psychotherapist must not disdain to make use of such drugs. Drugs can supply such relief, and even aid the physician in his efforts at psychotherapy. Let us consider some of the commonly used medicines, helpful in the treatment of neuroses and equally useful for relief in depressions.

BROMIDES: For many years bromides have afforded persons calmness in states of anxiety, some sleep in place of insomnia. Such preparations as sodium bromide, gr. 10 to gr. 20, in tablet form or dissolved in water or as a tincture; the effervescent bromide tablet (Burroughs Welcome Co.); bromide in effervescent salts (Bromionyl) are common forms. A personal favorite of mine is sodium bromide dissolved in elixir of phenobarbital. The amount of bromide can be increased or decreased as needed in a particular patient. The preparation is red in color and palatable. A prescription of C. W. Stone, combining the sedative action of bromides with the cathartic effect of cascara (for constipated patients), is the following:

    Sodium Bromide iv ʒ— 15 c.c.
    Aromatic Cascara i ʒ— 30 c.c.
    Elixir Simplex iv ℥—120 c.c.
          qs ad

Sig: one teaspoonful three times daily after meals
ʒ—symbol for dram   ℥—symbol for ounce

The dose of bromide is usually 15 grains three times daily, but this may be reduced or increased in accordance with the response of the individual patient. Bromides are beneficial but patients should be cautioned about the probable acne or other rash. Likewise, the possibility of a bromide psychosis should be kept in mind.

PHENOBARBITAL: Phenobarbital is one of the popular mild sedatives. It is used often in tablet form, gr. ½ (0.032 gm.)t.i.d. to gr. 1½ (0.1 gm.) at bedtime. The elixir of phenobarbital, which contains gr. ¼ of phenobarbital, is widely used in 1 to 2 dram doses q.4.h. As the dosage is small, I customarily add sodium bromide to it.

OTHER BARBITAL PREPARATIONS: Sodium amytal, gr. 1 to gr.3 in capsule form, is valuable for insomnia or for relief of tension. This should be used over a limited time, whereas bromides and phenobarbital can be taken over a long period of time—under the observation of the physician and with due regard to possible cumulative effects. Sodium pentabarbital, gr. 1½; nembutal, gr. 1½; seconal, gr. 1.½, are likewise excellent sedatives for relaxing a nervous patient, especially to provide sleep for one who is tense and wakeful.

CHLORAL HYDRATE in doses of gr. 10 to gr. 20 may give a prolonged sedative action for a sleepless patient. It can be dissolved in water or in milk and is commonly combined with sodium bromide:

  Chloral hydrate   ℥ i— 30 c.c.
  Sodii bromide   ℥ i— 30 c.c.
  Aqua qs ad   ℥ iv—120 c.c.
  Sig.: one teaspoonful in water or milk h.s. as needed.

BELLADONNA: Tr. belladonna, M. X. to M. XV, is helpful for relief of intestinal pain. It may be combined with elixir of phenobarbital:

  Tr. belladonna   ℥ i— 30 clc.
  Elixir phenobarbital ℥ iv—120 c.c.
  Sig: one teaspoonful with water t.i.d. p.c.

INSULIN: A patient who has a poor appetite and is undernourished will commonly gain appetite and weight if given insulin. This is administered in 10-unit dosage subcutaneously one-half hour before meal time. It is not rare for patients to gain five to ten pounds per month under an insulin regime.

MISCELLANEOUS: Nervous patients who show vitamin deficiency need extra vitamins; those anemic require iron; those fatigued and depressed obtain some lift from the morning use of dexedrine sulfate, 2½ to 5 mg. at breakfast and if necessary repeated at 10:00 a.m. and 12:00 noon. An adequate diet, well balanced to meet vitamin requirements, smaller meals several times a day or special foods are needed in gastro-intestinal cases. So too, in specific instances any drug in the pharmacopeia may have some use even in neuroses. The use of medication is as a supplement to, not a substitute for, the other steps in psychotherapy.

Suggestion

There are patients who concentrate upon a physical symptom and who are untouched by discussion, uninfluenced by medication. Indeed, the patient may not complain—yet he may have loss of vision, inability to use his arm, or may limp. Such an hysterical symptom is referred to as conversion, as though some idea, some inner conflict were converted into or exchanged for the symptom. If a patient does not respond to insight which is given him, or if, because of language difficulty or lack or time, an uncovering technique is not feasible, then suggestion may be employed. Suggestion is a technique in which the physician uses his authority (the power implied by his reputation and experience) to instill in the patient an acceptance, a belief in his recovery. The patient (the child) with complete faith accepts the assurance of his doctor (father) that he can see, can use his arm, can now walk.

Suggestion is more effective and its result more lasting if the patient also acquires insight. Yet it is a useful tool, a short-cut of real value. Suggestion may be simply a direct statement to the alert, wide-awake patient, or it may be given to the patient who is in a state of hypnosis. I have used suggestion effectively in patients made drowsy and more susceptible by the use of sodium amytal (gr. 7 to gr. 15 intravenously). Suggestion may also be fortified by a physical procedure, such as massage, faradic electricity, etc.

For patients who have some hysterical paralysis, suggestion is frequently successful. Hadfield in England relied chiefly upon suggestion to counteract the unfavorable autosuggestion of illness. My own personal experience in the treatment of gait disorders has been the use of suggestion under sodium amytal sedation.

Treatment of Corporal D. J. with Suggestion under Sodium Amytal

Corporal D. J. was an ambulance driver in North

Africa, whose leg had been injured by shrapnel. Though the wound had healed well, the leg became flexed at the knee and the corporal limped slowly and awkwardly. Likewise, he complained of nervousness, abdominal pain and backache. During several interviews and detailed examinations it was apparent that the bone and joints were uninvolved, that no nerve injury existed. The stiffness and marked limp which caused such a wobbly, slow walk, were not caused by organic disease. They represented an hysterical form of neurosis.

The patient related details of a fairly happy boyhood with the usual illnesses, injuries and upsets. He hadn't done well in high school, changing subjects frequently and finally quitting to go to work. He was concerned about illness, keeping a bottle of iodine at hand "to prevent infection." Then, at nineteen, he enlisted and was assigned to the medical department as a first-aid man and later as an ambulance driver. He was a diligent soldier and was promoted.

His outfit was sent to North Africa, where he went through the engagement at Kasserine Pass, and later participated in other battles of the Tunisian campaign. Many were the wounded he helped into his ambulance, many the soldiers whom he brought to safety. Of course the suffering and the mutilations he witnessed disturbed him greatly, but he maintained control – until the day a German plane dropped a bomb which crashed near him. "When I came to, I thought I was crippled for life. How I hated those damned Jerries! I could hardly keep from striking the first German I saw."

As this soldier unfolded his history in detail, he gave vent to a great deal of emotion against the enemy and also expressed the fear that he was paralyzed for life. Doctors had told him that his injury was bad, that certain nerves were paralyzed. It seemed as though all his attention was focused upon his paralysis. The mere telling of his symptoms, the physiotherapy he had received failed to modify his symptoms. So I decided on this additional step:

The patient was told that he would be given a special treatment which would straighten his leg and that he would be well. Then he was given an injection of sodium amytal, 15 gr. in 10 cc. of distilled water, intravenously. This was administered slowly and as he grew drowsy, the statement, "You will be well" was re-emphasized. As he relaxed into a state of semistupor I began to massage the muscles of his leg, and gently straightened the stiffly flexed knee. As I talked reassuringly and continued the massage, the bent knee yielded inch by inch and finally was relaxed straight on the bed. The patient was allowed to fall into a deep slumber. When he awoke an hour later, he was thrilled to see the improved position of his leg and proudly raised it and moved it around. With assistance, he stepped down and was able to stand erect. In several subsequent visits he was instructed to walk properly and he responded with an excellent recovery.

At this stage it was explained to him that the "paralysis" was *not* caused by severed nerves but was developed by a loss of control through pain and fear – and attention. The meaning of his symptom, its service, was made clear.

The patient was thrilled by the improvement and remained well for many months, during which he drove an ambulance for a motor pool in the United States. To the best of my knowledge his recovery has continued.

Some consider such treatment inadequate, however effective it may be at the time. True, we should not be content with the local improvement but should help the patient to understand the cause of the difficulty and to recognize its meaning. Even though suggestion is like patching a tire instead of buying a new one, we must remember that a patched tire can take us a long, long distance. As an example of duration of recovery, may I mention the patient with an hysterical leg paralysis, for which he had worn a brace for four years, who was treated by me in the 1930's, with a favorable result. Up to the time of my entrance into the service in 1942 this man remained well.

Treatment of Miss M. R. with Suggestion under Sodium Amytal

Another remarkably effective "cure" by suggestion aided by sodium amytal is that of M. R. Several years ago I was called to see this young woman, who was "paralyzed in bed." I found a pale, thin girl in the middle twenties, lying rigidly in bed, absolutely unable to turn from side to side and even resisting rising for a bed pan. She was actually in a pool of urine – too stiff to permit the bed pan to be placed under her. It was learned that she was brought up in an over-religious family, with undue emphasis upon preaching, printing and distribution of religious literature. Prior to the illness the young woman had spent a great deal of time in the choir, attendance at church, and in prayer. She had a gentleman friend but quarreled with him and broke her engagement. She took to bed, complaining of weakness in the arms and legs. At first she was able to be up and about for brief periods of time. Gradually she became weaker until completely bedridden.

At the initial examination, so marked was the rigidity and so sickly the appearance that I suspected severe organic disease. The young lady was placed in the Lakeside Hospital and many tests were done. A searching study was made, but no concrete evidence of organic disease found.

Away from the home, under routine psychotherapy, with aid of the nursing staff and physiotherapists, the young lady made slow progress. Inasmuch as, after two weeks, she still seemed unable to move about more than a few steps, I decided upon the use of suggestion under sodium amytal. This patient had explained to me that she believed her illness was associated with her religion, for, "whom God loveth, He chasteneth." When M. R. used this phrase, she conveyed the impression that suffering of this kind brought one nearer to God. It was therefore decided, by powerful countersuggestion, to attempt to overcome the suggestion of illness.

M. R. was put in a darkened room and given an injection of sodium amytal intravenously. As she grew drowsy, hypnotic suggestion was used. Both the nurse who cooperated with me, and I reassured her that she would awaken improved and able to walk. We stated that "God wanted His servants to work for Him and to minister to others rather than to be ministered unto." Reassurance and encouragement were repeated again and again until she fell into a deep sleep. When this patient awoke, she announced happily that she felt different. She said that she was hungry and eager to be active. She ate a hearty meal, got out of bed, and walked about quite steadily. From day to day she improved until she walked with a strong and elastic step and left the hospital feeling a great deal better. In the course of time she gained some twenty pounds in weight and even got a job. She regained full and complete use of all her musculature.

Of course the illness had prevented her marriage, had kept her nearer to her father and, in a symbolic sense, nearer to God. Likewise the illness had both punished her for her guilty (earthly) thoughts and purified her for a more angelic career. The brief treatment, supported by the hospital atmosphere and later discussions about a career, helped to bring about a marked improvement. She has made a fair adjustment for several years.

Narco-Analysis and Narco-Synthesis

Sodium amytal or sodium pentothal intravenously may be used not only as a means of rendering the patient more suggestible but also to make the patient speak more freely, uncover more readily. Under such state of narcosis, the patient can relive experiences repressed or hidden, can be led more quickly to reveal significant facts. The data thus gathered can then be discussed at the next interview when the patient is fully conscious. Such analysis and later synthesis have been used with striking success by Grinker and Spiegel in war neuroses:

"... By virtue of the dangerous and helpless situation, the ego has reacted as an infant might. It abandons the scene – stupor; refuses to listen to the noises – deafness; refuses to talk about it – mutism; or refuses to know anything about it – amnesia or in milder cases develops phobic mechanisms. During pentothal and shortly after, the patient will give up these defenses as long as the psychiatrist will furnish concrete evidence of his supporting presence."

Grinker recently detailed the case history of a captain in the Air Corps who was suffering from depression, anxiety, insomnia because of recurring battle dreams, and startling when someone turned on the light or made a sudden noise. The symptoms appeared at about the twenty-fifth mission, when a friend who had been flying on his wing went down in flames. In the course of one week this captain was remarkably improved. Under sodium pentothal sedation, the captain cried and sobbed when he excitedly went through the scene of warning his friend to "bail out" and "I hope I am not responsible for his death." The captain was assured that it was the Germans, and not he, who were responsible for his friend's death. In subsequent interviews he uncovered the story of his competitive striving, of his childhood ambitions under the exacting pressure of a strict father. In several interviews under the guidance of the therapist, the captain became conscious of his inner drives, sense of guilt, and fully aware that there was no basis in reality for his guilt. Grinker mentions several steps in this brief psychotherapy as "release of repressed emotions," "support of the patient's weakened ego," "instilling insight into the relationship between the neurotic reactions to war and the past character and personality trends," "encouraging the ego .. giving new confidence to the personality."

An example of a brief narco-analysis carried out by A. A. Weil is the following:

T. E. is a 27-year-old housewife, formerly an actress and dancer, who came to us in February, 1946, with the chief complaints of dryness in the throat, cold sweats, trembling, depression, and pronounced feelings of insecurity in all fields of psychosocial and psychosexual adjustment.

She gave the following history: She was the only child of maladjusted parents. She grew up in a home of constant argument and the parents were finally divorced. From her very early youth she had a great liking for the theater and took it up as her career. However, she was not a success professionally and she felt frustrated. She blamed this failure largely on her lack of push and made a meager living by playing in summer stock, tap dancing, etc. Her only great ambition, to go on Broadway, was not realized.

While in New York six years ago, she was aware of the first symptoms which she describes as palpitation, trembling, and cold sweats. She consulted a neurologist, who made a diagnosis of anxiety neurosis, administered superficial psychotherapy, and gave her sedative medication which produced a slight improvement. While in New York, she was quite attached to a boy friend who was an overt homosexual.

In August, 1944, she married her former childhood sweetheart, a free lance writer. This marriage is outwardly happy and patient claims to be very much in love with her husband. Three months ago she bore him a child. However, recently her home life has been colored by temper tantrums "which are her fault." She feels that the obstetrician "sewed her up too tightly" after the delivery.

On February 15, 1946, patient was reexamined, this time complaining of palpitation of the heart, dizzy spells, "a thick feeling in the head," fear of death, and she related dreams of caskets. Subsequently we started narco-synthesis, first striving to get some insight into her psychodynamisms and later using narcosuggestive measures to produce a faster emotional realignment. Patient had six sodium amytal sessions in all.

During the first session she spoke spontaneously of the shame and guilt she felt regarding the temper tantrums she exhibited against her husband. She stated that she had had no sexual relations with him for four weeks because such relations were painful to her. She also revealed that she had never reached orgasms and that she felt that she did not deserve her husband's love. "I am not a full partner in marriage."

Whereas during the first sodium amytal sessions we let the patient talk without interference on whatever subjects she chose, during the following sessions we tried to direct the analytical procedure by so-called lead questions in more or less chronological sequence. The following additional material was obtained:

T. E. grew up with a profound hatred for her mother. At the same time she was extremely fond of her father. She felt that her mother gave her father a "raw deal" and probably fortified the existing Oedipus complex of the child by her perfectionistic trends. Our patient was often punished physically by her mother but never by her father. The mother was always threatening. As punishment she cut off the little girl's hair, humiliating her even further. When the father did not immediately take a protective attitude towards her, she became very angry at him also. She remembers vividly the prayers she offered to the Lord that the parents should die. Immediately afterward she had a strong feeling of guilt and thought the Lord would punish her for these ideas.

Under sodium amytal, she remembered that one time at the age of 10, after a parental argument, her whole body suddenly felt paralyzed. During the quarrels at supper time she was unable to eat but her mother forced the food down her throat. Even at the age of 6, she made remarks to a playmate that her parents always quarreled. Her mother gave her a severe spanking and said:"That isn't true." I had a choking feeling in my throat at the realization that my mother could lie so shamelessly before the Lord.

She had her first contacts with boy friends at the age of 16 after high school dances. Her straight-laced, perfectionistic, domineering mother, however, told her that any good girl would stay away from boys and sex. At that time she had her first temper tantrums. In this connection she also remembers that her mother threw a fit of temper when our patient "explored her body" at the age of 5, slapping the child's hands and making her stand in the corner for hours.

After graduating from high school, T. E. left for New York, against her mother's wishes, and joined the theater. She had a hard time making the proper connections and developed the idea that this was probably punishment of some mystic nature for "thinking and acting badly toward her mother." She carefully avoided any sex contacts. "I felt as though I had been slapped when I kissed a man." The only boy friend she had and with whom she felt safe was an old homosexual. As soon as a man tried to show affection toward her, she turned against him. She despised convention since "my mother was conventional."

This patient finally accepted the fact that her rejection of any love was a form of self-protection and necessary for the preservation of self-esteem. "Whenever I wanted to love my mother, I was rejected in one way or another, ridiculed or even punished." She also accepted the fact that she experienced severe feelings of guilt since she "couldn't love her mother as a girl should."

Patient improved rapidly and was able to work fairly efficiently in spite of various financial handicaps until her mother made plans to visit her. She then assumed some of her former anxiety symptoms. But when the mother postponed her visit, the symptoms quickly subsided. Incidentally, the mother remarried but the second marriage was as unsuccessful as the first.

Patient's sexual situation has also improved considerably. The fear of death has been completely overcome and the anxiety has been largely replaced by a slight amount of fatigue.

One other point should be made and that is the fact that patient rejected her husband not only to preserve her self-esteem but also because he prevented her from realizing her vocational ambitions. In spite of her failures in her career, she still feels that she "has to give something to the world" and that her husband has cast her in the role of housewife. However, after suggestions were made to join amateur groups in another city when the husband's financial situation improves, she felt reassured on this point also.

Group Psychotherapy

The therapeutic approach which has been described thus far is carried out to a large degree in private between patient and doctor. Indeed, many patients insist upon the maximum of privacy before they will speak openly about the hidden and sometimes shameful or hostile impulses of the past. Yet experience has demonstrated that neuropsychiatric patients can be helped even in the presence of each other. The patient may be relieved to know that what is secret and dreadful to him can be discussed openly in front of others (Thomas). The attempt to treat several or larger numbers of patients together, or group therapy, has been quite successful and was applied in certain war situations.

The advantage of group therapy, particularly during the war, was the economy of time and effort when it was necessary for a psychiatrist to help a larger number of patients than he could possibly handle with individual interviews. Schilder feels that some individuals can be handled even better as members of a group than when treated singly.

The effectiveness of the method depends upon certain advantages which are derived from the group. The patient confesses his problems not to one representative of society but to a number of fellow sufferers as well as to the doctor. Secondly, the patient learns that his symptoms are not unique, that others have experienced similar bodily symptoms and hostile thoughts. Somehow the intensity of his bodily distress and emotional tension is lessened when his fellow men suffer equally.

The patient can learn more about the nature of his symptoms through hearing a recital by fellow patients and a repeated discussion by the therapist. On each occasion that the physician explains the symptoms to one patient, the others who are concerned in such problems get the benefit of such discussion. The patient, furthermore, is helped by the apparent improvement and the success which is reported by those patients who have already made progress. The so-called testimonial technique has been successful throughout the ages. Patients are suggestible and there is a contagiousness of ideas. Guilt, anxiety, despondency, and helplessness are individual problems which can be brought nearer to a solution when they are freely discussed in the group.

In the technique of group psychotherapy it is well for the physician to select patients after they have had an initial private psychiatric examination. The number of patients is limited, the range being from six to thirty according to the choice of the individual therapist. My own preference was for ten patients in a group.

Most therapists begin with general lectures on anatomy, physiology, and psychology, explaining the workings of the nervous system and giving general directions. Thereafter the patients are encouraged to unfold their problems, ask questions, and discuss each other's difficulties. The technique in certain groups is primarily analytical (Schilder); in others, the approach is repressive – inspirational (Pratt).

In every group there are several ready talkers who would

be eager to speak out and to criticize their fellow patients. One or two would be completely silent, listeners only. The group usually included one wit who would conceal his own distress by trying to make "wisecracks" during the session. As a rule, there would be a critical individual who would express displeasure and pessimistic prognoses. As the members talked, it was found that the listeners would nod their heads or shake them, expressing concurrence or disbelief and would later offer suggestions.

The patients thus became active participants, not merely passive listeners. Each seemed to gain not only a certain benefit from the general remarks of the therapist but also self-confidence and prestige in offering counsel, in relating how he or she overcame some symptom and some difficulty. The members had a sense of belonging, of expressing rivalry as in a family, expecting approval from the leader.

Following such a general discussion, the physician can then select one symptom such as anxiety, discuss its nature, offer suggestions on how it can be met, and give counsel of a practical nature which may reach a group of patients as well as the individual.

Pratt of Boston was a pioneer in the use of group therapy and began his treatment with a number of tuberculous patients. Later he extended this method to a group of hypertensive individuals and reported successful results.

Schilder has made an extensive study of this technique at the Bellevue Hospital and has summed up his views in these words: "It is obvious that an individual in such a group sees the fundamental identity of his problems with the problems of others. It takes him out of the isolation into which the neurosis has led him. The members of the group easily identify themselves with each other. The fact that one member of the group brings forward material which another very often tries to hide lessens the resistance and brings forward conscious as well as 'unconscious' material. Frequently it is easier to see one's own problem when it is brought forward by another. Any problem of money, occupation, or sex that may be met has its true meaning only in a social setting of which it is a part, and it cannot even be thought of apart from this. It is to be expected that the meaning of any detail of an individual life history will be better delineated if brought forward in a group and appreciated by a group."

In military life group psychotherapy has been used more extensively than in civilian life. Rashkis met with a group of 10 patients for an hour a day five days a week, and believes group therapy to be a valuable socializing mechanism. Foulkes applied this method to a smaller group of 7 patients, who were encouraged to speak freely on any subject and then he would interpret their ideas. He used individual interviews to supplement the group meetings.

Thomas has recently reviewed the literature on this subject and believes that group therapy is effective whether it be inspirational or analytical and should be more extensively used.

Certain phases of group psychotherapy may be utilized in the treatment of other than psychoneurotic patients. For example, in the ambulatory treatment of depressions it has been my custom to hold an open discussion of symptoms and treatment among a group of depressed patients. A selection is made to include several much improved patients with those who are about to begin treatment. The improved individuals are asked to relate their experiences. Invariably the encouraging statements which they themselves offer as well as their replies to questions put to them have a therapeutic influence upon those who are uneasy and fearful.

In the main, group therapy has its value because each patient is exposed to the general impact of his fellow men, inspired by examples of improvement, moved by the contagious power of ideas, enlightened by the discussions of the therapist.

Psychoanalysis

Psychoanalysis comprises both a body of knowledge about mental functions and a mode of treatment. This understanding of human behavior in sickness and in health, of instincts and acts, of wishes and dreams has been vital to medicine. As a technique of treatment, it has been limited – limited by the time involved, the cost incurred, and in some instances by its failures as well.

Psychoanalytic treatment is based upon the following fundamental concepts:

1. Symptoms are compounded of the past as well as the present; of unconscious as well as conscious material.

2. Past (infantile and childhood) experiences are dominant in their influence upon present behavior.

3. The attachment to certain powerful infantile patterns - fear of parents, a sense of guilt for aggressive and hostile ideas - results in a tendency to repeat such patterns in adult situations – even if the original vital experience be forgotten and forced back into the unconscious (repressed). For example, a child who feared and hated his father may be uncomfortable in the presence of any person whose position of authority represents a father substitute. As Stephen succinctly puts it: "All men and women who become important to him, in his unconscious fantasy are simply father and mother over again. All aggression tends to have the unconscious significance of murder of rivals or of frustrating love-objects, all disappointment the significance of weaning, early discipline, or the first frustration of love – the unconscious is still in the nursery. It is fixated there.

"But there is an important reason for this fixation and the repetition which it brings about, and this is that with all their pains and frustrations and disappointments, these early nursery emotional experiences remain for these people a type of sexual satisfaction, and they fly towards them again and again, inevitably, like a moth to a candle, always getting stunned and scorched, but perpetually returning to renew the attempt."

4. Certain childhood experiences that have been extremely painful were injurious (psychic traumata) to the development of the personality.

5. Recovery - or cure - is achieved when the patient gains insight – a sound perspective as to his symptoms.

6. Recovery is aided by the relief of emotional tension or abreaction of repressed emotional material.

7. Recovery is assisted by a therapist, who is looked upon as a father substitute towards whom the patient can rather freely express his love and hate – and from whom he obtains knowledge and ego support. The patient can approach the therapist like a boxer sparring with his trainer, gaining experience, understanding, confidence in an atmosphere of relative safety.

Kubie summarizes the aims and subject matter of psychoanalysis as follows: "(1) There are unconscious mental forces. (2) These always play an important role in determining human behavior. (3) Where they play a *dominant* role, such behavior cannot be influenced materially without altering these underlying factors. (4) In order to do this it is first necessary to find out what the unconscious mental forces are. (5) This makes necessary the use of a highly specialized technique, which is designed to overcome certain obstacles to the exposure of unconscious material. (6) This technique is at the same time effective in modifying the influence of the unconscious forces which are brought to light."

The procedures of psychoanalysis which make it possible for the patient to obtain benefit are:

(a) The patient is encouraged to tell about his present symptoms and to bring up material from the past. Kubie instructs his patient to "allow his mind to flow without guidance or direction, bumping along from thought to thought like a blindfolded man bumping from tree to tree. The patient is instructed never to withhold anything, never to reject one thought for another because the other seems more relevant, never to keep anything back because it seems impolite or because it seems trivial or unimportant" . . . (two ideas thus connected usually have meaning). Through free association he may connect present events and conflicts with the older, hidden patterns of the past. Psychoanalysis is thus an uncovering technique.

(b) *Dream Interpretation.* Recurring events in a dream, if interpreted by free association, may likewise furnish a clue as to past events highly charged emotionally. Horney advocates extensive use of dream analysis while Kubie advises that dream interpretation be employed sparingly.

(c) *Explanation and Discussion.* Though analysis depends upon the active working through of the material by the patient himself, he is guided in his evaluation by the therapist.

(d) *Transference.* In the analytic situation the patient relives (in miniature fashion) earlier conflicts. The attachments to the therapist (love) enables the patient to restore his sense of security (positive transference). Later there is independence or resistance to the therapist. As the patient improves, he develops freedom from the dependent attitude.

We may again quote from Kubie the following functions of the analyst: "Correspondingly, the psychoanalyst finds himself playing a dual role. In one he maps out for the patient a hitherto unknown psychic territory. He describes in a quiet, friendly, but impersonal manner the significant connections which he sees between the various components of the patient's free thoughts. This, strictly speaking, is the psychoanalytical approach to an understanding of the patient's life history. The patient soon discovers, however, that this work cannot proceed in an emotional vacuum; and that no matter how quietly encouraging and impersonal the psychoanalyst remains, no matter how little the patient knows about him in reality, the analyst soon becomes the storm-center of highly-charged emotions. This is the second role of the analyst; and in order to make it possible for the work on the biographical material to proceed successfully, these stormy emotions must be watched for and anticipated, described to the patient sometimes before he is fully aware of them himself, and resolved through making clear their sources. This is what is known technically as 'the analysis of the transference-situation.' "

Such procedures have been customarily carried out with the patient lying on a couch, the psychoanalyst sitting some distance away. Daily visits of an hour are scheduled for five days per week and the analysis may last a year or more. Recently several modifications have been introduced, such as that described in a new book by Alexander and French. They emphasize the value of briefer analyses with less attention to earlier infantile problems and more attention to reality, the analyses fitted to each individual as to number, frequency, posture, and depth. Their case histories attest to the practical value of their approach.

Some of the brief therapies mentioned in the earlier portion of this chapter are not psychoanalytic in the technical sense, yet they aim to uncover causes and to provide insight upon a reality conscious level. Alexander and French break with the orthodox procedures when they accept brief (one to ten interviews) psychotherapy as psychoanalysis.

An analysis is described in popular dramatic style in the powerful novel, *Arrival and Departure*, by Koestler. The hero, a refugee from his native land to North Africa, had developed inability to walk. A friendly physician analysed him. In the analysis the patient related the brutal experiences of torture inflicted upon him by his Nazi captors, from whom he had escaped. His ordeal and apparent courage in facing the tormentors raised him to the level of a hero. The analysis reveals that an inner sense of guilt accepted the punishment; indeed, his torture seemed welcome because it reminded him of his father punishing him for his own wrongdoing as a child. Encouraged by the analyst, the hero went farther back into his childhood and told of his jealousy at the arrival of his baby brother and how on one occasion he tried to blind the baby. About two years later the patient and his little brother were playing together, when the younger child fell, injured his eye and lost his vision. Henceforth the older brother had the sense of being responsible for this loss. Throughout his life he had exposed himself to punishment and suffering – in penance for his guilt. With this unfolding and analysis, the hero is "cured." He walks straight – but does not escape to America. He volunteers for his country's air force (still ready to sacrifice himself).

Kubie is emphatic in the need for deeper analysis of the roots of a neurosis, "the repetitive core of the neurosis." Patients whose troubles are at a deeper level and who do not respond to the simpler and shorter methods should be referred to a qualified psychoanalyst. His training and the time spent provide the opportunity to penetrate into the deepest recesses. Using free association, dream interpretation, as well as a discussion of everyday problems, the analyst attempts to uncover the deep roots of the neurosis. He tries to release repressed material, to give the patient a better understanding, an insight into his own personality. The patient is not merely passive; he must make sacrifices (payment), he must work toward recovery by bringing forth material, by analysing. He first becomes attached to the physician, devoted, enamored (transference). Later he becomes hostile, antagonistic. He is to be forewarned and guided through these stages and instructed to become self-reliant, to give up his symptoms, however they have served him, if he would become a mature person.

Psychoanalysis is limited because it is time-consuming and expensive, requiring about 18 months of almost daily visits. One of its limitations is the tendency in the past at least to avoid medicinal aids and to minimize the importance of reality situations. However, there are patients in whom other procedures of treatment have failed and in whom psychoanalysis alone can obtain a lasting recovery. Such individuals should consult an able, well qualified psychoanalyst who has had approved training and experience.

Shock Therapy

Shock therapy is used chiefly for psychoses (see Chapter VI) but has been employed in special cases of psychoneurosis, particularly psychoneurotic depressions. When other methods fail, and if depressive features with suicidal tendencies manifest themselves, electrocoma (shock) treatment may prove effective. The technique is discussed later.

What not to do in the treatment of neuroses:

Jelliffe once remarked that sometimes he did not know what to do, yet he always knew what not to do. He warned physicians against surgical procedures for relief of remote symptoms. Menninger has written a chapter dealing with the tendency of neurotic patients to request surgery – a request readily granted. He refers to this situation as polysurgery.

Experience has shown that the excision of some organ for relief of pain or other symptoms in a neurotic patient (except for positive surgical indications) usually fails to benefit the patient even though the immediate result may appear to be favorable. According to Menninger, the patient's sense of guilt demands punishment, "partial suicide," a demand met by the operative procedure. But the relief is usually temporary, since the problem persists and in addition the patient may be minus an organ and plus a scar, adhesions, and a hospital bill. Such patients may even insist upon another surgical procedure in the hope of getting relief from pain, adhesions or other symptoms. Surgery thus is not the method for psychoneurosis.

Another problem of psychoneurosis, particularly the industrial and war types, is that of compensation and pension. Disability from psychoneurosis may be severe and real and is, at first glance, as justifiable a cause for disability payment as other illness. Yet such compensation tends to solidify the symptoms, and removes a major incentive to recovery. The psychoneurotic has periods of disabling symptoms, which may be followed by phases of relative well-being, during which he can be productive and gainfully employed. Indeed, such work is the truest kind of occupational therapy. Hence, giving routine payments to a psychoneurotic is like giving morphine for pain – it is pleasant but habit-forming. Therefore in industrial cases I have urged lump sum settlement or other ways of terminating compensation for neuroses.

There are symptoms of psychoneurosis and periods in the life of the psychoneurotic patient when he is disabled, suffers acutely and causes suffering in those about him. The psychoneurotic and his symptoms require treatment. Such treatment is not simple nor limited to one technique. A combination of physical examination and mental searching are needed for the therapist and the patient to understand the nature of the illness and how to correct it. Then the physician uses a combination of analysis and discussion, physical and medicinal means, suggestion – any and all procedures to remove fear, restore confidence, and build well-being. It is remarkable that sometimes relief of one major symptom, adjustment to or removal of one disturbing situation may initiate a process of substantial and lasting improvement. Indeed, I have frequently seen brief psychotherapy accomplish sustained improvement. Unfortunately this does not apply regularly to patients with deep-set neuroses who require persistent treatment before they respond or who show but temporary improvement, only to resume their complaints in the face of any new stress and strain.

REFERENCES

Schilder, P.: *Psychotherapy*. Norton, New York, 1938.
Hinsie, L. E., and Shatzky, J.: *Psychiatric Dictionary*. Oxford University Press, New York, 1940.
Fetterman, J. L.: Correlation of Psychic and Somatic Disorders. *J. A. M. A.*, 106:26, 1936.
Alexander, F., French, T. M. et al: *Psychoanalytic Therapy*. The Ronald Press Co., New York, 1946.
Herzberg, A.: *Active Psychotherapy*. Grune and Stratton, New York, 1945.
Levine, M.: *Psychotherapy in Medical Practice*. Macmillan, New York, 1942.
Hadfield, J. A.: War Neurosis, *British M. J.*, 1:320, 1942.
Grinker, R. R., and Spiegel, J. P.: Brief Psychotherapy in War Neuroses. *Psychosomatic Med.*, 6:123, 1944.
Thomas, G. W.: Group Psychotherapy, *Psychosomatic Med.* 5:166, 1943.
Pratt, J. H.: The Influence of Emotions in the Causation and Cure of Psychoneuroses. *International Clinics*, 4:1, 1934.
Rashkis, H. A.: Some Phenomena of Group Psychotherapy. *J. Nerv. & Ment. Dis.*, 103:187, 1946.
Foulkes, S. H.: Group Analysis in a Military Neurosis Centre. *Lancet*, 1:303, 1946.
Stephen, K.: *Psycho-analysis and Medicine, a Study of the Wish To Fall Ill*. University Press, Cambridge, England, 1943.
Kubie, L. S.: *Practical Aspects of Psychoanalysis*. Norton, New York, 1936.
Jelliffe, S. E., and White, W. A.: *Diseases of the Nervous System*. 3rd edition. Lea & Febiger, Philadelphia, 1935.
Menninger, K. A.: *The Human Mind*, Knopf, New York and London, 1930.

Grinker, R. R., and Spiegel, J. P.: *Men under Stress.* Blakiston, Philadelphia, 1945.
Jones, M.: Group Psychotherapy. *British M. J.*, 2:276, Sept., 1942.
Schwartz, L. A.: Group Psychotherapy in the War Neuroses. *Am. J. Psychiat.*, 101:498, 1945.
Wender, L.: Group Psychotherapy—A Study of Its Application. *Psychiat. Quart.*, 14:708, 1940.
Horney, K.: *New Ways in Psychoanalysis.* Norton, New York, 1939.

Chapter IV

MANIC-DEPRESSIVE PSYCHOSES; WITH PARTICULAR EMPHASIS ON DEPRESSIONS

DEPRESSIONS are among the most common of all illnesses. They are varied as to cause, course, and cure. Some are endogenous, arising spontaneously, independent of the obvious external circumstances – called the depressive phase of manic-depressive psychosis. Others are intimately related to external factors, initiated by the hardships and humiliations of life's struggles, so-called reactive depressions. Some are distinct diseases. Others are but the depressive features occurring during fevers and other maladies or the depressions in organic brain disease. For in depressions, as in other mental illnesses, we can never ignore the complex threads, the interweaving of the personality, the disease changes and the situation, all of which compose the pattern and design and the fabric of the tapestry of illness.

Symptoms of a Depression

Whatever may be the cause and however varied the course, most depressions have a common pattern of symptoms, adorned and modified by the unique features of the individual and his setting. The cardinal features are a feeling of inner distress, a loss of healthful interest in surroundings, replaced by a mood of sadness, physical discomfort, and fear. The specific features are numerous.

The feeling of inner distress is a combination of physical difficulty and emotional misery. "I have a dark weight on my chest – you would call it despair – it's like a terrible heaviness. And with it is a dread and anguish. I have a burning in the base of my skull which produces a cloud that darkens everything – everything seems dim and I can't see or think clearly. My legs are heavy; my whole body seems leaden and all effort is futile because every task looms large and insurmountable."

The mood is sad. Patients describe the world as though they were looking at it through dark glasses. "My spirits are low. I find no joy in anything. Spring came and went. It's summer now – I know it by the calendar – but I missed completely the joyous chirp of the first robin, the swelling and bursting of the buds, the scent of lilacs, all the green growth springing from the earth. Every year I have loved spring and expectantly awaited the bloom of the forsythia – and how I thrilled inside! This year I saw, or half-saw is more correct, but my emotions did not respond. Things seem different, flat, sort of unreal."

Said another patient, "I have always loved life. The three things I enjoyed most were food, people – and love. Now I am led to the table; I see the meal and eat some of it mechanically because I am told to. I avoid people because I am uncomfortable. I feel so inferior. How I used to love conversation and meetings, but now I slip stealthily away lest I have to reply to the question of a friend. But the worst thing of all is women. You know, if Venus herself were alive and came into my room to share my bed, I would have to send her away. For why add to my humiliation? I have lost all desire, all potency. It's so different from the real me."

The sad mood permeates all thinking and all movements. Not only does the depressed patient state that he feels badly today, but he is certain that he will always be that way. It is remarkable that patients who have successfully recovered from previous depressions, and should know from such experiences that the mood will return to normal again, still feel hopeless when they are sick. Regardless of how often they are reminded of such previous recovery, the mood of present darkness envelops them and is projected into the future. They have lost all faith in themselves, in doctors, in life.

Depression usually leads to self-accusation. Patients recall all the unhappy experiences of life, describe themselves in unworthy terms. Some become prosecutors of their past, searching for some misdeeds of childhood and holding them up as a cause for suffering. This tendency is prominent in the melancholia of later life. Mrs. M. C., age 63, became sleepless, worried and cried a good deal. "I am afraid there is no hope because I committed an unforgivable sin. Yes, I am worthless and not fit to go on. I did the unpardonable. When I was 18 and was courted by my present husband, we were passionate – and maybe I became pregnant. We really didn't do anything, but it was wrong to let him make love to me. And I worried and I was late at the next menstrual period. So I did all kinds of tumbling exercises. It was wrong, wasn't it? I brought bleeding on – but I took a life. I committed murder! Of course I confessed, but maybe the priest didn't fully understand what a grave sin I was guilty of."

Such self-accusation may be an incident or may dominate the illness. Another woman, in the late fifties, had enjoyed good health and possessed normal confidence until she became depressed. The cardinal point in the depression was a sense of guilt, which first revolved about a misstatement or an insignificant error. Later the idea of wrongdoing radiated to self-blame for every tragedy in life: "I gave them a wrong age on my papers – I told them I was 40, but the truth was 41. That's a lie – I did wrong. Take me to the Judge and let him sentence me. I know it was all my fault." Day and night this patient berated herself and expressed her readiness to go before a court, make a clear "confession," and take the consequences. Later she became worse: "It's all my fault – I caused the war. I am responsible for all the bloodshed. Read the list of casualties and blame me – I did it all." Like a drop of ink dropped into a basin of water spreads and darkens the entire contents, so the self-accusation may begin with one plausible misdeed and spread to many troubles and many people. Still another woman in a depression remarked, "I did wrong and I will be punished. Yes, my husband also will be put in jail; my whole family will be arrested for what I did."

A vivid self-portrait of a depressed patient was furnished by a woman in the twenties, with literary ability, who usually was self-possessed and capable. In the depressed state she described herself as follows: "Like a cumbersome sea turtle waddling laboriously through the wet sand of the shore, each clumsy limb encased in a layer of sand to be shaken off or plowed through, its head furtively pulled in and out only enough to make a path of sand, but dodging the enveloping atmosphere, so do I heavily and figuratively encased in a layer of wet sand, move my limbs slowly and with laboring progress. Figuratively, I too pull my head into its skull, bringing it out only enough to guide my sense of direction, willing, by pulling it in, to dodge any interference into my all-enveloping sphere of self-reflection. My world revolves only in the tiny mass of my being." At another time she wrote: "My body seems a shapeless mass; a heaviness pervades my movement as though a weight were attached to my head, as though each foot were chained to a gummy morass from which each step had to free itself. My hands feel encased in mittens, powerless to grasp objects. Instinctively I shrink back from grasping, a fear that the object would escape me."

The disturbed sensations that arise from within as well as the dark outlook towards the environment may account for the complaint of unreality. Patients frequently remark: "Everything seems strange, things seem different; it's hard to tell if it is I that have changed or the world around me, but it's odd; something is unreal, maybe I am unreal." This feeling of unreality similar to a condition which has been called depersonalization, is a fairly common and uncomfortable experience with depressed patients. However, it seldom reaches the intensity of the other symptoms.

More troublesome, however, is the preoccupation with an idea which serves as the focal point of self-blame. The subject may be a business venture, severing partnership, moving into a different neighborhood. The patient frequently appears agitated, picks at himself, paces the floor, and talks somewhat as follows: "I have made an awful blunder ... I shouldn't have sold my business. My family will suffer from my stupidity; I'm afraid my children will go hungry.... There's no use my being here in your office. You can't help me; you can't give me back my business." The patient repeats these ideas again and again, talks about this subject incessantly at home and thinks about it at night during long hours of wakefulness.

Self-depreciation of varying degrees is commonly present. The patient feels small, insecure, inadequate. Every task looms large and insurmountable. "I can't go out with people, I don't know what to say ... I can't cook any more ... I am afraid I am making blunders," etc.

The depressed patient is often jealous of the apparent happiness of the rest of the world. She sees others dressing attractively, bustling with cheerful activities, and resents their well-being and success. It is as though others could enjoy the song of birds, scent of flowers, sunshine – for her only pain and anguish.

Physical discomforts are very common, particularly weakness, heaviness, and pain. Patients quite regularly stress tiredness, heaviness in the arms and legs, a slowness in action. "My hands are clumsy and I can't do anything with them. My legs are weighted down so that I can't walk." Patients mention odd discomforts in the region of the head: "It's a sense of pressure, a burning pain. It's like a cloud which starts in the back of my head and penetrates into my brain, for it makes me feel muddled. I can't think! I can't concentrate!" It is as though every sensation and every thought were interrupted by the recurrent intrusion of distress. Thus physical discomforts and mental distress merge or suffuse one into the other: "I have a pain in my head; no, it's really a pressure. I get it every time I think of my trouble – and I can't stop thinking about it." In some cases disturbed somatic functions and distress are the major symptoms of the depression.

The glandular system is disturbed. Saliva is dried, while tears overflow. Thus the mouth is dry while the eyes are wet with tears. Appetite is diminished and peristalsis sluggish; hence most patients lose ten to thirty pounds in weight during a month or two of illness. Some patients lose weight so rapidly that they present the cadaverous appearance of one who is in the terminal stages of a malignant disease. Several years ago I saw a depressed patient who was down to seventy pounds from her average of 130. (She regained all her weight after shock treatment.) Breathing is usually heavy and the person becomes conscious of a weight which oppresses him. One sighs while another consciously strives to take in air. Frequently a patient is disturbed by pain in the heart region or palpitation and this causes him additional anxiety.

Sleep difficulties are the most common of all symptoms. One patient can't fall asleep, while the other dozes off only to awaken many times during the night, startled by fears and troubled by unsolved problems. A third sleeps quite well until early morning, when his eyes open at 3:00 or 4:00 or 5:00 a.m. With this awakening is a re-entrance from peaceful oblivion into the worried world about him. "How I dread these awful nights! What torment to lie awake and toss and fret and keep thinking in circles. I can't stand another night of it. What a struggle – to get up three and four times, to smoke and pace the floor, and get in and out of bed, trying to find peace, trying to relax. But sleep won't come. . . . Yes, I sleep. Bed is the only escape, but I wake up at 4:00 a.m. when it's still dark outside and dark inside. What is ahead of me? One more long day of anguish? I just can't face it!" Thus patients tell of their unhappy experiences of what should be a refreshing, relaxing escape from the day's travail.

In this description of symptoms one cannot separate the psychic from the somatic. They not only influence each other – they merge again and again. Physical distress leads to inadequacy and vice versa. Fears, of course, produce all manner of physical reactions, which in turn engender fear. Depression and fear are cousins. The depressed patient fears himself and fears the world. He is thus concerned about bodily ailments. "I have a lump in my skin; maybe it's a cancer. I have such a muddled feeling, I know I am losing my mind." More frequently there is a disdain of the body: "I'd welcome some disease – appendicitis, a broken leg, pneumonia. Anything is preferable to this terrible feeling." But for some, concern over wrongdoing and social disapproval is dominant. "I've done wrong. People will blame me. But I know I am at fault and I am prepared to pay the penalty."

As a result of fear and physical distress, patients tend to draw within themselves, to avoid people and to dodge action. Many depressed patients show a marked loss of initiative, although they can do well once they are started. Mr. H. D. arrived at my office, haggard and hungry. When I asked when he had eaten, he replied, "It's about six o'clock (p.m.) and I haven't touched any food today. I have no appetite whatsoever—I can't eat." He was urged to go with me to a restaurant just to keep me company. As the food was served, he was coaxed to taste it. A meal was ordered for him and he finally completed a full course dinner. This patient lacked appetite and initiative. Once started, he did well. During the illness he became unusually thrifty, would not buy clothes and was too fearful to spend money for food. When he recovered, he was extravagant and bought four suits of clothes at one time, paying for them with fifty-dollar bills.

Certain symptoms are present in various types of depression and in specific patients. Among those who have involutional melancholia it is not rare to hear complaints of organ loss – so-called visceral nihilism. "I can't eat; I have no tube between my mouth and stomach. . . . There is an emptiness in my chest – my heart isn't there. . . . Please don't feed me any more – my colon is blocked and my bladder is gone, so I can't eliminate any more. If you tube-feed me, I'll die of poison." When this patient was given an enema and the copious results triumphantly exhibited to her by the nurse, she ignored the contents of the bed pan with the remark, "You can't fool me – that isn't mine. I *know* that nothing can pass through my colon." This patient was inflexible in her positive knowledge; hence her symptom was a fixed idea or delusion.

Depressed patients, haunted by an intense sense of guilt, develop ideas of reference. For example, a married officer had "an affair" while on leave and then felt that people were looking at him "knowingly." He became obsessed with the idea of his horrible wrongdoing, was certain that he would contract a disease, and was positive that others knew of his misdeed. En route to camp he jumped from the train to end it all.

Although most depressed patients are troubled by poor appetite, insomnia, and often inactivity, each individual may show a particular exception. One patient ate excessively, for he found that the occupation of eating kept him busy, and he therefore actually gained rather than lost weight. Another stayed abed because he felt protected only under the covers. This leads to a discussion of the behavior of patients, which combines the effect of the basic symptoms and the secondary reactions to them.

Secondary Symptoms: Behavior Manifestations

No two patients react alike to a depression, even though it be of the same degree. One surrenders, another struggles violently, while a third makes his escape. The usual concept of a depressed patient depicts surrender: a man or woman sitting with lowered head, sad expression, thinking slowly, disinterested in life's struggles (stupor type). His eyes, downcast expression, and sighing breathing tell an eloquent story of sadness. The next patient seems agitated; he picks his fingers, pinches his skin, paces back and forth, struggling to gain some relief from the overwhelming feeling of anguish (agitated depression). Yet the almost incessant repetition of the hand-rubbing, the pinching, the pacing show that this miserable feeling is inescapable. Other patients try walking fast, working hard, driving long distances in an automobile or even flying, for such motion helps some patients to free themselves for a time or to some degree from their troubles. Still others escape by the use of drugs, alcohol, etc. Sedative medication or alcohol, which is more available and socially more acceptable, enables some patients to gain surcease from sorrow. Indeed, certain cases of alcoholism represent escape symptoms from unendurable depression. Alcohol tends to silence (anesthetize) the scolding, self-accusatory voice of the super-ego. Thus used, alcohol serves well, although it may be used excessively or continued beyond the stage of self-therapy for depression.

But alas, many fail to obtain relief by such techniques and turn their thoughts to suicide. "To be or not to be" is a common soliloquy in the thoughts of a depressed patient, for he has more reasons than Hamlet why "not to be." Says a typical patient, "Why should I go on? All day long I suffer and my nights are but an endless torment. I am a burden to my family for my trouble wears them all down. I have no hope and I see none in the future. My family and I would be better off if I were dead. Please tell me what to do – don't stop me. It's the only way out." Thus the depressed patient thinks and talks. He may pause and ponder, "Maybe it will be painful or I won't succeed. Or I may bring tragedy to my family, and suicide will violate my vow to my church." So the depressed patient debates, like a man tottering on the edge of a precipice. If the method be available - a drug, a gun, an automobile – the patient may convert idea into action.

I have described the several steps to suicide under the headings of depression, debate, decision, deed and death. Nearly all depressed patients debate with themselves, yes even with their families or doctors, whether or not to go on living. The decision may be delayed by their regard for family or problem of technique. Patients have actually consulted me for advice on how to carry out suicide scientifically. The problem of method depends upon availability, upon what is stylish, and upon what is considered swift, painless, and irrevocable. Years ago bichloride of mercury was popular; today patients try sedative drugs. In the Army firearms headed the list of techniques. It is common for depressed patients to turn on the gas of their cars in closed garages. Sometimes the attempt is crude, as in the case of a patient who swallowed ammonia and of another who swallowed Lysol. Again, an engineer invented and constructed a special connection with which to bring the exhaust gas of his automobile more effectively into the car. Another patient in mid-winter lay down nude in a pile of snow, to contract pneumonia. He hoped the pneumonia would end his life yet preserve the honor of his name, for the illness was to be a concealed form of suicide.

Suicidal thoughts are thus a serious threat in many depressions. Less common and more difficult to explain is the impulse to hurt others. "Since I became depressed I can't stand being near a knife. I have the impulse to stab my daughter – or I have the desire to jump out of the window; sometimes it's one or the other impulse or both." This impulse "to push my wife off the balcony, to hurt my sister, to kill my family and myself" is often a troublesome manifestation of a mild or a severe depression. Sometimes it is done in effigy. A colored woman was depressed because of her husband's infidelity. She warned him again and again. One day she jumped from a balcony, carrying his dress coat and hat down with her. She was destroying him symbolically, as well as herself.

The majority of patients do not exhibit this tendency to destroy others, although it is an alarming threat when present. Yet some writers assert that self-destruction is but this same tendency inverted upon a portion of the personality which represents others. Freud's concept was that the ego has incorporated within itself the image of someone. The attempt at suicide is thus also a concealed method of destroying the other person. This impulse to hurt or kill is not concealed, indeed is overt in those depressed patients who tell of the impulse to stab parents, siblings and others. In the classical Greek tragedy, *Hippolytus*, Phaedra is markedly depressed to the point of suicide and states, "But on this day, when I shake off the burden of this life . . . I shall at least bring sorrow upon another . . . he will have his share in my mortal sickness."

The aggressiveness against others, dangerous as it seems, is rarely put into action. In most instances it is a fear, as was mentioned by a patient when he said, "Help me. I am driven by the thought of killing my daughter, but I love her and I am afraid of myself. I am afraid I might lose self-control and kill her."

Numerous variations in the theme of depression manifest themselves in the specific symptoms. When we consider how many different hands of bridge can be dealt from fifty-two cards, we can readily accept the enormous variety of symptoms arising from the innumerable combinations of age, sex, physique, illness, environment. Let us therefore leave specific symptoms to take a bird's eye view of the course of a depression.

The Course of Depression

In the typical case of a patient suffering from the depressive phase of a manic-depressive illness, the course follows a pattern. A person who has enjoyed good health for some years, following an earlier episode of depression, retires at night cheerful and well. Indeed he may thank God for his many blessings as he snuggles peacefully into bed. But in the morning things are different. He awakens before dawn with a feeling of heaviness, a dry taste, a sense of fear. As the morning wears on, he has no appetite, no zest, but rather a sadness overtakes him. From day to day he grows worse. He tries to find some cause, but there has been no change in his family's health, no financial setback, no frustration. Gradually it dawns upon him that he is sick again – another depression. However, the patient and the family attribute the onset of the illness to some obvious external event, sometimes apparently serious, again quite trifling. "My husband became depressed because he sprained his ankle, our son was drafted, his mother-in-law has cancer, the stock market went down yesterday," etc. The given cause may be an everyday incident of little moment – certainly insignificant as compared to the biological time mechanism that determines cycles.

In many instances the onset is abrupt and the early symptoms severe. There is no doubt that the person is really different. In other cases there is but a gradual change of mild degree. Indeed the depressive symptoms are moderate in depth and remain so for weeks. They are attributed to a cold, overwork, worry about minor situations, and would pass unrecognized but for the history of cycles. More commonly the symptoms grow worse from the time of onset until, in a matter of weeks, a depression is evident. This may be of varying depth or shade, from gray to deepest black.

Thus the patient remains for many months, the mood fluctuating somewhat during the day and from time to time. Patients describe themselves as most wretched upon arising, improved slightly during the afternoon, and considerably more cheerful in the evening. Also, the melancholy feeling does not remain equally dark throughout the months of illness. Some days are brighter, to the point where the family usually, and sometimes the patient too, expects recovery. Then quite unexpectedly the mood darkens to deepest black. Such an increase of symptoms is common in the premenstrual days for most women patients. The illness continues onward toward a spontaneous recovery, unless terminated by the good fortune of effective treatment or the tragic fate of suicide. Spontaneous recovery may occur after a period of weeks, months, or years.

There are patients who have brief depressions lasting a week or more which occur frequently – even every few months. Others have but one attack which is prolonged for years. The attacks in one person subject to recurrences may develop at the same season and continue for the same length of time. In another patient both the time of occurrence and the duration are unpredictable. Depressions which occur in the postpartum period are likely to be brief; those which develop in the involutional period are usually prolonged, may last for years, and there is less probability of a spontaneous recovery. Dayton cites figures from the State Hospital system of Massachusetts, indicating that one year is the average duration of a depression. Patients with histories of several previous attacks may forecast the approximate duration of their illness. Strecker and Ebaugh state that future attacks are often a repetition of the initial one, with a distinct tendency toward greater frequency, length, and severity. "The more 'reactive' the psychosis, the better the outlook. . . . The presence of definite schizophrenic elaborations appearing during the course of an affect disorder are unfavorable signs."

Manic States

A spontaneous improvement in depressive illness may not represent complete recovery. It may mean a cyclic swing from depression to manic phase. Gradually or abruptly the patient becomes joyous, exuberant in spirits, abounding in energy. A young woman who had been inactive, sleepless, weepy for months, quite suddenly became cheerful. She tripped into my office, her voice ringing with laughter, her ideas boundless. "I feel so good, Doctor. Your medicine did wonders – you ought to manufacture it by the gallons and give it to everyone. I feel *wonderful*. I don't talk – I *sing!* I don't walk – I *dance!*"

Another patient who had been depressed for ten months suddenly became aware of the world around him. "It's glorious again. I know what cured me – it was when I began to notice the flowers and trees and birds. I felt better right then." One week before, this same patient was discovered by his family in the act of tying a rope to hang himself. But from the moment he improved, he regained his confidence, mingled freely with people, and took on many civic responsibilities. The public looked upon him as a benefactor who did not take time out to rest, so zealous was he to do things for mankind. In this mood, during which he loved everyone and everything, he felt no fatigue and was full of ideas. He was in the hypomanic phase of his illness. Fortunately he did not go beyond this stage into a clashing, quarreling, difficult manic illness, as did another patient.

This second patient had his third depression at the age of forty. In it he lost all interest in people and could not eat or sleep or work. He would go without food because he was afraid to spend money for it. Quite abruptly the cycle changed. He talked incessantly and boisterously; he purchased extravagantly. When his family tried to control him, he became belligerent and fought them violently. He made expensive long distance calls in the middle of the night. He was driven by the urge to write books, apply for patents, start new enterprises. In the course of weeks until shock therapy was begun, he had become involved in quarrels, lawsuits, and serious financial difficulties.

Case History of a Manic Patient

Mrs. S. A. gave a history of nervous illness on the part of her mother, who had had a depression during the menopause. The patient herself had enjoyed reasonably good health until the spring of 1945 when she developed restlessness and sleeplessness. This previously quiet and timid girl became loud and argumentative. The condition grew worse in the course of time so that she talked incessantly day and night, refused all food, and assaulted her mother when the latter tried to assist her.

When I first saw Mrs. S. A. at her home, I found a slender woman in the early thirties who was busily jotting things on paper. The sheet began with the words, "Irving Berlin," and went on to say: "Irving Christian, Irving Hebrew, Irving Catholic, Berlin, Germany, what's in a name . . . ." There was a page full of notes with this flight of ideas and rapid association. She then began to talk somewhat as follows: "I don't like my family doctor any more; I never did; I am Mrs. ———, the late widow of Sir ——— overactive brain, insanity – Expectation is greater than anticipation – hypochondriac, hypocrite, screwballs." During the examination she sang several popular tunes, then burst into insulting remarks about her family and the medical profession.

Because of the intensity of the symptoms, this patient was placed in the hospital where she was observed for a period of time. Her condition became critical because of refusal to eat, so that electro-shock therapy was administered. As will be mentioned later under the heading of therapy, the result was successful after a large number of treatments.

The manic illness is diametrically opposite to the depressed state. There is elation, exuberance of energy and zestful action, overestimation of self, distractibility, flight of ideas. The three S's of the manic state are speaking, spending, and speeding. The manic has thrown off the yoke of superego. Stated in another way, the manic thinks of conquest, the depressed of inquest.

Although text books feature this cyclic tendency of manic-depressive illness, the tendency for a shift from depression toward average well-being is far more common than the swing into a manic state. The cycles are those of depression of months' duration alternating with longer periods (years) of average health. Manic illness is far less frequent than depressions.

In many cases the abrupt onset of illness in the midst of normal circumstances, the long duration and then the spontaneous recovery or swing toward the manic phase suggest an illness determined by unseen forces, a biogenic illness. I once likened this quality of onset and recovery to the going on and off of electric signs. Like an electrically lighted sign turned off by a time-clock, so the mood of a patient becomes darkened by a time switch wound by the fingers of destiny. (The fingers of destiny here refer to the constitutional factors.)

In some patients the depressive and manic phases are not separate cycles, one following the other. Rather they are concurrent; the illness is mixed or circular. The patient talks on and on, with restlessness, flight of ideas, yet weeps, feels sad and miserable. This admixture may appear simultaneously or there may be changes during the day. For an hour the patient may talk enthusiastically, jumping from topic to topic, move about in an excited fashion, then sit and sob and speak of feelings of hopelessness.

Case History of the Mixed Type

Mrs. C. B., a woman of 29, was referred to my office by her physician with a history of two short depressions several years previously. The present illness was of several weeks' duration, during which time Mrs. C. B. neglected her home and duties and busied herself writing and making haranguing speeches. She wrote on various scraps of paper and backs of envelopes.

An example of her writing is as follows: "Sensitive, alibi, explain, manage, don't courage (fear) – Attempt it – Do the thing you fear. Don't be afraid of failure or that people won't like you, i.e. criticism. God helps those who help themselves. – Sense of humor – Interest yourself – Boredom – Nothing is done finally and right. Nothing is known positively and completely. Every day something unknown becomes known." There were pages of similar notes on general subjects.

When this patient was examined, her eyes sparkled, her mood was cheerful, and she remarked: "I don't need a rest, I don't need much sleep. I have been fighting this way forever and ever because there is no such thing as time – – I was writing things and they were so beautiful when I saw them on paper and I felt they couldn't be true. I couldn't be true. I couldn't stop and I couldn't go on; I was like in the middle. We have so many things to do we haven't time to see a psychiatrist – there are so many things – so many people to see."

During another interview patient started to speak without provocation about national events. "The coal strike – do you know what it makes me think of – Strike Up the Band – but that don't settle a coal strike. If I could see that John L. Lewis, I don't know what I would say to him. I usually like fat people and he's fat, but I can't do anything about the coal strike, so why ask me?" Mrs. C. B. was quite proud of her comment and gay and happy about all the world.

When she appeared at the office several days later, she was markedly depressed. Her husband described her as follows: "She is calm, below normal, can't do anything, sits around a good deal." The tone of her conversation was now sad: "I feel responsible for not doing the right thing. I have been a failure. People commit suicide because of the fear of failure and I know that I will fail."

Within about two weeks there was a profound change from overactivity and bubbling enthusiasm to a retardation of thinking and a melancholy mood. In the subsequent weeks there were similar fluctuations occurring more rapidly, with periods of relative good health in between. During one visit she would begin to talk quite cheerfully and then gradually shift into ideas of sadness. "I must find out if I am crazy or not. Then I'll know what to do. I'm afraid you can't help me; it's too late. Did they want to help me? No, they just wanted to make me partly well.

I don't know how it happened, only I think that God is – He is just a little round snowflake in a whirl. But I am afraid that God can't come down to help me. Maybe it is just the devil in me. He never should have made a devil. I can see only the bad in people; I guess I'm bad. I guess I'll die pretty soon because if I die, I'll take the people that love me out of the place where they are. Let's play a game or something. It is all down in a book somewhere but I have never had a chance to read it because it hasn't been written yet. Will you please write a book for me and let me read it."

During this visit there was still flight of ideas but the euphoria had changed to sadness and there was a feeling of utter failure.

Clinical Examples of Depression

Mrs. L. S., a woman of 45, became tired and sad. She could not eat well and her sleep was troubled. Everyone knew the "cause," for it was so obvious. Her two sons were overseas and one was a prisoner of war. Mrs. L. S. brooded more and more – perhaps the son was dead. In fact, she became sure he was dead. Thus she sat mourning, refusing all food, crying. Even when mail arrived from both sons, she refused to believe anything but that the one was dead. She lost all interest in her appearance, in her home, and in food. She talked only of the catastrophe. No amount of reassurance could change her. Therefore, one day she swallowed Lysol to end her miserable existence. This suicidal attempt was discovered and she was given first aid, successfully. When she was placed in a sanitarium and while waiting for the chemical burns in her throat to heal, she continued her weeping and wailing. Even an official letter from the War Department did not comfort her. Indeed, she told me that many others were dead and warned me that a like fate would overtake all of us: "We are doomed. The end of time has come." Thus four months after the onset of her illness, Mrs. L. S. was physically emaciated, her voice rough and her throat scarred. Her depression had extended from the delusion of personal loss to encompass universal death. At this point a course of shock therapy was administered. The recovery was complete and she was overjoyed to greet her son when he came home on furlough. A year later she has remained perfectly well.

Mrs. O. W. was 48 when she was referred because of a depression. The history indicated that she had been depressed some ten times over a period of twenty years. Each attack came on gradually and without cause. She grew worse, remained at a level for about four months, and then the depression cleared. At the worst phase Mrs. O. W. was unusually quiet, lacked initiative in planning meals or selecting her wardrobe, avoided people and entertainment, and felt "blue." At times the idea of suicide entered her mind, but she was too apathetic to act. She did not lose any weight and showed no agitation. Few of her friends knew that she was ill.

Mr. E. P. had been a dynamic, intelligent man until the age of 50. Then his sleep was troubled and he awakened at 3:00 or 4:00 a.m. He was tense, uneasy, not knowing what ailed him. He lost interest in reading and in the radio, although previously he had been intensely concerned with world events. He avoided business responsibilities, sitting aimlessly around. The appetite for food left him. He declined invitations. When asked how he felt, he would reply, "I can't tell, it's a miserable feeling. I am afraid to say or do anything. I seem dull and incompetent and can't grasp anything. I can't concentrate on any subject." He grew worse to the point of a suicidal attempt with a small number of amytal capsules. He was then placed in a hospital which did not use shock therapy at the time of admission. He remained there some three years, his condition unchanged.

A Typical Example of Manic-Depressive Psychosis

The case history of N. Z. is quite typical of the life story of certain patients who have recurrent depressions. N. Z. consulted me early in 1931 with a history of inability to sleep and to eat, symptoms which had been present for several weeks. An inquiry into the family history revealed that this patient's father had become markedly depressed in his late forties and that, during this depression, he took his own life. The patient himself had been fairly healthy during childhood and young manhood, had been an excellent student, and took an advanced course in a science school. In his early twenties, while he was studying engineering, N. Z. became discontented, moody, lost interest in his studies, and was ready to quit, stating: "This is no profession for me; I'm bound to be a failure." He developed insomnia and loss of appetite. This state continued for several months, after which he made a complete, spontaneous recovery.

The illness that occurred in 1931 progressed onward. A few weeks after onset the patient became agitated, stating that he couldn't get well. He cried a good deal, tossed objects around the house. "I'm no good. My memory is poor. My mind doesn't work. My profession is no good. This is a hell of a world." Two or three months later he talked of suicide and then was found experimenting with methods. The family caught him one time turning on a gas jet; on another occasion he had prepared a noose in the basement. We talked about these suicidal attempts and he said that he would already have taken his life but he feared the pain, that perhaps the act might be incomplete, or what might happen after death. Because of these suicidal attempts, he was placed in a mental hospital. He remained there for a period of many months. About a year after onset there was a remarkable spontaneous improvement.

Upon his return from the hospital, the patient presented a picture entirely different from that during his depressive illness. He walked with vigor, talked with enthusiasm, and spoke of remarkable plans for the future. He participated in many activities and was looked upon as a dynamic, successful individual. He was full of energy, spoke enthusiastically about his self-confidence, and even boasted of his health. He was elated – he had regained a sparkle in his eyes, he laughed loudly, talked carelessly to all he met. For a short period he was hypomanic, then he became calm and enjoyed average health.

Four years later, in 1935, he had another depressive episode which lasted some five months and from which he made a complete recovery. He was well, without overenthusiasm, for a period of some years, until 1942. In the spring of 1942 he became uneasy. "I must get away from the house." He complained of feeling broken down. "I am no good. Everything has gone to smash. I can't go back to my business." He stopped eating, was agitated, and avoided people.

He felt that he was making blunders in his business, causing his partners to lose a great deal of money. "I am no good. I am no more intelligent than a dog." During this depression the patient consulted a psychoanalyst and an analysis was begun. Some six weeks later a sister found him looking tense, pale, and disturbed, saying: "I am no good to anyone. I don't want to get well. I am the cause of losses to my family and to my customers." A bottle of poison was discovered in his pocket.

This patient discontinued the analysis and was then placed in the Windsor Hospital, where he was given a course of electrocoma (shock) therapy. After five major reactions (coma and convulsion), N. Z. made a splendid recovery. During the past few years he has been at an even keel, apparently well.

The significant items in the case of N. Z. are the family history of a psychosis with suicide, recurrent attacks in

1924, 1931, 1935, and 1942. The most severe was in 1931, following which the patient showed a moderate hypomanic phase. Electro-shock therapy was remarkably effective in bringing about a recovery in a matter of two weeks.

Case histories like these give one an idea of the varying intensity and duration of the illness. Let us now consider briefly the nature and relationship of the various kinds of depressions.

Types and Causes of Depression

Everyone has felt depressed, yet such a feeling is no more the illness – depression – than an everyday cough is pertussis (whooping cough). Of course, the depressed feeling gives similar symptoms (temporarily) and perhaps utilizes similar mechanisms, just as the apparatus of the cough is the same in the two instances cited above.

Depressions range from a temporary dejected feeling resulting from disappointments to a progressively downward melancholia terminating fatally by starvation or suicide. They produce the uncomfortable visceral distress, they modify thought processes in the direction of failure, and darken the mood. Let us dismiss the common depressed feelings which arise from discouragement as something brief, readily modified by changing circumstances, responding to the comforting of friends and the calming influence of sleep, activity, and time. These are but the everyday experiences of life and need not detain us now.

But what about the more serious condition, the illness that is called a depression? There are several types: the depressive phase of manic-depressive psychosis, reactive depression and its closely allied psychoneurotic depressive state, involutional melancholia depressions in schizophrenic patients and depressions in organic diseases. The standard classification is:

Manic Depressive Psychosis
  Manic type
  Depressive type
  Circular type
  Mixed type
  Perplexed type
  Stuporous type
Involutional Psychosis
Reactive Depression (Psychoneurosis)

Each of these has certain distinctive features which can be listed on paper, but in the patient distinction may be difficult. For example, we separate the endogenous from the reactive depressions, by the point of difference that the former occurs from within and the latter arises from external causes. Yet again and again patients become depressed over experiences which we accept as more or less normal. It has been customary to attribute the depressions of women whose sons are in service to the factor of worry about them. But if the departure of a son into the service be a sufficient cause for depression, then millions of American mothers would have acquired depressive illnesses. There has been no such epidemic of depressions in the United States nor in Russia nor in the British Isles. The inference is that those who remained depressed had some additional internal factor. Mrs. L. S., for example, was diagnosed "reactive depression" when her illness occurred at about the same time she learned that her son had been captured by the enemy. Yet we saw that the positive statement of the War Department as to his safety failed to ease her mind and furthermore her delusions spread from the certainty of her son's death to fear that all Americans would be killed.

One cannot entirely dismiss reaction to tragedy and to failure as an important cause, for all of us know of the wave of suicides which occurred after the stock crash in 1929. It has also been observed that depressions constitute one of the commonest causes for admission to psychiatric wards of service hospitals. Men and women in the service, exposed to frustrations and to conditions which are intolerable to them, develop depressive illness. It seems that man cannot endure a continuous frustration, although he can more readily react to one catastrophe, however painful.

Another problem is the closely allied psychoneurotic depression. Is the depression a distinct illness in a psychoneurotic or but one major symptom? Theoretically one distinguishes endogenous depressions from psychoneuroses with depressive features by the following criteria:

	Psychoneuroses	Endogenous Depressions
1. Somatic Symptoms	Dominant	Present but may be secondary
2. Mood	Neutral or depressed	Depressed (severely)
3. Blame	Others usually	Self usually

4. Modified By	Frequently influenced by contacts	Not significantly influenced by contacts
5. Escapes	Often enjoys rest, reading, attention	Unable to rest or relax
6. Suicide	Suicidal impulses, infrequent	Suicidal impulses, frequent
7. Time of Day	Usually worse in evening	Worse in morning
8. Weight Loss	May be present	Marked
9. Family History	Psychoneurotic tendencies	History of manic-depressive illness in family
10. Past History	Psychoneurotic trends	History of good health but interrupted by periods of manic-depressive psychosis
11. Treatment	Partially influenced by shock therapy	Readily and successfully treated by shock therapy
12. Mood Swings	Slight or none	Periods of elation alternate with depression

These are some of the criteria which I use in distinguishing between the average psychoneurosis and a depression. The borderline case is a difficult challenge.

Involutional melancholia has many features of a depression, tends to occur in the fifth and sixth decades and is likely to run a progressive downward course. Titley has emphasized that the strict, oversensitive, overconscientious type of person is more commonly affected. Bodily symptoms, hypochondriacal complaints, and sometimes visceral nihilism ("I have no heart, no stomach, no colon") are common. The patient is usually agitated, picking his nails, wringing his hands, pacing. Major ideas are of self-accusation with a feeling of utter futility and suicide as the only escape.

Noyes offers the following description of the type and mechanisms in those who develop involutional melancholia:

"Pre-psychotic personality shows an inhibited type of individual with a tendency to be serious, chronically worrisome, intolerant, reticent, sensitive, frugal, even penurious, stubborn, of rigid moral code, lacking in humor, overconscientious and given to self-punishment. Interests narrow, habits stereotyped, cared little for diversion, avoided pleasure and has but few friends. The pre-psychotic personality is characterized by a deeply seated sense of insecurity.

"At this period, more or less conscious recognition that early dreams and desires cannot now be fulfilled, that the zenith of life has been passed, that ambition and life's forces are waning: ebbing potency in the male, and the realization by the female that her period of childbearing is over. Thoughts of death appear . . . . with decrease in physical strength, unconscious forces, old conflicts and complexes threaten and torment. The menace to the ego is ceaseless."

There may be no history of previous attacks; indeed, the addition of paranoidal ideas points to a probable schizophrenic basis in some cases. From a practical viewpoint, we will place the involutional melancholia close to depressive illness because of the close resemblance of symptoms and the favorable response to electrocoma (shock) treatment.

Combinations of depressive mood and schizophrenic thinking are not uncommon. Sometimes a depressed patient develops ideas of reference or persecution, becomes suspicious to the point of watching and listening. Later a veritable delusional structure is fabricated. Also, some schizophrenic patients become depressed because of the overwhelming sense of futility in not attaining delusional goals or in a feeling of desperation because of their inability to cope with omnipotent enemies. Or it may be a coincidence that the two illnesses are combined into one. Everyday experience shows that they are not antagonistic. This applies particularly to patients in the late thirties or forties who have developed a mental illness for the first time.

For instance, C. U., a woman of 42, became fretful and worried. She had a dream in which an attacker had broken into her bedroom in the middle of the night and raped her. She became puzzled whether this was a dream or had really occurred. There were pains in her abdomen and she had difficulty in voiding. "The attack must have occurred." She began to cry and could not eat or sleep; she thought of nothing but disease. At about the same time she observed a cold sore on her lip." *It must be syphilis!*" This idea now dominated her thoughts. "I, who had been so honorable, have a horrible, loathsome disease. People seem to avoid me – they too must know." She gave up working, became agitated and wept. A feeling of hopelessness pervaded all her thoughts.

I saw this patient after she had been ill some ten months. She looked worn and wrinkled, agitated and depressed. She insisted that she could hear people talking about her "disease;" she said that they entered her room at night, changed her bedclothes, yes, even attacked her during the night. The illness could properly be labelled schizo-affective. Treatment by the electrocoma (shock) method proved efficacious. This woman made a complete recovery in 1942 and has maintained excellent health since that time.

Depressive symptoms may be present or may even dominate the clinical story of a patient with organic brain disease. Cases of arteriosclerosis and of syphilis may appear as depressions. The change in the brain seems to uncover the basic personality trend and this may be depressive. Mrs. C. M., a housewife, lost interest in her home. She seemed unable to cook or keep the house in order. She became weepy, nervous, and sleepless. A sense of failure and fear overcame her. One day she was found near the water's edge, about to drown herself. At first glance her symptoms suggested a simple depression, but she presented physical evidence of organic brain disease. A blood Wassermann and spinal fluid tests showed conclusive evidence of syphilis. The diagnosis was paresis and treatment with fever and tryparsamide resulted in recovery.

The exact nature of endogenous depressions is not yet known. Thus there are several schools of thought, especially those who consider the illness psychogenic and those who believe it to be physical. The latter concept, namely that depressions are caused by physical or physico-chemical changes, appeals to me. The reasons are as follows:

1. The frequency of a constitutional tendency.
2. The spontaneous onset and spontaneous improvement.
3. The alternating cycles of manic and depressed states.
4. The high percentage of cases in the menopausal period.
5. The fluctuation of symptoms during the daily cycle.
6. The failure of psychic methods to effect a distinct recovery, as opposed to the consistent improvement obtained by physical means (shock therapy).

The cause is believed to be physical. We are all familar with the influence upon mood and direction of thought exerted by alcohol. A person, silent and bitter and depressed by troublesome situations may, after a few drinks, become talkative, pleased, and look hopefully at the same situation. A better parallel to the chemical (glandular) influence upon mood is the experience of many women in the pre-menstrual stage. Many a woman becomes tense and depressed, is overly sensitive, uneasy, inclined to weep, and feels neglected by her husband and less fortunate than her friends. Two or three days later, without a single change in her husband, home, and the world, this same woman becomes light-hearted and self-satisfied. This brief cycle repeats itself with monthly regularity. The influence of hormones upon mood appears clear.

The Treatment of Depressions

Prevention of depressions is highly desirable but can hardly be attained in the endogenous types, except through strict eugenics, hardly practical in this day of love and romance. The prevention of reactive depressions is also theoretical and would consist of removing unhappy situations and training persons to adjust in a more plastic way to fate's decrees. The rigid personality is fragile in the face of the inevitable blows and collisions of life.

Once a depression sets in, several methods may be used to ease the patient's distress and to make him more comfortable until he recovers, if not actually contributing to the recovery. Let us take up first psychotherapy and then individual methods, which are similar to those employed in the therapy of neuroses.

Psychotherapy of depressions consists chiefly in permitting the patient to free his mind of his problems and to provide some measure of reassurance. The depressed patient must tell someone of his misery, his discomfort. Indeed, he talks to anyone who will listen to the story of his suffering. As he furnishes his physician the history of his illness, he gains some temporary ease, some relief by confessing his guilt. He has some hope, even though he has lost faith in himself, that the physician may help him. It is amazing how depressed patients come to the doctor ready to recite their symptoms, asking for "something to sleep," and yet doubting themselves and the world. Some, of course, do not go the physician willingly, but are coaxed or coerced into consulting him. So deep is the depression that the patient is positive he is beyond the help of the doctor – "I know my case is beyond help." Even such a patient will relate the story of his unworthiness, his growing suffering – but without relief. Most patients do get some relief, however, by talking. As the patient sighs and weeps and tells his story, the physician obtains the data which are helpful toward a correct diagnosis.

When he has obtained sufficient information from the patient and his family, and after a physical examination has been completed, the doctor is in a position to guide, offer counsel as to necessary steps, and provide reassurance. The weight of the burden of guilt is often lifted, even if only for a short time, by the physician's statements to the patient: "You have not performed a criminal act; the episode you describe is a common, everyday experience. You have not sinned – of course you are forgiven." So too the patient's mind is often relieved when the nature of his fear is explained to him. "This spot on your face is only acne and not syphilis. You have absolutely no signs of syphilis." "You have no cancer – this swelling is only a fatty tumor, a lipoma." Patients frequently are much happier when they leave the doctor even if this freedom lasts only for an hour or a day. In severe depressions discussion and logic are of little avail in stemming the tragic tide of dark thoughts. But if the depression is not too black, the patient may take some hope in repeating to himself the helpful words of his physician.

Positive counsel must be given as to residence, work, and activity generally. Such advice may need repetition, as does the reassurance, because of continuity of symptoms. Therefore, in subsequent visits the patient is encouraged to bring up his problems. This material need not extend deeply into the infantile period nor need it uncover unconscious material. The patient needs guidance in a practical way about immediate and concrete problems.

There is a temptation to minimize the complaints of the depressed patient with such a remark as, "Forget about it . . . . there is nothing wrong with you. All my physical and laboratory tests were negative. Smile – forget it." Such words cheer the giver but chill the receiver. For the usual reaction of patients to such a pep talk is: "I guess he doesn't understand me, or he doesn't believe me, for how else could he say there is nothing wrong. I'd rather have any dreadful disease, any broken bone, than endure this agony." The statement commonly given by phyisicans after a physical examination, "There is nothing wrong with you," is incorrect as therapy and as diagnosis. The patient feels too ill to accept it, and the illness is too real in a physiological sense to be so flimsily dismissed. Invariably patients are worse rather than relieved by such a statement. Thus the physician himself and the family whom he has instructed must show a sincere sympathy in the patient's suffering – there is something wrong, even though existing tests fail to reveal it. Such a sympathetic attitude, accompanied by encouragement and expressions of hope, may prove more comforting.

Medicinal procedures are of direct service to the sick person. His symptoms may be alleviated by the use of such drugs as may be needed. To aid the patient's appetite I advise wine before meals. Two to four ounces of sherry or other wine before mealtime may change the dry taste and poor appetite to one of more cheerful interest in the food placed before him. In psychoneurotic depressions I administer insulin, 10 units one-half hour before meals; an improved appetite and weight gain may result. An elixir containing thiamin chloride, a dessertspoonful at mealtime, may take the place of wine. Small amounts of alcohol often prove relaxing.

Sedatives are usually helpful. Bromides in adequate doses or phenobarbital in similar amounts aid the patient to obtain relaxation.

Disturbed sleep is another serious symptom which requires attention. Patients are instructed to take long walks in the evening, to try warm baths, to drink warm milk. Such suggestions usually help, but to an insufficient degree. The patient still has trouble in falling asleep or in remaining asleep. It is advisable to prescribe some barbiturate: seconal, gr. $1\frac{1}{2}$; nembutal, gr. $1\frac{1}{2}$; or sodium amytal, gr. 3 may be given at bedtime. Each may be tried in succession; for a long illness may demand a change in the medication. A second capsule is allowed if needed. In cases of extreme insomnia a rapidly acting barbiturate capsule may be reinforced by a longer acting sedative such as chloral hydrate, gr. 10 to 20, and sodium bromide, gr. 15. At first glance one may revolt against the apparent overmedication. Yet sleeping medicine, to be worthwhile, must be adequate. Secondly, although it is granted that such doses of sedatives continued night after night carry some danger, the wear and tear of sleepless nights, the pacing and smoking and agitation, the struggle with suicidal impulses are greater hazards. There is an impression that sedatives will make the depression deeper. Experience shows the opposite result; the anxiety, the tension, the inner struggle of decision and doubt, of impulse and inhibition are lessened. Finally, patients who recover from the depression do not crave more sedatives and not a single instance of addiction from such dosage in depression comes to my memory.

Just as sedatives are valuable for sleep, so stimulating drugs are often helpful in the morning. Benzedrine or dexedrine sulfate has proved of value in some cases. It is prescribed in 5-mg. doses at breakfast and at 10:00 to 11:00 a.m., the amount to be increased if no effect is obtained. Some patients report an increase in energy and an awakening of interest. Unfortunately, many patients are troubled by jitteriness, uneasiness, sweating, and other visceral reactions to such a degree that they object to continuing with benzedrine. However, it is worth trying.

A third accessory form of treatment is activity. The depressed patient is inclined to become idle or to wear himself out with worry and agitation. He should be directed to keep working, even if to a limited degree, as long as he is able to do so. If he cannot work, then walking, gardening, golfing, and other outdoor sports should be urged. Most patients obtain some ease when outdoors if engaged in activity. As a rule, they tell you that even when walking or working or weaving, troubled thoughts fill their minds. This protest notwithstanding, depressed patients should be kept busy. Prescribed occupational therapy, weaving, painting, clay modeling, all are valuable. Occupied time is the best occupational therapy.

Vacation trips are considered unwise because the patient is usually idle, cannot enjoy the changed surroundings, and may miss the support of his family and the protection against suicide which he needs.

Suicide is the major hazard in depressions and must be prevented if possible. The family may learn and the doctor certainly should estimate how intense is the suicidal impulse. How far down the steps of the downward D's has the patient gone?

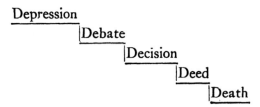

Observe carefully the tenseness, the desperate discomfort of the patient who can no longer endure his illness. Inquire by gentle, subtle questions how the person feels about ending it all. Be particularly wary of those whose gestures (buying or concealing dangerous drugs) or whose attempts signify the will to die. In all cases apprise the family of the potential danger and instruct them in regard to taking precautions. Constant vigilance is the motto which represents the family's duty in many cases.

In severe cases, or if in doubt, hospitalize as soon as possible. In other instances, ease the tension by sedatives, remove poison pills, poison liquids, knives, firearms, the automobile keys, or any tool that may invite self-destruction. One must be cautious about the amount of sedative medication that the patient can lay his hands on. For instance, I examined a Mrs. S. S. who had been depressed for three months. Four years previously she had gone through a moderate depression. At the present time she complained of burning pains in the legs, inability to sleep, loss of appetite, weight loss of twenty pounds, inability to read, and utter self-depreciation. So worthless did this otherwise beautiful and capable woman feel that I suspected the danger of suicide and advised constant vigilance, along with sedatives, until a hospital bed could be secured. The family physician prescribed sodium amytal, gr. three to gr. six at bedtime, but ordered 24 capsules. The patient slept well for two nights and then told her husband she was better. He left her alone in the house for half an hour. Upon his return, she was unconscious; she had swallowed the twenty unused capsules. Luckily she was resuscitated by gastric lavage and intravenous picrotoxin and later was successfully treated by shock therapy. The large number of capsules was an invitation to eternal sleep, welcome to this severely depressed woman.

Hormones have been used, with doubtful results, in endogenous depression. For many years theelin was popular and several authors reported success with small or large doses. Others, such as Bennett, tried it on a fairly large series of cases, with negative results. My experience agrees with that of Bennett, and I would not recommend its prolonged use in severe depression, although it may be tried in milder menopausal depression. Also, in depressed male patients, testosterone has been recommended, but as yet the evidence in its favor is far from convincing. A short trial of several weeks may be in order, but continued use in the face of a progressive illness is unwise. The dosage advised by Sargent and Slater is 25 mg. i.m. three times weekly.

In depressions as in psychoneuroses an adequate diet should be given. Unfortunately there may be anorexia or refusal to eat so marked that tube feeding or shock therapy may have to be used.

Shock Therapy – Electrocoma Therapy

Like a beacon light which signals a safe harbor to a storm-tossed sailor on a dark night, so shock therapy is the haven for the endogenous depressed patient. For this method has proved consistently useful. Properly administered, shock therapy is safe and effective. Some ninety per cent of patients with endogenous depressions will respond favorably in a brief period of weeks. Indeed, in some instances there is a noticeable improvement immediately following the first treatment. For example, Mrs. W. H. had been depressed for some ten months. One of her major symptoms was loss of appetite. When this patient awoke from her initial coma and was given a small breakfast, she volunteered the statement, "This is the first food that has tasted right in ten months." Mrs. F. R. was depressed some three months. Her major complaint was a burning sensation in the back of the head and a clouded feeling around her head. Here too, there was an amazing clearing of this symptom after the first reaction.

Effective electrocoma therapy consists of a course of treatment which averages 10 to 12 major reactions. In some instances this compact series of treatments is followed by an occasional additional or maintenance dose. The original series is administered three times weekly, but the spacing is adjusted to the intensity of the symptoms and the physical and mental status of the patient. Because of the tremendous importance of this mode of therapy for psychoses in general and particularly for depressions, the subject is covered in detail in a subsequent chapter.

Depressions constitute one of the commonest ailments in the realm of psychiatry and thus they are not infrequent in the experience of the general practitioner. In most instances the weeping and stupor and morbid ideas quickly reveal the nature of the malady. In other cases, physical complaints, with marked emphasis upon the soma, persist for weeks and months. Such patients may be mis-diagnosed and operated on – with no benefit. Then, too, the hazard of suicide requires early recognition. The attempt at suicide is usually a symptom of a depression which, promptly and adequately treated, can be relieved.

Treatment may be started along several lines: medicinal, occupational, and psychotherapeutic. If the condition grows worse, the patient should not be allowed to go through the intense torment of his melancholia but should receive a course of electrocoma (shock) therapy. This acts as a specific. It can be administered as an ambulatory procedure or in a hospital. The results are highly satisfactory.

REFERENCES

Dayton, N. A.: *New Facts on Mental Disorders: Study of 89,190 Cases.* Thomas, Springfield, 1940.

Strecker, E. A., and Ebaugh, F. G.: *Practical Clinical Psychiatry.* 5th edition. Blakiston, Philadelphia, 1940.

Titley, W. B.: Prepsychotic Personality of Patients with Agitated Depression. *Arch. Neurol. & Psychiat.*, 39:333, 1938.

Noyes, A. P.: *Modern Clinical Psychiatry*, 2nd edition. Saunders, Philadelphia, 1939.

Bennett, A. E., and Wilbur, C. B.: Convulsion Shock Therapy in Involutional States after Complete Failure with Previous Estrogenic Treatment. *Am. J. M. Sc.*, 208:170, 1944.

Sargant, W., and Slater, E.: *An Introduction to Somatic Methods of Treatment in Psychiatry.* Williams & Wilkins, Baltimore, 1944.

Chapter V

SCHIZOPHRENIAS

SCHIZOPHRENIA, or better the schizophrenic reaction types, includes a group of mental illnesses which have in common a splitting off from reality, a dissociation from normal thought and action. These illnesses were formerly labeled as dementia praecox, a term which, though smooth sounding, conveys the dismal connotation of early occurrence and tragic termination. Today we look upon the schizophrenias in a more favorable light and we recognize that they may begin early in life or even in the latter decades, that the illness may come on abruptly and clear up entirely, although we are well aware of the chronic progressive forms which end in deterioration. We know that there are many types, whether they begin early or late, which have as a common denominator a preoccupation with self to the exclusion of reality, a dissociation of thought and feeling, peculiar behavior ruled by delusions. The following introductory case history will illustrate a common type of schizophrenia:

Pfc. P. F., age 32, was hospitalized in England when his conduct and odd remarks disturbed others in his outfit. His family history was negative except for the fact that his mother had been confined to a mental hospital for several months. P. F. was one of eight children, who had a healthy boyhood and was a good student. He was considered overconscientious, spent a good deal of time by himself, avoided women, and had few friends. He was inducted in 1942 and assigned to the Radio School. His intelligence and assiduous efforts led to his promotion to private first class.

In England he began to notice "irregularities" and concentrated on "watching." He became suspicious of the personnel in the radio operator's department. It seemed to him that code messages were not delivered correctly, that planes did not report in the usual manner, and that there were too many emergencies. He became convinced that some American soldiers were saboteurs and that British officers were mixed up in it. Then he searched the desk of his colonel "to find out whether the colonel was on the beam." In going to and from his barracks, it seemed as though he were being followed by a British officer who was involved in a sex crime. He was terrified lest he be a victim. So he locked his window, but found it broken in the morning. He reported to his superiors that he was going to be killed "for knowing too much." As his condition did not improve, he was transferred to the United States.

Under observation here, he continued to have similar ideas. "I am sick," he said, "too tired to read or do anything. It's from the dope the nurse put into my food. She is acting under orders from the higher-ups in the War Department. If I get out, I'll shoot the s.o.b.'s." At times P. F. seemed calm and at ease. More frequently he remained abed or stood aloof, because "those men look at me in a funny way; they must think I'm a fairy. They are trying to get control over me – they seem to know what I am thinking even before I do – I hear them talking of things which run through my mind."

Symptoms of Schizophrenias

The schizophrenic acts oddly because his thinking is abnormal – it is delusional. The major delusion revolves about the theme that the patient is uniquely all-important to the world as well as to himself. People look at him with particularly significant glances (ideas of reference); others are whispering insulting remarks (auditory hallucinations) or are writing and broadcasting slurring statements, yes even plotting to do him harm (persecutory delusions). It occurs to him that perhaps he has committed a grave sin (delusion of homosexuality) or that he is some very important personage, close to God, being persecuted by certain non-believers. Such ideas dominate all sense impressions and are not subject to correction by logic or reason. Bleuler calls it autistic thinking (auto – self), a reverie projected into reality believed in, carried through. The individual's thinking is dissociated, cut off from reality – in a word, schizophrenic.

The schizophrenic is likely to interpret the actions of all as directly related to himself. "People leave the streetcar when I enter – It's because an odor of decay comes from my body and offends them – I can tell by the way they sniff." Thus spoke a young man who bathed twice daily, who rinsed his mouth, and who took enemas in the endless and futile effort to clear away the olfactory evidence of bodily decay. "I must have something diseased and horrible in me – people open windows; they walk across the street to avoid me; some persons even leave a movie shortly after I take my seat. I can smell this odor myself" (olfactory hallucination). The idea of bodily decay had no physical basis, was not relieved by the assurance of physicians after many examinations, and persisted as a false fixed idea or delusion.

Another patient had become uneasy after he had denounced lawbreakers. One day as he was shopping for bread, two unknown men entered the store. He looked at them and his interpretation was: "Perhaps they are bootleggers and are here to take me for a ride." He hurried out of the bakery without completing his errand. Several days later he was in a store selling some articles when he noticed a man peering in the window. Again there flashed into his mind the thought that he was being spied upon and followed. Quickly he closed his sample case and hurried out of the store. It then occurred to him to go out of town and he got into his car and began to travel. As he toured toward another city, it seemed that he was being followed, and so he detoured and hastened home. He stayed home some days, quite relieved of his frightening experiences. Then one day someone knocked at the door to inquire about an address. The stranger certainly looked suspicious. "What if they attack me in my own home," he thought. As he sat uneasily, an automobile turned in the street, its lights flashing in his windows. Frightened, he hid himself in the basement. "I am positive that not one, but a gang of bootleggers is after me. They are going to try to destroy me. I would like to call the police but I am afraid that they are mixed up in this affair too. Please, Doctor, try to protect me."

This man's wife explained that the patient had been a meek, withdrawn individual who had no contacts with and no enemies in the world of liquor and lawbreaking. Indeed, he was an abstainer, rather seclusive and religious. The ideas were obviously fears of persecution – indicating the paranoid type of schizophrenia.

The common hallucinations are auditory, tactile, visual, olfactory, and gustatory. Indeed, any sense impression may be distorted and interpreted as of some special meaning to the patient. Auditory hallucinations are among the most common. They can be a distinct voice, speaking clearly to the patient, denouncing, accusing, warning. It is usually a private matter concerning only the patient, although he may be convinced that the sound is so clear as to be audible to all in the room. The voice may be recognized as belonging to some particular person, or it may represent a babble coming from a group. Sometimes the voice comes from some close friend, known to be dead. "I hear it – it tells me to be careful. I recognize it as my father's voice. It's hard for me to explain this, for I know my father is dead." In some cases the voice is not clear and the patient is perplexed. "I can hear words. Sometimes my dear grandmother speaks, but usually it is my own thoughts. The voice is faint; it's an echo of my thoughts. Maybe I merely think it and don't hear it. But I am certain I do hear it!" Again it is not a voice but a sound – "It's a crackle, like parchment. It's in my head, and when I hear it I think of John. He loved me but I didn't marry him. This sound is a signal from him. Can you hear it too?"

Visual hallucinations occur in schizophrenia, taking the form of someone closely attached to the patient or of some religious being. "I was sitting in meditation when I saw Him appear on the wall. He seemed sad and He beckoned to me." Such a vision of God may be accepted as a spiritual experience and within the scope of normal religious ideas of a devout person. Yet this particular patient continued to sit, awaiting further orders, and refused to work or eat, stating, "Now that God has chosen me, I no longer am earthly or mundane. I don't need food or money. I won't die. I'll go to heaven." This patient had given away her money, had refused all food, and was in a state of dehydration, so that it was obvious that her vision was an evidence of a pathologic mental state, not a spiritual uplift.

Tactile hallucinations are described as pinching, burning, pricking, or electrical sensations. They are intimately associated with a delusion as to cause. "I felt my skin prickling; electricity was entering my body – it must come from my bed being wired. I got up and looked to see if there were wires connected with it but I couldn't find any. Perhaps it's in the form of electrical waves. I am not sure who is doing it, but I think a labor union is up to it. I got a notice from a union and didn't join."

Olfactory hallucinations are usually unpleasant. "It's a kind of smoke or chemical, like sulphur. It's in the air. It stifles my breathing and poisons my mind." One of the first patients that I treated with insulin in 1937 had pronounced olfactory hallucinations, sometimes holy, sometimes vulgar. "My room had a peculiar smell. It was like the incense in a church, like gardenias and other flowers at a funeral – in fact it made me feel I was at a funeral. But sometimes the odor changed. It was like fecal material – a foul stink – coming from somewhere." Another patient who had been in an isolated ward for several years, considered as an almost hopeless schizophrenic, mentioned an odor "like the ejaculated fluid of a male orgasm. It's everywhere – it's filthy!"

Gustatory hallucinations are usually connected with food or beverage. Quite commonly the food is believed to be tainted or poisoned by the evil-doing of some person or group. Thus a schizophrenic will bring a bundle which he will quietly open before the doctor, remarking, "Please have this analyzed by a chemist. I am sure it's poisoned. My wife is trying to harm me." For example, L. G. attended a clinic for stomach illnesses, complaining of indigestion. One day he announced to the doctors that he had discovered the cause of his stomach trouble. "It's my wife – she is putting poison in my food." His remark passed unheeded, but not so his actions – several weeks later he fired a bullet into her heart, killing her!

Such hallucinations and many others are interwoven with delusions and also with the inner drives, wishes, and fears of a patient. This is clearly seen in the olfactory hallucinations of a young man of 17 who had given up school and who sat around lazily looking at movie magazines. "Doctor, don't you smell that perfume? It's so sweet and fragrant – it's like narcissus. I recognize it – it's Hedy Lamarr's perfume. See, this is her picture. She must be outside waiting for me. I know she is there because I can smell the perfume." So this youth walked the streets in search of the beautiful actress who was to be his date. Such an hallucination is an obvious extension into reality of a wish, of a daydream.

Patients are inclined to apply to themselves items which they see in newspapers or hear broadcast over the radio. "I saw the picture of a woman holding a baby in her lap – it means I should have a baby." Said another patient, "When I was in Hawaii and I heard the broadcast, I knew it was a signal for me. Even now there are warnings to me over the radio. One program said, 'Be careful not to offend.' They must know about me – I'll not leave the house."

The thinking of a schizophrenic is abnormal since it does not conform to the laws of logic and reason but represents the translation of wishes, the language of dreams, the ideas of childhood and of primitive man. This applies to the ideas that are at the core of the illness. It is incorrect to say that a schizophrenic thinks as an infant or as a primitive man on all subjects. He may think and talk as an adult, mature and educated, about many subjects of daily life. He can be well versed in music and current events and science, yet in the sphere that concerns his personal striving, his relationship to people and to the world, the abnormality appears. Like the infant who does not distinguish the world from himself, so the schizophrenic may incorporate the world in his own body, rule it, lead it. "I have swallowed a pearl, which is the world." "I move a ring on my finger and it controls the movement of the sun." "Leave me – I am the source of all tragedy and all suffering." "Look up at the sky; see those clouds? See, the white fluff is separating into letters. Read them – P O W E R – it means I am to have the power to rule everything."

Another patient, S. M., the son of a tailor and barely able to eke out a living as a taxi driver, stated: "I am not just an ordinary man. You will soon find out who I really am – I have talent, greatness; I'm not just a local leader but you'll soon find out my international position when you read about me at the United Nations Meeting."

It is not always that the schizophrenic believes that he dominates others; indeed, it is common for patients to feel that others control them: "It seems as though people can read my thoughts and they know what I will say even before I express it. . . . In fact I believe that they make me think and do things whether I want to or not. They seem to have control over me."

Such false ideas, or delusions, are not only false, they are intense and absorbing. The patient is so preoccupied with them that he can think of little else. For why should S. M. be content with an ordinary existence as a cab driver when he expects to be called on to rescue the world. Thus one patient believes himself to be a savior, another a sinner – "Don't come near me," he cries, "I am the cause of all illness and death." A third patient is perplexed – "What is life, what is nature, who am I?" Like an adolescent suddenly aware of the universe and his place in it, the schizophrenic tackles the vast unanswerable problems of life. But unlike the adolescent, who can dismiss these thoughts to eat and sleep and dance and study, the schizophrenic cannot let go – and continues to ponder and puzzle and usually arrives at a delusional conclusion.

The thinking of schizophrenics is not always so definite. In the early stages some patients are aware of the incongruity of their delusions, yet cannot dispel them. "I am so puzzled by it all. I heard my father talking – his voice was faint, but he called my name and he told me to be ready for something wonderful. I know that he means I am going to put an end to the war. I even heard Roosevelt telling me this. But my father is dead, and I know that a dead person can't talk. Yet I am positive of what my father said. He warned me to be careful so I haven't dared to touch any food – it isn't safe." This patient was bewildered, since his life's experience proved to him that his father was dead and could not speak, yet he "heard" the voice of his father. This puzzled him. He pondered over the impossibility of the experience but at the same time was positive that it had occurred. Hence he was perplexed, doubting, questioning himself, yet unable to free himself of the conviction of the hallucinations.

Later in the course of schizophrenia there is bizarre association of ideas. Thoughts and words are scrambled (word salad), or there seems to be a dearth of ideas. In the chronic stages the patient is neglectful of his person, indifferent to reality, and even lacking inner drives. The structure of the personality has crumbled, thinking has become dilapidated.

The alternation from the expansive delusions of the adolescent schizophrenic to the withered inactivity of the chronic stage has been vividly described by Storch as follows: "The biologic revolution of puberty often forces the disease towards its first manifestation. In this period of life, experiences take place which may plunge the human being into a shoreless maelstrom of uncertainty. Whether to follow his enthusiastic impulses and give himself free to the world, or to withdraw gloomily into the self. In this tense mood, leading at one moment to overflowing desire, at another to autistic reserve, the pathological process not rarely establishes itself; all the dams which reason has erected then give way and the psychic experiences unfold themselves unimpeded in the boundless sphere of the unconditioned. There is an intoxicating cosmic consciousness, a grandiose world fantasy; the person feels himself the center of the universe. He is the master of wonderful magic power; he expands into the cosmic whole; he wars with the demons of his fate; in the mystical ecstasy of his introversion, he attains to a knowledge of the infinite – he is God.

But this fabulous effervescence and ambitious growth is transitory. Usually only a single phase of an ominous disease process, the flowing experience is dissipated like a vapor. The return to the world of reality is barred; there remains only one way out and that leads through rending torments, rambling confusion, apathetic waste, to imbecility or empty torpidity."

The emotions of a schizophrenic patient are likely to be abnormal. The classical description pictures flattening of emotions. Recently I saw a patient who told of strange bodily sensations and hallucinations: "My chest and stomach are cold - strange. I feel faint. I hear voices talking about me. It's the nurses saying they are going to experiment with me – maybe do away with me." During the entire examination the patient smiled and giggled. Even when talking about a dream of seeing a corpse, she continued to smile and laugh to herself. When she described the delusion that the nurses were plotting to destroy her, the inappropriate smile was on her face. Thus also did a young schizophrenic who had attempted suicide continue to smile and laugh in a silly way. (This is an example of inappropriate emotion – or rather, the emotion may harmonize with inner ideas, but certainly not with the expressions or with external reality.)

The behavior of a schizophrenic is usually dominated by his delusions and not by the demands of reality. Thus the patient who was a traveling salesman spent his time hiding from the bootleggers whom he feared. L. G. took medicines and went to clinics, seeking relief from his gastric symptoms until he "discovered the cause" (his wife). Then he watched her every movement, like a detective piling up "evidence" of her wickedness. Finally, when he was "convinced," he decided to take the law into his own hands and purchased a revolver and killed her. When I saw this patient in the County Jail, he sat blankly, seemingly unaware that his wife was dead or that he had killed her.

Patients will listen intently to the faint voices of hallucinations and will act in accordance with them. If these voices tell them not to eat, they may refuse all food for days at a time. Thus such patients are brought into the hospital, lips dry, pulse rapid, bodies emaciated and feverish from starvation. When food is offered, they may clamp their jaws; if tube-fed, they will try to vomit. For if their delusions be correct, it's safer to starve than to be poisoned.

Some persons withdraw into silence, while others speak to win applause or approval. Some draw away to escape "tormentors;" others call the police, write to the newspapers, or attack their persecutors. Several years ago a woman killed the proprietor of a store whom she accused of hoaxing her. At about the same time a young man, studying peacefully in the New York Public Library, was struck in the head with a hatchet wielded by a paranoid individual who was seeking his "enemies."

The language of some patients is unique – full of symbols which have private meaning. For instance, F. M. wrote: "Y to b 4 Zu – S not an of S (N. W.) offensive ... J can hear you say what ... make me—." It was a combination of code, shorthand, and correct English – unintelligible to the outsider but undoubtedly reflecting her thinking. She would also make sketches – brief cartoons between lines of her writing. Other patients are busy painting. The result may be a messy blotch of colors or an artistic classic. The writing or the painting may be unclear to the reader, but reflects the inner thinking of the patient.

There are schizophrenics who maintain seemingly normal relations with the world, working steadily, dressing neatly, conducting themselves appropriately. It is as though the schizophrenic ideas ran parallel with a course of normal conduct, neither influencing the other. Such a person may hear voices, believe himself "different," and only in the silent hours of being alone answer back, write private codes, and plan special deeds. Yet such ideas are privately expressed and do not have the power to destroy seemingly correct behavior.

A woman of 35 was employed as secretary to a professional man. She dressed neatly and attended to her duties faithfully, doing an efficient job. Those who met her believed her to be a normal individual. Yet, outside of work, she had a restricted social life and no recreation. She went to doctors complaining of burning in the vagina which led to repeated masturbation. A recent letter which she sent affords an understanding of what really goes on in her mind:

"My dear Dr.————:
Only God could have sent me to you after Dr. D. U. saw me and *posed* as someone interested *in me*. I am quite sure it is he who planned all of this abuse of me. I have not had one moment free from some sort of abuse, and it seems *now* that *all* that my body

gained thru the fear shock I received when my dog was supposedly poisoned and died.

"Such suffering! *Now* I am built into some sort of queer something or other. In order to find comfort - I am *forced* to abuse both my vagina *and* my rectum and there is immense feeling in both places. My vagina has been made *very* small."

There are schizophrenics who even attain prominence and success as a result of their illness or in spite of it (Nietzche, Nijinsky, Van Gogh). Nietzche wrote eloquently during the intervals between serious illness and at times even when his mood seemed abnormal. Indeed, certain of his writings such as *Thus Spoke Zarathustra*, have the ring and clash of manic outbursts. Nijinsky, the talented Russian ballet dancer, achieved world fame even though he manifested serious symptoms towards the end of his dancing career. Van Gogh showed deviation of personality early in life and then exhibited more serious manifestations such as cutting off his own ear and uncontrollable behavior which brought him to sanitaria. Despite these disabilities and perhaps because of them, he was able to draw on paper sketches which stir the observer's sympathy. Few of my patients have attained the fame of these three artists. Nevertheless there are many individuals who can maintain themselves at a useful social and industrial level despite the fact that they also exhibit schizophrenic mental processes.

Yet the majority of those whose illness persists deviate seriously from normal interests. They disregard their duties for they are preoccupied by the delusions which rule their behavior. One patient continued to draw the blinds, spent hours spying on her neighbors whom she suspected of peeping at her sexually. In other matters she was keen, well informed, and apparently intelligent. Another patient may stand staring into space, then suddenly yell, shriek, jump, strike out in frenzied uncontrollable excitement. Or some patients lie abed, all clothes off, defecating and urinating, completely unmindful of all proprieties; refusing all food—spitting it out when offered; inattentive to any remarks, either ignoring the questioner or replying in unintelligible gibberish.

One could go on to mention numerous other symptoms, but enough has been covered so that we may proceed to a consideration of the course of schizophrenia.

Course of Schizophrenia

The mode of onset may be silent, gradual, insidious. So subtle are the changes in the actions and ideas of the patient that the family may not be aware for months that schizophrenia has set in. A young man may express the idea that fellow workmen are critical; he may even change his job because of this. Yet for months he continues to live quite normally. Then one day he refuses to go to work at all, explaining, "It's more than the workers; it's a union. It's the Catholics. They talked about me and accused me of sabotage. The F. B. I. are following me because my parents came from Germany. I won't leave the house." In another instance the disease begins abruptly, almost without warning, like a tropical storm. S. N. had been a hard-working, studious high school boy, interested in the serious side of life. One day he refused to go to class, saying he was being tested. He paced up and down, listening to sounds. When it rained, he suspected that he was being tested by God. Later he refused to go to bed – he *must* stay awake to figure out all these peculiar things.

Once the symptoms of the illness have become manifest, what is the course and ultimate status? Fortunately the prognosis today is more hopeful than in the days of Kraepelin when dementia precox (schizophrenia) usually meant a chronic, hopeless mental disease, running a long course and often terminating in a deteriorated mental and dilapidated physical condition. Now a broader experience has revealed many different courses. For example, the illness may begin abruptly, run a short, favorable course toward recovery. Such was the case of P. B., whom I saw in service.

> P. B., age twenty, came from a healthy family and was a successful student at college. He enlisted in the Air Corps and for several weeks awaited orders. The delay was disturbing and so he drank moderately. Then the orders came and he was en route to Miami, Florida. He sat up all night, tense and worried. At the reception center he was given several inoculations, as well as his uniform.
> "I went to some movies," he told me later. "One was *In Which We Serve*. The others were G-I stuff about venereal disease. It was warm. I seemed worried. I couldn't sleep and stayed up all night. Then it seemed as though everyone was hyponotized, as if they were waiting for me to say something. I thought I was Jesus. I predicted the end

of the world. I was trying to reform them. I thought everything was tumbling down and so I shouted, 'Hell is going to freeze,' and I was in it. They took me to a hospital. I thought I was in a cell and that I would be massacred. I thought it was Hitler and the Germans; I could hear them talking about killing. I thought things were burning – I was burning. I yelled because Hitler was coming after me – to kill me again."

The air cadet was thus disturbed for twelve days and was then transferred to a hospital where I saw him. By the time of his arrival he had fully recovered. He remained well during the period of observation.

If we view such an illness at the time of its intensity, we must consider it as a serious psychosis. Yet viewed from the life story of the patient, his good health, the abrupt onset after induction, the stormy course, the favorable outcome, we may look at it differently.

Another case studied recently is that of S.N., a patient of 16, who had been a healthy youngster, somewhat studious, highly intelligent, a Grade A student. He had been more devoted to his classroom work than to social and athletic activities. In the family history we find that two members, his mother and an uncle, have had recurrent depressions.

In the fall of 1945 this patient began to act oddly in school. He asked the teachers if they had changed the books. "My books seem different. There is something funny in the Latin and the German books. Some words are capitalized and others are not. I believe the teachers and the authors of the books have changed them to help me or to test me." Gradually his doubts extended to other persons and other activities. While sitting in a restaurant, he asked his parents, "Who are those people? They are looking at me rather funny. I wonder what they're up to." The boy became restless, sleepless, perplexed, and asked innumerable questions.

At the time of the initial examination, while I was doing a physical study, he kept asking, "Why do you do this? Are you sure you know what you are doing? Are you my doctor? Maybe you're not the doctor." It began to rain and he became startled and asked, "Is it raining? Am I making it rain?" The patient was asked to describe certain of his observations and he remarked, "There's something funny going on. I don't know what it is. The radio in our car is different; it has been changed – it's telling me things. People have been treating me in a very queer way."

He heard a sound in the hallway and asked if it was a real noise and what the meaning of it was. Apparently he was hallucinating because, while listening, he said he heard a voice which was saying: "Boy, you've got something there." The voices seemed to have some control and seemed to know what the patient was thinking. His behavior became more and more difficult; he refused to eat, became overactive, and was sleepless. The condition reached the state where it was necessary for his family to place him in a mental hospital.

During the initial study at the hospital, he laughed in a silly manner, asked odd questions such as, "Is this the radio in the car (pointing to the radio in the room)? No, it must have been changed; it was changed to help me." He paced back and forth with an expression of bewilderment on his face. Within five days during the period of observation, there was a remarkable improvement. He announced: "Everything is so different now. I thought everything that happened was because of me. When it rained, I believed that I was causing the rain, that I could control it and make it stop at my will."

Gradually his condition improved, and within ten days after admission to the hospital the young man was considered sufficiently improved to be allowed to go home. He was observed at my office at weekly intervals, during which time he developed remarkable insight into his condition. "How could I have imagined those things? I interpreted the noises. I thought everything that happened had some meaning especially for me. I imagined things on the radio. I heard different people talking – two people, two voices. Each represented an idea. One wanted me to give up; the other insisted that I go on. I could identify those voices; one had a British accent and the other was American. It seemed that whatever I thought came back over the radio."

As the patient slept well, enjoyed a good appetite, and developed good insight, he was permitted to return to school. His condition has been followed for a period of about one year and he is at present well.

The condition had all the features of schizophrenia; the remarkable clearing up in a matter of several weeks justifies the diagnosis of an acute schizophrenic reaction. The fact that there are two members of the family who had recurrent depressions suggests the possibility that this illness may be cyclic even though the obvious symptomatology is that of schizophrenia. Indeed, with the silly laughter, the age of onset, one's initial impression was that of a malignant psychosis. Yet the improvement, even though it may be temporary, is remarkable.

These two cases belong to the group of acute schizophrenic reaction. This group of illnesses, seen not infrequently in the Army, has been explained in various ways. One view is that the symptoms merely resemble schizophrenia and are in reality a psychogenic reaction to unbearable stress of service life. Another explanation for the acuteness and recovery is that the illness is basically manic-depressive with manifestations of schizophrenia, clearing up as quickly as cyclic illnesses sometimes do. Yet one sees schizophrenia begin, clear up for a time, only to reappear later. Noyes mentions that some 40% of the chronic schizophrenic subjects had previous admissions with apparent recovery, which was but a temporary improvement. In other cases, as for example Z. J., the onset was slow and the course more or less continuous.

> Z. J. had been a fairly healthy, well developed youngster and had gone through puberty quite normally. During her junior year in high school, she became somewhat withdrawn, did not mingle as freely with her fellow students and avoided dates. Then she seemed to become preoccupied and would stand and stare. Next, quite abruptly, she made a suicidal attempt by swallowing some roach poison. She was given first aid and made a quick recovery from this attempt. Her behavior continued to be abnormal and she was therefore placed in the Windsor Hospital.
>
> At the hospital Z. J. would lie in bed or stand in the center of a room staring. When spoken to, she was likely to repeat the examiner's words and would often use the same phrase again and again. For example, I might say: "How is everything here in the hospital?" and she would reply, "The nurses are nice; Z. J. is nice; I am nice; everyone is nice." At times she would listen intently as though hearing someone. She would leave the interviewer, explaining, "Someone is calling me. They said, 'Z. J., come here.'" Once or twice she mentioned olfactory hallucinations: "There's some peculiar odor outside the building. It sickens me." Her behavior became disturbed and on one occasion she tried to run away; another time she bit one of the attendants. When she was asked about the voices, she replied: "I don't think I really heard them. Maybe it was the radio. A man's voice said, 'Z. J. is nice; Z. J. is very nice.'" When asked about the odors, she replied, "Oh, I

smelled something around the house. Maybe it was gardenias."

Concerning her suicidal attempt, she explained: "I wasn't doing so well at school, so I thought I would like to end it all. I took Peterman's and swallowed it. They rushed me to the hospital and gave me lime water. I don't think I should have done it. Let me go home and I will be all right."

As Z. J. recounted her earlier childhood, she emphasized the fact that she had been afraid of her father because of his tendency to fly into rages, chiefly over her homework. She told about her hopes to finish school and get married. However, she expressed a marked fear of syphilis, but had no adequate explanation for this fear.

Z. J. was first seen in the hospital in the spring of 1942 and a course of electro-shock therapy was started. During the earlier phase of the treatment Z. J. would stand by herself, occasionally smiling in a silly way, and again repeating phrases with marked perseverance. On several occasions she would stand like a statue, completely unresponsive to questions. As the course of shock therapy was continued, there was a decided betterment to the point where she was permitted to go home on trial.

After a period of several weeks of fairly good behavior, she became difficult and unmanageable and had to be readmitted to the hospital. Upon readmission, she was somewhat fearful lest her father and mother were being harmed.

I entered the Army for a period of two years, during which time Z. J. remained in the hospital, her condition relatively unchanged. When she was reexamined in the spring of 1945, she had gained physically but showed absolutely no interest in reality. I pointed to the snow outside and asked her to describe what she saw. She stood staring and finally, after long delay, answered, "It is my snow." I showed her a watch and she had difficulty telling time. A course of insulin-shock therapy was undertaken, again with temporary improvement.

However, in February of 1946, a matter of some four years after onset, Z. J. is confined to the disturbed ward because she is assaultive and neglects her person. When spoken to, she may not reply at all or may answer in an incoherent manner.

This is a serious type of schizophrenia with hebephrenic and paranoid features, the prognosis poor. Shock therapy has failed. This case showed temporary improvement but the symptoms soon recurred and have persisted with malignant tenacity.

Types of Schizophrenia

To speak of dementia preacox as though it were one disease entity fails to do justice to the many forms, varying as they do with the age of the patient, the course, and the response to treatment. It is more exact to use the term "schizophrenic reaction types" and to acknowledge possible combinations, with mood disturbance, under the heading of schizo-affective disorders. For I believe with Singer that manic-depressive illness and schizophrenia need not be mutually exclusive – "It is not a question of one or the other, but more or less." Certainly cases respond to shock therapy which have the surface appearance of schizophrenia, but the course of recurrent depressions.

There are several recognized distinct types:
Schizophrenia, simplex.
Schizophrenia, hebephrenic type.
Schizophrenia, catatonic type.
Schizophrenia, paranoid type.
Schizo-affective disorders.

In my own practice which, unlike that of State hospital psychiatry, deals largely with earlier cases, I have found it useful to employ the following subdivisions:

SCHIZOPHRENIA SIMPLEX: These occur relatively early – in late adolescence and about the age of twenty. The individual may be of asthenic build and introvert personality, withdrawn, studious, failing to develop a complete social and sexual adjustment. Deviation is evident early in the odd traits of the growing young man or woman – seclusiveness, over-religiosity, excessive daydreaming expressed in words or writing and drawing. There is an avoidance of social contact and a withdrawal of interest.

The individual lacks energy, does not strive towards a useful goal – and tends to neglect himself and his responsibilities. For instance, A. K. was a slender, highly intelligent boy who was quite normal until puberty. Then he became abnormally self-conscious, gave up sports. He spent an excessive amount of time reading and daydreaming. He attended high school, but did not achieve the level expected of this previously bright, successful boy. All invitations to social affairs were rejected because he was too tired or not interested. He took to writing poetry and tracts on man's purpose in life. After completing high school, he tried and failed at several jobs. He was either too tired or complained that fellow workmen avoided him. Then he gave up work altogether, spending his time at home, daydreaming, writing poetry, or just sitting around. He has become untidy, neglects to shave or bathe. When left alone, he is good-natured, but when corrected, he becomes angry and abusive. For the past year he has rarely gone out of the house of his own volition.

Such patients continue on and on, with complete failure to develop interest in a career or in life (the so-called surrender type of C. MacFie Campbell).

THE HEBEPHRENIC PATIENT has progressed further and has attained a better adjustment. Then he becomes preoccupied with himself – as did our patient, C. M., who noticed a few acne spots. He began to apply lotions, look at himself in the mirror, lie awake nights. He gave up his job and sat at home smiling to himself. When the physician inquired about his thoughts, he remarked: "These spots represent a disease; I've been immoral; people look at me and know I have it. God wants me to die." While he expressed such tragic ideas, this patient sat smiling to himself. The smile was certainly in contrast to the words uttered. This patient improved for a time, then again became agitated – yet always grinning in a silly manner.

THE CATATONIC GROUP has two features or phases, one of which may merge into the other. The longer and more characteristic phase consists of a period of silence, of immobility, of utter disregard for place, problems, and life's needs. The patient may lie abed, unresponsive to any stimulus, disregarding any person, indeed, ignoring bodily functions. Another patient may stand for hours or days, as immobile and silent as a statue in a museum. Quite suddenly, however, there is an abrupt change to the phase of overactivity. The patient may shriek, jump, run and strike. This state of frenzy, referred to as catatonic excitement, may continue for hours or days until the patient once more sinks exhausted into the condition of negativism. E. M. has been lying in bed for months, making no voluntary statements nor answering any questions. She resists pleading or physical attempts to move her. Tube feeding has been necessary to keep her from starvation. On several occasions, however, she has leaped out of bed, struck and bit attendants, yelled and shrieked wildly.

THE PARANOID VARIETY is much more common. It may occur

early in life, before the age of twenty, but is more likely to develop in the third and fourth decades. In some instances its course is chronic and continuous; yet the person retains a keen mind and sufficient grasp of reality in impersonal matters to make a reasonable adjustment to life. Mrs. M. A. worked diligently, felt fine, cooked, and kept her home spic and span. At the age of 45 her persistent accusations and queries became intolerable so that her husband finally sought psychiatric help. It was then learned that this woman became suspicious of her neighbors when she was first married, at the age of 24. She was considered a lively, intelligent, capable woman. However, she did not respond sexually and had never had the experience of an orgasm. She then began to suspect her husband of having illicit love affairs as his sex demands declined. At first she would accuse him jokingly, but in the course of years these taunts were more persistent and her accusations were directed against specific women. Indeed, if a woman's voice called on the telephone (wrong number), Mrs. M. A. was positive it was a call for a rendezvous. If a woman sat in a parked car near their home, it was her husband's sweetheart. Her son grew up and became a gifted violinist. She accused him of playing seductive music so as to procure female partners for his father's sexual pleasures. Recently she threatened to kill a neighbor whom she accused of being her husband's mistress. Yet her husband is a gentle, devoted, industrious man who actually has given her no basis for her accusations.

Even more serious was the case of Mrs. W. W., who was referred to me at the age of forty, after she had had symptoms for about two decades. She was an attractive, intelligent woman, neatly dressed and quite charming in manner. Certainly she did not look the part of one who had a serious mental disease. But this is what she said: "I can't stand my neighbors – they are awful. They look into my house. Why, they like to spy into my bathroom whenever I bathe or urinate. They must have special tricky apparatus to do this. You know, I put up thick curtains, but they could see through them. I felt their eyes upon me, so I had dark blinds put on all the windows. But even that doesn't keep them out – they must have periscopes. I thought they were hiding in the bushes around my house so I had flood lights attached to every window and I fooled them. But they still keep at it. I saw one of them talk to the postman and look in my direction. She must have told him what she saw, because they both smiled. I called her up and threatened to do something if they didn't stop annoying me. I can't stand it any more!"

The husband of this patient had accepted his wife's statements at first as fact and later as an idiosyncrasy. Yet when the symptoms persisted even though they had moved their residence, and when she invested in the lights and made threats of violence, he became concerned.

L. G., who suspected his wife of poisoning him and then shot her, was a typical paranoid. His criminal act was to him a logical and correct deed, a fact which makes paranoids dangerous.

THE SCHIZO-AFFECTIVE DISORDERS are rather common, including schizo-depressions and schizo-manic behavior. They run cyclic courses, respond well to shock treatment, and thus have a favorable outcome. I prefer to use this combination term rather than to call them either schizophrenias or depressions, because both features are present and prominent. Those cases which fail to respond and ultimately require confinement to State hospitals are usually true schizophrenias. Thus a psychiatrist whose patients consist of State hospital cases is likely to stress this diagnosis. However, many get well and their illnesses may be affective disorders with schizoid features. Since only time can make the final diagnosis and we are accustomed to applying a label, I find it convenient to use the combined term schizo-affective.

Causes of Schizophrenia

The exact nature of schizophrenia is a problem that awaits solution. There are many concepts: organic (brain or gland (Schilder)); psychogenic, in the Freudian sense of a fixation of libido in an infantile narcissistic state; in the sense of Adolph Meyer's concept of parergasia or energy diverted from objects to one's self; psychogenic in the sense of an hysterical escape from an intolerable situation. These theories, seemingly in conflict, may each be correct in specific types of cases. Certainly schizophrenia simplex, beginning at adolescence and continuing onward, impresses me as an organic defect, even though a gross study of the brain shows no obvious abnormality. Acute schizophrenic reactions may be either psychogenic or organic. In the Army there were frequent examples of both types. Two varieties of schizophrenic symptoms which were presumably psychogenic are, briefly, as follows. A latent homosexual whose well controlled tendencies have kept him out of trouble is inducted into the Army. In the barracks he sees fellow soldiers undress, and he, himself, is exposed in the nude. Dormant fantasies are awakened. One day he hears fellow soldiers speaking, and perhaps they have used the word ferry. It seems to him as though they are looking in his direction, and he translates the word as "fairy." Inner thoughts and self-accusations are projected outward. He becomes panicky and cries for help. Another type may be the escape of a timid, over-protected youth from the fancied hardships of war. Soldiers who do not know the language, who don't feel accepted, who are self conscious, become suspicious, depressed, and bewildered. In some, the reaction of escape is that of a temporary psychosis. The paranoid forms combine features of failure in sexual development and psychogenic mechanisms. For the most part I hold with Singer and with Schilder that schizophrenia is fundamentally organic.

At this point I should like to detour from the subject of schizophrenia to discuss schizophrenic-like reactions which are psychogenic:

Faced with engulfment by the sweeping tide of circumstances, man may react with symptoms whose features are those of a psychosis. A person confined to prison; a youth of retarded intellect transplanted from the routine of a farm to the unaccustomed and to him difficult task of learning to be a soldier; a soldier about to be sent overseas, anticipating submarine sinkings and the hazards of combat; a soldier confronted by the dire deprivations and dangers of warfare will obviously react to such threats. The reaction may not be constructive, may not be for the good of the group. Rather it may become an uncontrolled exhibition of fear, helplessness, and confusion. As such, it will exhibit the weakness and confusion of panic, although in our organization, protective of the weak, it will serve as an escape from the threatening situation.

The form of the reaction, the avenue or exit chosen by the individual will vary a great deal. Some exhibit visceral imbalance of intense degree: nausea, vomiting and diarrhea, a rapid pulse with palpitation, dyspnea, weakness. It may take the form of neuromuscular abnormality: tremors, weakness, staggering. Emotional symptoms may predominate such as weeping, crying. Sleeplessness, inefficiency, and dependency characterize every type.

Of particular interest to us at the moment are those disturbances of consciousness, those periods of confusion, the failure to distinguish fantasy from reality. In such instances the patient exhibits the bizzarre behavior of a psychotic. He may lose his identity or believe that he is now someone else. Beliefs and aims about himself, hitherto concealed and appearing in daydreams or in dreams at night, seem now attained. Fears kept in check by self-control now seize the patient and overwhelm him. Inner voices of self-regard, and especially of self-accusation, become projected outward. They sound real and frightening, seemingly being spoken by inimical persons just outside the door or broadcast over the radio. The patient reacts to these voices – hallucinations which interest or terrify him. Occurrences in the environment take on a new meaning, vital to the patient himself. Or another patient reverts to an apathetic state of infantile indifference to the serious dangers around him.

In the main, the symptomatology, the delusions and hallucinations, and the behavior impress the examiner as indicative of schizophrenia. Then quite suddenly the picture changes. Sometimes the condition clears spontaneously and the patient becomes fully cognizant of all events, with or without the ability to recall this episode. However, more frequently a change in circumstances is required before the process improves. Again and again, soldiers have been examined overseas when they developed such symptoms and a diagnosis of schizophrenia made. Such soldiers were sent back to the Zone of the Interior and when they arrived, the symptoms had vanished or the illness was in remission.

Treatment of the Schizophrenic Patient

Whereas diagnosis stresses the abnormalities, the pathology, treatment is directed toward the intact functions, toward the man. What can be done to help him meet life, face reality, be productive in the face of his psychopathology – or better still, how can we eradicate the abnormality?

A physical examination, as is the case with depressed and psychoneurotic patients, enables the physician to make a friendly contact with the patient and often permits the schizophrenic to feel that he has an ally in the doctor. This is followed by a searching study of the mental processes so that the physician becomes familiar with the deviations in thinking and is able to judge what is intact and what has been lost. Many patients, however involved they may be in delusions, still possess intact functions. Likewise, the physician can compare the basic qualities and endowments of the individual with the present status. Indeed not only the program of therapy but the prognosis will depend upon what type of person has become sick.

One can thus evaluate what is preserved and what is lost, what can be modified by instruction or explanation and what is too fixed to be influenced. Some effort at explanation may be attempted, with the appreciation that one must be on the patient's side in his struggle against a hostile world. Hence we cannot ridicule, deny or denounce his hallucinations or delusions. They are above reason and more real to the patient than reality itself. We can only guide the intact portion of the personality, direct the patient to be occupied, keep him interested or busy in spheres of endeavor away from his troubled zone.

Some schizophrenics can maintain themselves in society and continue to work despite a structure of paranoid delusions. Somehow the force and radiation of these ideas do not crash into the total personality and do not wreck the daily routine of work. Indeed, the patient may push the schizophrenic symptoms into the background as he keeps occupied with his work on the farm, keeping books, or grinding lenses. Or he may pursue his schizophrenic goals, dancing (as did Nijinsky), painting, preaching to a socially acceptable degree – earning both approval and a livelihood. But some day the symptoms may become violent, the actions extend beyond the normal, and so striking is the peculiar behavior that something drastic must be done.

Certain symptoms require prompt care. Some patients are sleepless because of restless behavior, suspicious alertness, or dreadful fear: "I know that our house is being watched; two men are in an auto spying upon us. If I fall asleep, they'll do something dirty. We must keep awake all night or we'll be dead pigeons." Wakefulness requires sedatives. If the patient trusts the doctor and his family, he will take a sedative (such as sodium amytal, gr. 3) and get some hours of sleep.

The patient's nutrition should be kept up. He should be encouraged to eat and if he refused all food, he must be hospitalized and tube fed.

As a rule, the acute schizophrenic, one who is suicidal or homicidal or who presents any serious problem of behavior, should be hospitalized. Here he will be under a regime of diet, medication, occupational therapy, and shock therapy.

Shock therapy is the one method which in many cases offers some prospect of recovery or improvement. It is useful in calming an assaultive patient, relaxing one who is fearful, and converting a patient who presents a feeding problem into one who takes nourishment. Shock therapy thus serves as a symptomatic measure in most patients and as a specific procedure for recovery in some. Here we will briefly discuss insulin coma therapy, leaving for a later chapter a consideration of electrocoma therapy.

INSULIN COMA THERAPY
Written in Collaboration with
Dr. Maurice B. Gordon

Introduction

Sakel had used insulin in large doses for the treatment of morphine addiction. He observed quite fortuitously that the occurrence of deep coma from such doses of insulin proved beneficial rather than harmful. Out of this observation there grew the use of insulin for purposes of producing coma as a therapeutic measure for psychoses. From its earliest administration in 1932 and 1933 it proved to be a remarkable advance which aroused an active approach on the part of all psychiatry. No longer were physicians in a hospital content to catalog illness, nor was it sufficient to trace symptoms back to childhood complexes. Insulin coma therapy meant action, an awakened interest in a positive effort to bring the mentally ill patient out of custodial care towards the world of well-being. The introduction of insulin also led to other methods; metrazol was first tried and later electrocoma therapy became more successful.

I began to use insulin in the treatment of psychoses in 1937 and found it extremely beneficial. However, in the course of time electrocoma therapy proved simpler, safer, and easier to administer. Furthermore, insulin coma was more or less limited to the treatment of schizophrenic patients whereas the electrical method could be employed for the large group of depressions as well as for schizophrenia. In my experience, in line with that of Kalinowsky and Hoch, an adequate series of electrocoma therapy yields a recovery rate which is close to that obtained with insulin. Because of this personal experience and preference, I have devoted considerable space to the discussion of electrocoma therapy and will mention insulin shock therapy briefly. The reader who wishes to employ this method in hospital treatment will find complete details in the books by Kalinowsky and Hoch, and Jessner and Ryan.

Technique of Administration

A. GENERAL: The aim of treatment is to bring about an improvement in mental state which may be of lasting duration. Experience has shown that although temporary improvement takes place with a small number of shocks, enduring results require an extensive series of coma reactions, say fifty or more. The dosage of insulin and the handling of each patient is an individual problem.

B. DOSAGE: The initial dose of insulin is ten to twenty units administered intramuscularly early in the morning, breakfast omitted. Each succeeding day this dose of insulin is increased by five to ten units or more until signs of hypoglycemia become evident. The patient is observed for three to four hours and then is given food. Such treatments are given daily five to six days per week. This constitutes an introductory or trial period, sometimes referred to as phase I.

During phase I, the patient shows the early changes of sweating, hunger, rapid pulse, and drowsiness. As the dosage during phase I is stepped up, the drowsiness deepens and unconsciousness develops in the third hour of hypoglycemia. The occurrence of coma represents the more significant therapeutic stage referred to as phase II. During the first episode of unconsciousness, it is advisable to terminate the coma in 15 minutes. As a rule, however, the patient is permitted to remain in the coma stage for half an hour unless complications arise.

The drug is standard insulin, given as a rule at 7:00 in the morning to a patient without breakfast. During phase I the treatment is terminated some four hours after the injection by permitting the patient to drink some type of sugar solution which contains as many grams of glucose as units of insulin given.

Additional sugar in the form of fruit juice or weak tea is allowed and a full course of food is given at the next mealtime.

C. MANIFESTATIONS DURING COMA: Signs and symptoms during the comas are as follows: During the first two hours there are drowsiness, languor, perspiration, and salivation. The patient frequently complains of hunger and thirst. Gradually consciousness becomes clouded and sleep overtakes the patient. Yet, during this period there may be restlessness, shouting, and excitement. The speech becomes slurred, words may be mumbled, actions are clumsy. Involuntary muscular movements appear, such as tremors, twitchings, sucking and grasping movements. The temperature of the body falls and the pulse rate changes. The patient then becomes unconscious and no longer responds to any stimuli.

The more severe features appear during the third hour after the injection and are often allowed to remain for half an hour to an hour. However, if the coma becomes more profound, the face becomes flushed, the pupils dilate, the pulse gets rapid, and more severe hyperkinetic symptoms develop. Unless the coma is terminated, there may be tetanic spasms, a marked rapidity of pulse rate, and disturbance of breathing. Such "deep coma" is avoided if possible.

D. TERMINATION OF COMA: Each coma is permitted to last up to an hour if the patient's status is satisfactory. When it is desired to bring the patient out of the unconscious state, a stomach tube is passed nasally. The proper position of the tube is assured by aspirating the stomach contents and testing with litmus paper or by listening over the stomach area while forcing air through the tube. Then a sugar solution such as dilute Karo syrup is poured in.

The awakening after the administration of sugar is a gradual process which takes some ten to thirty minutes. Slowly the patient opens his eyes and becomes aware of his environment. At the end of about thirty minutes he is fully conscious, comfortable, and is ready to take nourishment and resume activity.

Frequently it becomes necessary to terminate the coma more rapidly. If there is any complication such as circulatory or respiratory difficulty, then the therapist can administer up to 100 cc. of $33\frac{1}{3}$ per cent dextrose solution intravenously. When the patient regains consciousness from the intravenous glucose, he is given beverages containing sugar by mouth. Later, when he is fully awake by whatever mode of termination, a well balanced meal fortified with additional carbohydrate is allowed.

E. Course: As a rule phase I continues for a matter of about one week, since it takes on an average of 50 to 150 units of insulin to produce the stage of coma. Phase II or the coma period is then continued for a period of six or eight weeks for a series of some fifty coma reactions. The treatments are given daily for five to six days per week with a rest period on Sunday. When the patient has improved and the coma episodes are no longer desired, some physicians discontinue all treatment, while others taper off with smaller doses of insulin for a period of several days.

Complications

Insulin coma therapy is a much more drastic procedure which requires considerably more time, nursing staff, and involves more hazards than electrocoma therapy. There are certain complications, some of which can be prevented by adequate precautions and others which are often unavoidable.

A. Convulsions: It is not infrequent for the patient in the stage of coma to develop a severe convulsive reaction. As a rule this is not critical and does not interfere with the therapeutic result. Some physicians prefer to terminate the coma by intravenous glucose immediately after the convulsive reaction. Other psychiatrists do not terminate the coma on this account. However, it is advisable at subsequent periods to give such patients phenobarbital, gr. ½ t.i.d., in order to prevent convulsions. The reason for such a recommendation is the tendency for fractures to occur during such seizures.

B. Circulatory Disturbances: Quite commonly the pulse is slow during the early stage of the coma but may become irregular or rapid. The occurrence of consistent tachycardia and particularly development of irregularity such as auricular fibrillation call for prompt termination and several days rest from therapy. Likewise, any indication of circulatory collapse demands immediate termination by intravenous glucose and the use of such drugs as strophanthin.

C. Respiratory Difficulties: Any disturbances of respiration also call for termination by intravenous glucose, the injection of lobeline, and the administration of oxygen.

D. "Hunger Excitement": This may appear during phase I

and is characterized by loud crying out for food. When this occurs, the hunger should be satisfied by sufficient nourishment to terminate the treatment on that particular day. However, a larger dose of insulin is given on the following day and this may bring about drowsiness which effaces the hunger excitement.

E. PROLONGED COMA: This is a more serious complication. The patient fails to arouse or to remain conscious after he has been awakened. Deep coma persists even though the blood sugar may have returned to normal. Any such persistent coma demands immediate measures which include potassium chloride (two grams), betalin, adrenal cortex extract, and whole citrated blood intravenously.

Sometimes the patient fails to respond to such measures and remains in deep coma for days. Any indication of persistent coma is a warning against overly prolonged treatment.

F. DEATH: Death has occurred from insulin shock therapy. The average death rate is about one per cent, one author quoting a range of 0.5 per cent to 2 per cent (Müller).

Results

As a rule there is early improvement physically in most patients. Appetite is increased, there is a gain in weight and a general betterment of bodily vigor. Likewise, in many instances there is improvement in mental functions. The intensity of preoccupation diminishes and there is a renewed interest in the outside world. As the coma therapy continues, all delusions and hallucinations are pushed into the background. The patient may recall his previous abnormal ideas but speaks of them in a detached way as though they had occurred some time in the past.

The recovery rate from insulin therapy is fairly high. Many authors have reported that as high as eighty per cent of patients with early schizophrenia have recovered while some sixty per cent of those with more chronic forms show improvement. However, not all who improve remain well and there is a tendency for the schizophrenic manifestations to recur. A careful study of state hospital material by Ross and Malzberg gave the following results in a comparison between a control group and those treated with insulin: In the group who did not receive insulin there were 3.5 per cent who recovered, 11.2 per cent much improved, and 7.4 per cent improved. The total of improvement was 22.1 per cent. In contrast, the patients who received insulin showed a recovery rate of 11.1 per cent, considerable improvement in 26.5 per cent, and improvement in 26 per cent. The total who were benefited reached 63.6 per cent. Apparently three times as many patients showed improvement with insulin coma therapy as compared to the improvement in the pre-insulin days.

Bond and Shurley reported the results of a ten-year study of a group of schizophrenics treated with insulin. At the end of treatment 48 per cent of their patients were recovered, and at the end of a five-year period 37 per cent were apparently improved. These figures are certainly greater than the 16 per cent for control cases under hospital treatment without insulin or other shock therapy.

Shock methods are valuable in the management of the patient even if they do not change his ultimate fate. Picture several disturbed patients violently striking at hallucinated enemies, refusing all food because it is poisoned, or exhausting themselves crying for aid from tormentors. The control of such patients, in the interest of their safety and that of the ward, is a challenge. Shock therapy meets the need. A few treatments usually convert the assaultive patient into a more cheerful and cooperative person, the starving, suspicious one into a person who relishes his food. This benefit may be temporary and the serious evidences of the disturbed mind may recur. Nevertheless, the changed behavior itself is valuable. It was particularly needed in the Army if a psychotic patient was to be transported by plane or ship, when violence would endanger him and those who were to look after him.

Illustrative Case Histories

CASE I. *R. I.*

The first patient whom I treated was a young woman in the twenties who withdrew from her job as a seamstress and sat meditating in her home. She would frequently glance out of the window looking for some man whom she referred to as the philosopher. In the course of time she mentioned certain odors which were sickening. "It seems that I am in a dark room; I smell incense; I think it's a funeral. No, come to think about it, the odor is different, it's decay; it reminds me of death; maybe I'm dead." This patient had spent a good deal of time watching passersby, suspicious of a certain man whom she called the philosopher, who was dominating her thoughts.

Insulin coma therapy was given in 1937. The patient

reached phase II, the stage of coma, with seventy units of insulin. After she had had some ten comas, she stated: "I am better; I can now think without interference from the philosopher. I used to have visions and smell certain odors but I don't any more." Patient was given additional coma reactions and then treatment was discontinued. She remained mentally clear for a period of years.

CASE II. G. R.

A youth of 22 was referred to me in July, 1940, because of peculiar behavior over a period of weeks. One cousin was confined to a state hospital with a diagnosis of schizophrenia. While in a camp, the patient himself took sick with "nervousness and mental confusion."

During the initial study in the hospital, he sat about in a perplexed manner. "Am I 18 or am I 22? Something has happened to change me from 18 to 22." He had delusions about God. "I am closely connected with God; I am concerned with the cosmos." While talking about these experiences, he would go through various mannerisms, especially handshaking. He would place my hand in the hand of a nurse and say: "You are my father and mother." We considered the illness as predominantly schizophrenic, although there were some manic features.

This man was observed for a period of several weeks, during which time he would sit by himself laughing. At times he became noisy and uncontrollable. Early in July insulin coma therapy was begun. Phase I lasted some ten days. In August he had his first successful coma reaction with 120 units of insulin. The coma treatments were continued, each carried on for one hour. Towards the end of August he remarked: "These treatments are making me feel better. I believe I will be entirely well." He was given a series of some 50 I. C. T., and treatments were discontinued in the middle of September, at which time the patient was allowed to go home. From 1940 until 1946 he has remained relatively well. Early in 1947 he had a recurrence of mental symptoms in a milder form.

Conclusion

Schizophrenia has constituted a major problem for psychiatry. When we consider the youth of many of the patients at the onset of the illness, and, consequently, the many years of invalidism, when we consider the frequency of the disorder and, thus, the large number of schizophrenics confined in hospitals, we become aware of the magnitude of the problem.

Fortunately, we have made remarkable progress in the therapy of this disease, even though we do not know the cause. Of course, we realize that there are different types, some organic, others psychogenic, some chronic and more or less hopeless, others acute, with sufficient intact personality and emotion to be greatly influenced by psychiatric efforts. Electrocoma treatment has cleared the symptoms and brought about apparent recovery in many. Some, who failed to respond adequately to the electrical method, have been helped by a prolonged course of insulin coma. There are others who have failed to improve with either electrical or insulin coma therapy and who have continued to be disturbed, assaultive or negativistic. A certain percentage of such difficult cases have been restored to useful lives by the procedure of a lobotomy, which was introduced by Freeman and Watts. The severance of fibers from the thalamus to the frontal lobes removes aggressiveness and hostility and leaves the patient more calm and cheerful, even if, at times, duller than he was. With one or a succession of such positive methods along with occupational or psycho-therapy, it is possible to bring about a certain degree of recovery in many patients. There are many who recover completely. In my files are the case histories of a good number of characteristic schizophrenic patients, a few of whom have improved spontaneously and many of whom are better after some variety of coma therapy. Others are not entirely well but are able to adjust adequately to a life within their homes and in the community. They may require maintenance doses of shock therapy, but nevertheless, they are more or less useful citizens.

Unfortunately, there are those whose recovery is but slight and who return home only to lead restricted, protected lives.

Finally, there are unfortunate individuals whose symptoms are of such disturbing degree that their presence at home disrupts the household routine and even endangers the lives of those around them as well as themselves. Such persons must have more or less permanent institutional care. Even some of these very tragic chronic cases do occasionally show brief or prolonged periods of improvement.

My own personal experience permits me to close this chapter on a hopeful note. Of the many patients whom I have seen over the years diagnosed as schizophrenics, a considerable number have succeeded in making fairly good adjustments to life outside of hospitals, and some are apparently well.

REFERENCES

Bleuler, E.: *Textbook of Psychiatry*. Macmillan, New York, 1934.
Noyes, A. P.: *Modern Clinical Psychiatry*, 2nd edition. Saunders, Philadelphia, 1939.
Singer, H. D.: Psychosis and the Central Autonomic Nervous System. *J. A. M. A.*, 110:2048, 1938.
Schilder, P.: *Introduction to a Psychoanalytic Psychiatry*. Nervous and Mental Disease Publishing Co., New York, 1928.
Bond, E. D.: Continued Follow-up Results in Insulin-Shock Therapy and in Control Cases. *Am. J. Psychiat.*, 97:1024, 1941.
Kennedy, A.: Convulsion Therapy in Schizophrenia. *J. Ment. Sc.*, 83: 609, 1937.
Kalinowsky, L. B.: Electric Convulsive Therapy with Emphasis on Importance of Adequate Treatment. *Arch. Neurol. & Psychiat.*, 50: 652, 1943.
Kalinowsky, L. B., and Hoch, P. H.: *Shock Treatments and Other Somatic Procedures in Psychiatry*. Grune & Stratton, New York, 1946.
Sakel, M.: The Nature and Origin of the Hypoglycemic Treatment of Psychoses. *Am. J. Psychiat.*, 94 (Supp.):24, 1938.
Freeman, W., and Watts, J. W.: *Psychosurgery*. Thomas, Springfield, 1942.
Jelliffe, S. E., and White, W. A.: *Diseases of the Nervous System*. 6th edition. Lea & Febiger, Philadelphia, 1935.
Kraines, S. H.: *The Therapy of the Neuroses and Psychoses*. Lea & Febiger, Philadelphia, 1941.
Bond, E. D., and Shurley, J. T.: Insulin Therapy and Its Future. *Am. J. Psychiat.*, 103:338, 1946.
Storch, A.: *The Primitive Archaic Forms of Inner Experiences and Thought in Schizophrenia*. Nervous and Mental Disease Monograph No. 36, 1924.
Vigotsky, L. S.: Thought in Schizophrenia. *Arch. Neurol. & Psychiat.*, 31:1063, 1934.
Sakel, M.: Neue Behandlung der Morphinsucht. *Ztschr. f. d. ges. Neurol. u. Psychiat.*, 143:506, 1933.
Jessner, L., and Ryan, V. G.: *Shock Treatment in Psychiatry*. Grune & Stratton, New York, 1941.
Cleckley, H., and Templeton, C. M.: Prolonged Coma in Insulin Therapy of the Psychoses. *Am. J. Psychiat.*, 97:844, 1941.
Freudenberg, R.: The Use of Vitamin B and Preparations of Suprarenal Cortex in Insulin Shock Therapy. *Am. J. Psychiat.*, 94 (Supp.): 317, 1938.
Muller, M.: The Insulin Therapy of Schizophrenia. *Am. J. Psychiat.*, 94(Supp.):5, 1938.
Ross, J. R., and Malzberg, B.: A Review of the Results of the Pharmacological Shock Therapy and the Metrazol Convulsive Therapy in New York State. *Am. J. Psychiat.*, 96:297, 1939.

Chapter VI

ELECTROCOMA THERAPY OF PSYCHOSES

Introduction
by
Foster Kennedy, M.D.

THERE is in the following pages a concise yet detailed account of present experience in our use of the electric current, fully controlled in dose and in time, for the amelioration and, most usually, cure of many abnormal mental states; and my experience since early 1941 has been in complete consonance with that of the author.

Such abnormal mental states, now cured in a few weeks' treatment, as lately as a dozen years ago placed patients in mental hospitals for many years and maybe for a lifetime. Many delusional melancholias occurring after childbirth have been cured by this method which often never recovered in former days. I have had many patients whom I cared for by the old methods whose agony of spirit, twenty or more years ago, lasted three and five years; they have each had an identical attack occurring in the past seven or eight years, cured in three or five weeks.

This is an event of prime importance; as I've written elsewhere it shows that we stand today, in the treatment of "mental" illness where, in surgery, Lister stood when he made his first carbolic spray.

The miracle of these results has not been readily accepted despite the steady accumulation of favorable results; no such prejudiced resistance was seen to the introduction of sulpha drugs or penicillin. These were put quickly to use by doctors without cavil probably because we all have been by training accustomed to the idea of putting something beneficial into the body to kill in it something noxious. But this physical process was a new departure in almost another dimension of thinking. Such innovations are not quickly accepted by men especially if they seem to defeat all those men's previous philosophy of the origins of "mental" illness. These "origins" have always been thought to lie in environmental circumstances – "he went into a depression on losing money in Wall Street," "when he was jilted by his lady love," "when, most wrongly he entered into an unfortunate and irregular relationship with a married woman," "when he had been involved in that awful hotel fire where so many people were killed." These emotional strains were believed to unhinge the mind, though the stress of modern war gives rise to no more of the psychoses which fill our mental hospitals than would have occurred in the same number of civilians in peace time. The truth would seem to lie in this: that our emotional and mental health is determined by the inherited balance existing between the tide of energy in us which stimulates and the opposing tide of energy which retards. We doctors think too much of the pathology of fibre and too little of the pathology of forces. This balance is subject to the universal rule of rhythm – systole lives by diastole; Planck's Theory shows that even in the Cosmos, energy is sent forward in bursts and not in continuity. The regulating organ of our energies is apparently by hypothalamus. Structural disease of this organ has been shown to produce changes in the behavior of the total organism. The hypothalamus is not only our pacemaker of vegetative function but of emotional rhythm as well. We are all in the last analysis energy-organisms and an energy agent like to ourselves has been found capable of redressing the balance of the energic forces in us. As Sir John Mandeville, seven centuries ago, was wont to say, "And this too is a very great marvel."

The most important development since the remarkable introduction by Sakel of insulin shock treatment for schizophrenia is the use of the electrical method for the induction of a convulsive reaction. The electrical method has almost entirely replaced metrazol and insulin for depressions and is frequently used prior to or in place of insulin for schizophrenia. This preference for electrocoma therapy is based upon the relative safety and ease of administration. For this method I have proposed the term, electrocoma therapy, a term which conveys the idea of a drastic procedure (coma) induced by electricity, and yet one which is free from the disturbing connotations of the word, electroshock. The term, electroshock, unnecessarily and erroneously frightens patients who expect a painful electrical sensation, whereas no such sensations are experienced, since consciousness is lost instantaneously.

Other names such as electrofit, electroconvulsive, electrosleep are not as euphonious nor as accurate as the term, electrocoma.

Indications

Electrocoma therapy is almost a specific for psychoses featured by depression, is of value in lessening the intensity of the manic stage, can benefit schizophrenia, and is of temporary help in controlling the assaultive and combative patient. It is not a procedure of substantial value in psychoneuroses, except for those cases with marked depressive features. However, in some instances electrocoma therapy can make the neurotic patient more accessible to psychotherapy (Moriarty and Weil).

The depressive phase of manic-depressive psychosis responds favorably. It is amazing to see the mood altered from dejection to cheerfulness, insomnia give way to sound sleep, anxiety and distress replaced by calmness and well-being in the brief space of days or weeks. Several treatments tend to relieve self-accusation, eliminate ideas of hopelessness, and turn the patient's thoughts from introspection outward. As the course continues, there is usually further progress towards improved appetite, gain in weight, restored confidence.

At the end of the treatment schedule there may be unpleasant forgetfulness, yet the patient is now cheerful, his vigor has been restored, he has a sense of well-being. The treatment has operated in the direction of the recoverability inherent in the illness. But it has accelerated the recovery from a period of months and years to a matter of weeks; it has relieved the distress and suffering of the illness; it has reduced the incidence of suicide.

Such favorable outcome may occur in the old age group as well as in younger persons.

Mrs. S. M., a woman of 69, who had been depressed for 18 months, complained of many somatic difficulties. All physical examinations were negative except for moderate hypertension and arteriosclerosis. She had lost interest in her home and in the outside world. She accused herself of wrongdoing and begged to be taken to the police so that she would be arrested and punished. Gradually she lost appetite and energy and sank into a state of apathy. When I first saw this patient, she appeared sad, emaciated, pathetic. Her weight was down to 82 pounds. So sickly did she appear that one hesitated in advising drastic treatment.

Yet there was no alternative program. Electrocoma therapy was, therefore, begun.

After six treatments over a period of two weeks, Mrs. S. M. developed a good appetite so that she demanded extra portions at mealtime; she took an interest in fellow patients at the hospital. One week later she enjoyed visits from her family and worked skillfully in occupational therapy. At the end of one month Mrs. S. M. left the hospital improved, weighing 100 pounds! She has been seen on several occasions at my office, a sprightly, dynamic little woman, dressed smartly, and absorbed in her family, in world events. She is fully restored to health – her mood cheerful, her manner self-confident.

Similar results are common in many cases of involutional melancholia. Such patients have been going downhill for months. The symptoms include distressing somatic sensations such as burning in the head, incessant pains or emptiness in the abdomen, profound weakness. The patient is tormented by sleepless nights, suffers through days, praying for death as release.

The manic phase of manic-depressive psychosis does not yield as readily to electrocoma therapy as does the depressed phase. Nevertheless, electrocoma therapy can reduce manic overactivity, bring about sleep and calm. When used properly (Kalinowsky), electrocoma therapy can abbreviate the duration of a manic illness considerably

M. E. had become overactive, jumpy, sleepless. She talked on and on about sex, babies, children. She laughed gaily, planned programs, wanted to run and do – without reason or judgment. She exhibited marked evidence of manic behavior, speaking ceaselessly, spending extravagantly, and speeding carelessly. When her family tried to curb her overactivity, she became resentful and combative. After many sleepless nights, she was brought to the hospital. As she yelled all day and night and refused nourishment, we began a course of E.C.T. Two treatments were administered daily for three successive days. M. E. became calm and pleasant. Later, the manic features reappeared but were again checked by further treatments. She was given some 20 treatments in all. This patient made a good recovery and has remained well for the past 18 months.

Certain patients with schizophrenia also may respond well to this treatment. This applies more to the schizophrenias which appear in the late thirties and forties than to those of adolescence. It is more true of the schizophrenias loaded with affect, in those patients in whom depressed mood and schizophrenic ideas coexist, so-called schizo-depressions. On the other hand, the deviations which appear early in life, such as those referred to as dementia praecox simplex fail to respond to electrocoma, therapy. An example of a schizo-depression successfully treated comes to mind:

C. U. was a professional woman in the early forties who became tired, weak, and unable to do her work. Prior to this illness, she had been a cheerful, highly efficient administrator, well adjusted to life. In the course of weeks she became sleepless, lost appetite, and developed some menstrual irregularity. A gynecologic study showed some questionable enlargement of the uterus and thus a hysterectomy had been performed. During the convalescence patient continued to have nervous symptoms and she was sent to Florida. The rest and sunshine were of no avail and she was sent to relatives in Cleveland.

During the initial examination, the patient seemed tense, anxious, and was preoccupied by delusional experiences. "I cannot sleep at night; it seems as though my bed is being jiggled; I know I was being followed in Florida; there were many crooks around; they have been pursuing me; I don't think I can ever get well; I'm sure I have syphilis; my brain must be affected by this disease; I must have been raped."

Inasmuch as the symptoms had extended over a period of about a year without improvement, I decided upon a course of electrocoma therapy. Treatment was begun in July, 1941. Quite promptly she showed an improvement in mood. She became free of physical complaints and slept better. After some eight treatments, she no longer mentioned the subject of syphilis. After 10 treatments this woman stated voluntarily that she was feeling better; she turned her thoughts to reading and to the world around her. Some 14 treatments in all were given, and she was discharged from the hospital, cheerful and apparently free of symptoms.

For a period of weeks she complained about some soreness in the mouth, mentioning: "I am afraid I have contracted the hoof and mouth disease." Several additional treatments were then given.

I have had the opportunity of observing this patient over a period of 6 years. During this time she has maintained remarkable wellbeing and has achieved renown in her field of work.

Electrocoma therapy is of value, though only as a temporary measure, in most forms of schizophrenia in converting a belligerent excited patient who is disturbed, into a fairly agreeable and cooperative individual. This improvement may be merely temporary.

E.C.T. may be administered in psychoneurotic depressions, and in some psychoneuroses, to render the patient more susceptible to psychotherapy. However, it is of little or no use in obsessional neuroses. Nor is it advisable as the essential procedure in the usual case of psychoneurosis.

It is not a remedy for psychoses of organic type. However, certain patients who appear to have a senile psychosis of a progressive, hopeless type are brought to recovery by electrocoma. The explanation is this: A patient in the late sixties or early seventies becomes preoccupied by somatic or even paranoidal delusions. He shows striking loss of recent memory, a significant sign of organic disease. The patient has lost considerable weight and this adds to his senile appearance. Consequently he is thought to be a hopeless senile case.

This was the concept applied to J. W., a man of 65, when a psychiatrist certified him for State Hospital care. But the surface appearance concealed the reversible emotional nature of the illness. However, I was influenced by the profound evidence of depression – "I am a poor man, I will lose my home, my family won't have anything to eat." These statements were contrary to the actual situation. Furthermore, when J. W. did respond to certain questions, his fund of knowledge and his memory were not as deficient as they were reported to be. Consequently I deemed it advisable to proceed with a course of E.C.T. The result was excellent. The patient recovered. He resumed his position in a highly technical field and now, some two years later, is physically well and holding his job efficiently. He even appears younger, as do many patients after treatment.

Obviously electrocoma therapy is not a method for use in toxic psychosis, which can be quickly benefited by intravenous glucose, saline, insulin, and thiamin chloride (Strecker et al). Nor should it be used in other organic psychoses whose cause is known.

What are the contraindications to this mode of treatment? Theoretically, we consider physical disease such as cardiac disorders, marked hypertension, pulmonary lesions as contraindications. However, in the specific case one must weigh the potential risks of treatment against the hazards of the spontaneous course of the disease. Certainly it is prudent to withhold electrocoma therapy from a mild depression with a history of brief cycles in a patient who has serious valvular heart disease. Yet for the patient with a chronic and progressive melancholia, who is agitated, sleepless, and suicidal, who is wearing himself out pacing the floor, striking himself, treatment is advisable even in the face of known organic disease. One must ask the question – Which is harder on the bodily economy – Which is a bigger strain upon physiological processes, a series of brief convulsive reactions each lasting one minute, or seemingly endless days and nights of restless torment? Usually the answer is in favor of treatment – and the improvement is often astounding. Over a period of years I have yet to regret active treatment and have been sorry that I declined to treat certain patients. The following two examples furnish two different experiences which lead to one answer.

A woman in the middle fifties had coronary disease and had undergone an operation for this by Dr. Claude Beck. She had improved from this procedure and was reasonably well until she developed involutional melancholia. She was treated for months – without avail. She was exhausting herself and her attendants because of her agitation and sleeplessness. She was getting worse when it was decided, with the approval of Dr. Claude Beck and Dr. Harold Feil, to try electrocoma therapy. Seven treatments brought about a recovery. This patient has remained well for six years.

In contrast to this successful result is the case of a male patient who had had an attack of coronary disease three years prior to the depressive illness. Because of this history and some changes in the electrocardiogram, we hesitated to employ electrocoma therapy. This patient attempted suicide. He survived, but acquired an incurable encephalopathy from inhaling exhaust gas.

General Aspects of Treatment

APPARATUS

Electrocoma treatment can be given by a high frequency apparatus, of which several commercial types are available. These vary as to the particular features of dosage and minor differences in delivering the current. In most machines an alternating current of some 500 m.a., 100 - 120 volts is administered for the brief period of 0.3 to 0.7 of a second. Two electrodes are applied to the head of the patient. The conventional places were the forehead, between the angle of the eye and the ear. Now we apply one electrode over the center of the vertex and the other over the brow. Among the commercial makes available such as the Offner, the Rahm, the Lektra, the actual differences are slight so that an experienced psychiatrist can use any machine. My own preference is for the Offner apparatus whose accuracy and reliability over a period of years has in my experience proved safe and dependable.

Recently there has appeared the Reiter-Wilcox-Friedman apparatus which uses a unidirectional current. The proponents of this apparatus assert that much less current is needed to produce the desired reaction than with the previously conventional alternating current. We have employed the Reiter-Wilcox-Friedman and can corroborate this statement. As a rule, patients awaken more quickly and exhibit less memory clouding than when the sinusoidal current is used. With this apparatus we apply one electrode over the motor area of the scalp and the other in the usual position over the brow, above the angle of the eye.

Another modification has been introduced by Liberson, and has been used also by Goldman. In our experience with this method, the Brief Stimulus Technique, it is our impression that it constitutes an improvement. Although the current is allowed to run for one or more seconds, it is interrupted and becomes pulsating so that the actual milliamperage is much smaller than in the conventional method.

One may state that, though the principle of electrocoma therapy has remained quite standard, the technical phase, especially in the matter of apparatus and application, has undergone modification. The actual make of apparatus is not of vital significance, nor the specific requirement as to whether the amperage, voltage, or time should be changed – as certain manufacturers argue. *What is of vital importance is an adequate reaction in each treatment and a complete course. Expressed differently, it is not only the machine but the man who operates it that is important.* Merely because one possesses a violin and a bow does not guarantee beautiful music. Merely possessing an electroshock machine does not assure results. There is needed an experienced psychiatrist who knows his patient, the dosage and course of the illness – and how best to employ electrocoma therapy along with psychotherapy.

Dosage

Kalinowsky emphasized the importance of an adequate course of treatment. This means a major (coma and convulsive) reaction whenever the treatment is administered. The amount of current necessary is smaller in younger patients and greater in the older group. The factors of time, voltage, amperage vary with age and with the type of apparatus. Experienced psychiatrists have long avoided minor (petit mal) reactions as undesirable. Some consider them worthless, others actually harmful. Thus, if the initial current used in any session produces a minor response, then the dosage must be increased to a substantial degree so that a major reaction is obtained. For example, if a current of 0.3. of a second, with 500 m.a. produces a minor response, then increase to 0.5 of a second, or raise the voltage substantially. A slight stepup of 50 m.a. usually results in another failure. The experienced therapist does not hesitate to step the dosage up at the one session so that a full reaction takes place. Furthermore, it is good policy to increase the current at the following session, even if a successful major reaction has been obtained, when there has been a delay of five to fifty seconds between application of the current and the onset of the convulsion. Use a sufficient dose to obtain a prompt major reaction. Kalinowsky promptly sends a larger current if the initial dose fails to produce an immediate convulsion.

Time Factors

It has been the custom to administer treatments every other day, usually in the morning. Though this time interval is usually satisfactory, it is advisable to adjust the frequency of treatment to the requirements of the individual case. For instance, older patients who show an early improvement in mood but exhibit clouding of memory should then receive treatments twice weekly or at less frequent intervals. On the other hand, patients who are markedly disturbed, especially manics, require more frequent treatments. It is my practice to administer two treatments, "double header," in the same session, as the initial dose. One treatment follows the other by a brief time interval of ten to thirty minutes. Then single or "double header" treatments are given daily for several days until the patient becomes calm. As a rule, a series of some six treatments, closely spaced over a period of several days, is sufficient to bring about an improvement. Then the customary every other day schedule is followed.

COURSE OF TREATMENT

Recovery rather than any stated number of treatments is the goal of the therapist. Thus, I do not follow any fixed rule of a specific number, nor is the desired procedure a certain minimum or a state of confusion. It is my practice to give a steady series of treatments, which averages six to twelve for depressed patients and twenty or more for schizophrenics. The number of treatments for depressions is less for those patients who show prompt and lasting improvement early. When the patient reports himself better, I give one or two additional treatments as reinforcement. Then I omit a treatment and wait until the next session. If the condition remains satisfactory or improves during several days' vacation, then no treatment is given. Close observation is continued so that any downward change may be detected early and treatment promptly resumed. For patients whose response is slow or who relapse, I do not hesitate to give fifteen, twenty, or more treatments.

The number of convulsions to be used in a schizophrenic patient is greater—a minimum of twenty. Although I had good recoveries some five years ago when I employed ten to twenty electrocoma reactions, I now follow the suggestion of Neymann and of Kalinowsky and employ a minimum of twenty in the initial series. One is apt to obtain a more sustained improvement when using this number than if one stops at the initial improvement.

For psychoneuroses in whom electrocoma therapy is used to render the patient more amenable to psychotherapy, we employ a small number, say three to six, and follow these treatments with sessions of psychotherapy.

MAINTENANCE TREATMENTS

In many cases one compact series will not bring lasting improvement unless it is followed by occasional subsequent treatments. Indeed, such treatments, given once a week or once a month—a so-called maintenance dose—may prevent relapse and help to increase the favorable results.

Mrs. D. C. had been severely depressed. She was hospitalized and given some ten electrocoma treatments with a favorable result. Yet, about two months later she became depressed again. Three treatments were administered and resulted in a marked change for the better. Weeks later there was another recurrence of moderate apathy. At this stage two treatments were given over a period of a week, with significant recovery. Several months later the condition slipped backwards – and required two treatments. Now it is a year or more since the last session and Mrs. D. C. remains cheerful, industrious, and apparently well.

I recall a hypomanic patient who improved with a series of some thirty electrocoma treatments in the hospital. She improved sufficiently to return home. Then she became overactive, but was given two or three treatments during a period of several days. Such a brief series was readministered several times in six months. Two years have elapsed since the last series and this patient remained well.

A professional man continued to exhibit occasional depressed phases following a prolonged severe depression, successfully treated by electrocoma treatment. This patient became sleepless, doubted himself, avoided people, and sat around sighing. He was given one treatment and then another several days later. These maintenance doses were repeated again and again for several months until they were no longer necessary.

As regards the length of treatment and number, I have gone up to 75 treatments without any harm, indeed with improvement. This number is brief compared to the long series of about 248 successfully employed in a patient in a California State Hospital (Perlson). The author reported that the patient had finally made a recovery from a severe schizophrenia. Intelligence tests show a fairly normal mental status.

The Practical Administration of Treatment—Specific Steps

PREPARATION

No special preparation is needed other than some explanation to the family and to the patient. These will be presented in the section on handling the family. Just before the treatment the patient is urged to void, so that the tendency to involuntary urination be minimized. Then all dentures are removed. The patient is undressed, except for underwear for men and under garments and slips for women.

As to the matter of food before treatment, it had been the custom to omit breakfast. In certain hospitals some patients are not treated until 10 or 11 a.m. They are often parched, hungry, and uncomfortable. Consequently, I tried giving some food in the morning. Our patients were more comfortable and no ill effects have been encountered. We allow fruit juice, coffee or milk up to an hour before treatment time.

MEDICATION

(1) It is our custom to use sodium amytal, gr. $3\frac{3}{4}$ to gr. $7\frac{1}{2}$, intravenously for all patients who are tense, worried, and apprehensive. Such an injection is safe, it lessens the anxiety, and also serves to make the awakening period more natural. Patients who have received amytal return to wakefulness more gradually and with less bewilderment.

(2) Intocostrin—We employ intocostrin in short, stocky patients and in any patients who complain of pain in the back. Our customary initial dose is about two cc. as a test of sensitivity, and an increase in subsequent treatments to three and four cc. as needed, depending upon the weight of the patient and the reaction. As has been established by Bennett, the intocostrin should be injected slowly, forty to sixty seconds I.V. Bennett uses a larger amount, but we have found the smaller dose to be safe and quite effective. Though it does not seem to alter the convulsion, apparently it lessens the violence of the first muscular contractions and of the clonic movements sufficiently to reduce the likelihood of trauma. Yet its potential danger requires caution.

(3) Coramine—two cc. of coramine I.M. are used some eight minutes before treatment in those patients who have shown marked apnea and cyanosis in the previous reaction. It is even more effective given I.V. directly before the current is passed.

THE TREATMENT

The patient is placed upon a firm table, thinly covered by a blanket. A bed whose springs are covered by a board to reduce "springiness" and bed "bounce" has been found equally useful. A folded sheet or small sandbag is placed under the back at the level of the shoulder blades so as to hyperextend the spine. There is a tendency to neglect the proper position of this sandbag—since patients feel more comfortable when it is placed under the small of the back. So I caution the attendants to place the bag in such a position as to throw the chest out—"to make Bali Girls not Hottentots."

One attendant then protects the mouth, using a soft mouth gag placed between the under surface of the tongue and the lingual aspect of the lower teeth. The left hand holds this gag in position while the right hand everts the lower lip and also exerts upward pressure on the chin. The type of gag used must be changed to accommodate the dental condition. If only several incisor teeth are present or these are loose, a folded handkerchief shaped like a "U" can be fitted around the teeth in such a way that this kerchief receives the impact of the jaw compression and removes any pressure from the teeth themselves.

Another attendant holds the shoulders towards the table and the arms to the sides. I instruct this attendant to rest the balls of his thumbs on the chest of the patient and to place his fanned fingers in such a way that the thumb rests on the center of the clavicle and the little finger on the insertion of the deltoid. This provides maximum protection with minimum direct pressure on any one spot.

A second attendant holds the hands of the patient and exerts mild pressure on the pelvis and thighs. Except for some firmness at the beginning of the treatment, the attendants are cautioned not to use great force, but to allow free play of muscles during the clonic phase of the convulsion.

A minor item which I have used for some six years is the slogan, "One, two, three—pleasant dreams!" This is my signal that I will press the button and for the staff to be ready. Patients have often commented that the last words they recalled were "Pleasant dreams."

After the convulsion is over, the patient is carefully watched until his respiration and color return to normal. Many patients begin to breathe promptly, and soon the pallor or cyanosis which had developed during the convulsion gradually gives way to a normal pink. However, some patients remain apneic and dusky in color for a minute or more. For such patients we assist a return of respiration by artificial chest compression and by upward pressure of the tongue at the angle of the jaw. If there be considerable bubbly mucus in the throat, the patient should be turned on his side or face. In the event intocostrin has been used, we have available one cc. prostigmin in a syringe, a tongue forceps, and an airway. These are used if there be obstruction to breathing or paralysis of the respiratory muscles. Indeed, the treatment team is drilled to act promptly and automatically in any such eventuality: One attendant starts artificial respiration immediately, another holds the airway which the physician has inserted, while the doctor himself gives prostigmin intravenously. Thus far our experience has been favorable and, though we met some unpleasant reactions, we have not encountered any disasters.

Post-Treatment Care

When the color of the patient is improved, he may be placed back into his own bed, watched by an attendant. Some patients remain quiet and deeply asleep for many minutes. Others thrash around in bewildered confusion, twisting, groaning, unresponsive. These should be guarded and kept from falling out of bed. It is prudent to allow such patients to turn about and seek a comfortable position, without offering restraint. For restraint may provoke more resistance. However, protective guardianship is necessary.

Most patients emerge gradually from the unconsciousness to an awareness of the world around them. At first they are hazy and fail to recognize their surroundings and may fall asleep again. Later, they identify the place and people but ask: "Did I get a treatment yet?" Within some 15 minutes the average patient is fully awake and well oriented. However, there is a blotting out of memory for the treatment itself – the patient does not know, yes even denies, that he had a treatment.

A few patients are nauseated, some complain of headache, others call attention to muscle soreness. As a rule, the patient feels quite well, asks for food and wants to be active again. Many patients return to their usual state for the remainder of the day.

During the short period of recovery from the stage of coma, little care is required except for watching. We give aspirin, five to ten gr., to those who complain of headache. We allow patients to get up and have the remainder of their breakfast as soon as they ask for it.

After the patient is fully awake and has had food, he is permitted to do as much as he is able and cares to do. Some feel tired and prefer to rest, the majority feel comfortable and are eager to resume activity. In the hospital they participate in occupational therapy and outdoor sports or in visiting and playing cards. On the following day they carry on their customary routine.

Ambulatory Electrocoma Therapy

Although electrocoma therapy was originally administered to bed patients in hospitals, experience has amply demonstrated its feasibility as an ambulatory method. Myerson, Wender et al., Patry, Fetterman have reported on its successful administration in outpatient departments, in clinics and well staffed offices.

The advantages of the ambulatory method are
(1) Economy.
(2) Saving prestige.
(3) Sparing hospital beds.
(4) More normal activity between treatments.
(5) Ease of administering maintenance doses at subsequent intervals when necessary.

The disadvantages of the ambulatory method are
(1) Added responsibility on the part of the family.
(2) Some difficulty in completing a long course.
(3) Hazard of suicide.

The advantages are so important that I would recommend the ambulatory procedure if it is feasible. This means adequate facilities for the handling of the patient and the proper selection of cases.

To provide adequate facilities means sufficient room, fairly isolated for the treatment proper, and space for rest and recovery. Many hospitals can provide such room in their outpatient departments. Most clinics do have such facilities and some doctors' offices are spacious enough to meet these needs. The next requirement is adequate personnel. The minimum would be the psychiatrist himself, one trained nurse, one or more attendants. Additional staff are of help in the event of any problem patient or any emergency. Likewise, the size of the staff is determined by the number of patients to be treated. *Of course, experience with treatment is even more important than number. I would advise any psychiatrist who wants to use this method successfully to train with one who is thoroughly familiar with the apparatus, the pretreatment medication, the dosage, the timing. Merely procuring the apparatus and an instruction sheet is inadequate preparation in the use of a method whose potential for good is so great. Properly administered, electrocoma therapy can contribute tremendously towards recovery. Electrocoma therapy used in a haphazard fashion, minor reactions, incomplete series of treatments, neglect of after care will lead to a higher percentage of failures than need be.*

To reduce the disadvantages of ambulatory electrocoma therapy, a careful selection of patients is necessary. Those who are strongly suspicious, who are combative, who refuse food, who are obviously suicidal are better off in hospitals. Depressions are more easily handled by the ambulatory method than schizophrenias – yet I have treated many schizophrenics successfully as ambulatory patients.

Equally significant in selection is *the family*. They must be understanding of the patient's symptoms and be both sympathetic and firm. They are required to provide companionship and safeguards. Hence, they should be intelligent and positive enough to provide persuasion and muscle power, if need be. Success depends upon a complete treatment course. Some patients are apprehensive and displace their fears upon the treatment. It is common to hear patients who previously feared cancer and heart attacks forget these ideas and express apprehension of the treatment. The family must be able to convince the patient and to bring him for the next appointment.

It is necessary that the family possess the understanding and the capacity to face problems such as the safety of the patient. The neglect of suicidal precautions because of lack of understanding may be dangerous. In one instance, a wife failed to watch her husband and he took his life. To reduce this danger we instruct the family to remove from reach guns, poisons, the automobile key, and to provide constant vigilance for the potential suicide case. Fortunately, the first treatments tend to reduce the impulse to suicide.

The usual family, who have lived and suffered with the patient, are eager to provide the care and attendance which are necessary. Indeed, they have expressed gratitude for the opportunity of doing something actively. We have less difficulty with families of those collaborating in electrocoma therapy than with those who sit passively and anxiously at home while the patient is in the hospital.

It was my earlier impression that, with proper selection, fifty per cent of those needing electrocoma therapy could be handled in an ambulatory way. As we have gained wider experience, I find that over seventy per cent of patients can be thus handled.

Handling of the Family

To obtain the best cooperation for the patient, it is my custom to outline to the family exactly what the nature of the treatment is and what to expect. The drastic nature of the treatment is mentioned, the potential danger pointed out. However, the hope and benefit and actual safety of the method are also stated. Then we obtain the written authorization of the family for the treatment. Though this may no longer be necessary, since electrocoma therapy is now an approved and accepted procedure, it has the value of assuring assumption of responsibility, both moral and economic, by someone other than the mentally ill person.

In addition to the personal discussion with the family, I supply them with a mimeographed sheet of explanation. This tends to comfort the family of a patient sent to a hospital. Such is the fear of mental hospitals, magnified by age-old pictures of cruelty and neglect, that a written explanation serves to relieve the family. Furthermore, it anticipates some of their questions and saves their uneasiness and many harassing telephone calls. The first instruction sheet is the one which I supply to the family of a patient sent to a mental hospital and the second is that furnished for ambulatory E.C.T.

INSTRUCTIONS TO THE FAMILY OF A PATIENT GOING TO
........HOSPITAL

An appointment has been made for a member of your family to enter.. ......Hospital. Attached is a folder from the hospital giving you directions about visiting hours, etc. Please try to bring the patient to the hospital from 9:00 to 11:00 a.m. or 1:00 to 3:00 p.m., as these hours are most suitable for the admission of new patients.

At the time of the entrance of a member of your family to the hospital, you will be expected to sign certain forms. Rest assured that the hospital will take care of the patient in the best way possible and that the forms which you sign are your guarantees of cooperation.

The hospital has several divisions, from an isolation ward for very disturbed people to an open ward which is as free as any country club. The patient is placed in that ward which is required by his condition and will be moved if there is any change. Improved patients, as you see, are permitted to be outdoors, to go to occupational therapy with perfect freedom. Those who are very sick are confined so that they can be kept under more careful study and observation.

Visiting should be a source of comfort to you and reassurance to the patient. As a rule, it is advisable for you not to visit for at least a week until he gets settled, unless you are instructed otherwise. These sick, nervous patients ask that you take them home. Should you carry out their wish, you have undone what you and the doctors have planned for quite a while. If you refuse, it makes you and the patient feel badly.

When you visit a member of your family in the sick wards, you may notice that other patients are nervous and perhaps even carrying on by gestures or speech. Such activity is not contagious. Do not fear that the ideas expressed by one patient will hurt or contaminate the thinking of another. No doubt the member of your family was put in the hospital because of sickness in thinking or feeling and acting. The treatments which will be given as a rule will help a great deal towards his recovery. It is this hope which you must have in mind and not the fear that the hospital atmosphere is harmful.

Some patients will receive electrocoma therapy. These treatments are very beneficial for those patients who require them. However, the treatments produce a clouding of memory so that for a period of time there may be forgetfulness. Fortunately, when the treatments are completed, the memory returns in a matter of several weeks.

It is suggested that you come in to see the doctor at intervals of once a week or less often, if the condition is getting along satisfactorily, for a personal discussion of the progress.

A similar sheet of instructions is given to the family of a patient who is to receive ambulatory electrocoma therapy. It anticipates their questions and provides directions which they can follow. Since I have employed this instruction sheet, the family reassures the patient when he expresses fear of memory loss, and has a better approach to the problem.

INSTRUCTIONS TO FAMILIES OF PATIENTS RECEIVING AMBULATORY ELECTROCOMA THERAPY

A member of your family is to be given a course of treatment at the......... Hospital. This treatment is usually successful in bringing about improvement or recovery from his nervous symptoms. Your cooperation will prove helpful towards his recovery. The following instructions may assist you in providing the best possible help:

1. *Appointments:* The patient is to report on the mornings of Tuesday, Thursday, and Saturday at 9:00, 9:30, or 10:00 a.m., as will be designated by the doctor.

2. *Attendants:* A member of the family is to accompany the patient, stay until the treatment has been completed, and then escort the patient home. This member of the family is to act as bedside companion during the period of awakening from the deep-sleep state.

3. *Care to be Given:* The patient may have a small breakfast, such as fruit juice and a cup of coffee before 8:00 a.m. on the morning of treatment. At the bedside, the patient is to be watched until he is fully awake. Then he may be permitted to dress and return home. Most patients are comfortable and need no special care afterwards. A few are troubled by headache, muscle soreness, or drowsiness. They may rest as desired, take aspirin, five to ten grains, as needed. Those who feel well and are eager to be occupied, may help around the house, take walks, and do as much of their accustomed work as they desire.

4. *Memory Defects:* Many patients develop a clouding of the memory during the course of treatments. They may forget having the treatment, but this clears of itself a few weeks after the treatments have been completed.

5. *Necessary Supervision:* Some patients, who are nervous and very depressed, are troubled by morbid and self-destructive thoughts. As a rule, a few treatments relieve such thoughts and the danger is reduced. Nevertheless, if, during the patient's illness, he is obsessed by such unhappy thoughts, *it is imperative*

that he be closely observed. Any articles that may invite tragic action, such as drugs, should not be available.

6. *Explanations and Attitude Towards the Patient:* The patient who is ill enough to receive a course of treatment is usually in need of companionship and encouragement. He may be depressed, worrisome, and fearful. One should not make light of his distress, but give as much hope as possible. Sometimes patients doubt the value of the treatments, or may feel temporarily improved. As a consequence, the patient may refuse to continue with his treatment program. It is important to insist by persuasion or strong urging that he continue his course of treatment as advised by the physician. I explain in advance to responsible members of every family that patients frequently develop opposition to therapy. For example, one will object that he is not a bit better after several treatments, a second has developed intense fears, a third feels distinctly improved. Thus, for one reason or another, the patient is reluctant to return. It is made clear that we must go forward until the goal is reached. Columbus would not have discovered America had he turned back too early. Success depends upon a complete treatment program.

Results of Electrocoma Treatment

The immediate results of electrocoma treatment are usually excellent. Such treatment tends to relieve anxiety and tension, allays fears and introspection, and permits interest in external affairs. Patients sleep better, eat with improved appetite, and become more cheerful. It is a common experience to see patients, even schizophrenics, improve strikingly after one to several treatments. What is even more significant is the calming effect upon manic patients who had been pacing, tearing, shrieking. After several "double header" treatments administered daily, the patient becomes quiet, sleeps longer, and cooperates better.

The question often arises as to how soon a patient shows evidence of improvement. The answer is that patients vary in all phases of recovery as they do in symptoms. As a rule, in the successful case, the patient will show a prompt response to the initial treatment or two, and then steady progress from session to session until complete well-being is attained. In other instances, there are fluctuations, ups and downs on the road towards good health. Then again, there are instances in which no significant alteration is achieved during six or eight or even ten treatments. Then, quite abruptly, there is a striking change for the better, which may be lasting. Thus the speed and course of recovery are individual matters.

Some eighty to ninety per cent of depressed patients show a recovery sufficient to return to normal living or usual activity. Some depressed patients remain completely and permanently well. I have made follow-up studies of patients whom I treated in 1941 and 1942. Many have remained well throughout this period of time, despite the vicissitudes of war and the mishaps in their families.

Some, however, have shown early relapses which can frequently be corrected by several followup or maintenance treatments. Thus, if a patient shows a regression weeks or months following an apparent recovery, he is given one to several treatments in a week. Then he is seen at frequent intervals and, if he fails to remain well additional treatments are administered. They are usually successful in raising the percentage and permanence of recovery. This merely signifies that an effective course is not limited to a compact series, but must be followed by occasional or maintenance doses over a period of weeks or months, so that the patient remains well. One patient may require but one or two such treatments; another may need six or eight at intervals of two per month. Then there has been one patient who has returned for additional treatment at irregular times over a period of a year. As a rule, such after-care was not necessary.

Aside from the early relapses which represent insufficient treatment, there are patients who recover fully for the particular attack. But their illness is cyclic and they develop recurrences at intervals of every year, or every two or three years.

> For instance, Mrs. E. O. gave a history of depressions lasting some four months, occurring at intervals of one to two years. I treated her in 1941 with four electrocoma reactions. She got well and remained well until 1943. Then she took sick again and was treated by Dr. Foster Kennedy of New York. Once more she made a prompt recovery. But in 1945 the cycle recurred and a third attack developed. Again electrocoma therapy was promptly effective.

In such cases the patient and the family are aware of the recurring nature of the malady and they have been told that electrocoma therapy does not alter the tendency to recurring cycles. Yet, each depression (or manic attack) can be promptly met and abbreviated with a course of electrocoma therapy.

Treatment may consist of one compact course only, it may require one course followed by supplementary maintenance doses, or repeated series are made necessary by later cycles of depression. There is a high percentage of satisfactory results in depressed patients and those with involutional melancholia, especially when the treatment program is adequate. When compared with the therapy of preshock days, one may state that suicides have become rare in treated cases, suffering reduced, recovery accelerated in a substantial number of cases.

Furthermore, manic states following recovery from depressions are rare – even though brief periods of elation occur commonly.

The depressions which occur with psychoneurosis also respond favorably to E.C.T. However, the improvement is temporary and largely a mood change and not a basic alteration. Hence, supplementary psychotherapy is in order.

The manic phase of manic-depressive psychosis is considerably benefited by E.C.T. Yet, the course is longer than with depressions and maintenance doses are often needed for follow-up therapy.

A substantial percentage of early schizophrenics do improve, though the lasting results have not been so common. The malignant nature of schizophrenia in many instances is responsible for initial failure, or recurrence of symptoms even after some initial improvement. Yet we do encounter recoveries which endure. My five-year follow-up study has shown that a considerable number of patients whose diagnosis was schizophrenia have remained well. Several examples are included in the section on illustrative case histories. In these recovered cases one may ask whether the diagnosis was correct. Bennett of course asserts that improvement generally means an affective disorder. Nevertheless, there are patients, especially in the third, fourth, and fifth decades, whose symptoms are clearly schizophrenic and who respond favorably to treatment. Of course, neither E.C.T. nor insulin contributes a lasting recovery to any substantial number of the chronic hebephrenic and simplex types of schizophrenia.

The remarkable and lasting recoveries in cases of involutional melancholia are outstanding. For this is an illness in which there is intense and prolonged suffering. Few diseases produced such anguish as the somatic distress and the mental torment of this malady. The disease tended to continue onwards; spontaneous recoveries were not the rule, suicide was common. Electrocoma therapy frequently brings prompt improvement in many cases and lasting recovery in a high percentage.

For example, C. O. was a professional man in the late sixties who developed the self-accusatory idea of sin. He could not sleep, refused all food, paced and groaned. He felt hopeless and prayed for death. His symptoms had progressed downward for eight months, at which time he was gaunt, agitated, seemingly hopeless. I saw this man in April, 1941, and administered ten treatments. He recovered and has remained entirely well up to the present.

Few therapies can approach the speed and safety and success of electrocoma therapy in a disease which was formerly so difficult to treat.

Complications

The remarkable improvement achieved by electrocoma therapy is attained at the risk of certain complications. Fortunately, these are not as serious as was first believed and they can be minimized in some instances by proper techniques. Furthermore, the complications represent hazards which are unavoidable in specific instances and must be accepted because of the hoped-for benefit in serious situations. The complications are (1) clouding of memory, (2) traumatic effects such as fractures, muscle injuries, (3) toxic mental reactions, (4) the possibility of permanent mental damage (unlikely), (5) the possibility of death (very rare indeed).

Memory Disturbance

Memory disturbances are common during the course of treatment. Practically all patients have no recollection of the incidents related to the treatment proper and awaken bewildered, wondering how they got where they are. As the course proceeds, forgetfulness for events that preceded the beginning of therapy sets in. Patients are unable to recall people they saw and experiences they had for hours, days, or even weeks before. They may become forgetful of incidents which take place between treatments. This amnesia is slight in most patients, so that they are little disturbed by it. In others, especially when the number of treatments is high, the loss of memory is so profound that the patient and the family become greatly concerned. This clouding grows worse as treatment progresses, so that many therapists discontinue treatments or space them farther apart.

As a rule, memory returns when the treatments are discontinued. Indeed, within one to three weeks most patients can recollect many past events and certainly recall recent experiences well. In a few cases, patients have forgotten events and capacities which they had acquired over the years. For example, one woman had difficulty in remembering cooking recipes for weeks after a successful course of therapy. The great majority of patients may fail to recall the situation just at the beginning of treatment, and thus may not realize when they get well how sick they had been. Yet they soon become alert and re-acquire the capacity for recent memory very well.

Thus, my patients have been able to go back to their original activities and perform efficiently. For example, a trained nurse who had been sick for one year was given a series of 14 major reactions. She seemed dull and confused, but her spirits were elevated. She resumed her work, attended classes, and did creative writing a year after her recovery. A man, editor of a magazine, received 15 major reactions until he recovered. He proudly stated that his memory was not affected adversely. On the contrary, he asserted that his memory was improved. This may have been actually so, because his depression had been so deep, that all attention was feeble and recall impoverished. As the treatment made him more alert he could pay attention, and thus was able to remember better. At any rate upon the completion of the treatment program, he took a brief vacation and then resumed work. He reported his usual ability as a writer and was able to utilize a fund of past information.

So, too, a lawyer won a major suit involving intricate details of a technical nature several weeks after a course of six treatments. An export merchant was capable of resuming a business enterprise, global in extent, in less than two months after a course of ten treatments.

The function of recent memory is soon regained. The earlier fears of permanent loss of intellectual resources have been swept away by the experience of years. I do not recall any patient who lost mental qualities or abilities that he possessed prior to the treatment.

Furthermore, the newer techniques and apparatus (Reiter-Wilcox-Friedman, and the Brief Stimulus Therapy) tend to spare patients memory loss to a considerable degree. Such methods employ less current, and consequently produce less clouding of consciousness. For example, a physician had received seven treatments using the conventional method. He obtained relief but moderate clouding of memory. He resumed practice and was well for three years. Then he developed a recurrence which required another and longer course of electrocoma therapy. On this occasion he was given 15 treatments with the R-W-F apparatus, employing the motor application. Despite the longer series of treatments, he volunteered the statement that his memory was less blotted.

Such memory disturbance is accompanied by physiologic evidence of a change in cortical function, an alteration in brain waves which corresponds with the number of treatments. Such changes of brain waves tend to return to normal in several weeks or months.

TRAUMATIC COMPLICATIONS: FRACTURES, MUSCLE INJURIES

The convulsion which accompanies the coma reaction is usually of about forty seconds' duration. It begins with a violent extensor reaction followed by strong clonic thrusts of all extremities. So powerful are these contractions that muscle strain and even fractures may occur. Following the treatment patients frequently mention pain in the back and soreness in the jaws, arms, and legs. In some instances, certainly less than five per cent, compression fractures of the spine may occur. These are localized to the bodies of the midthoracic vertebrae and appear as moderate narrowing of the anterior margins. Such compression fractures may be single or multiple. They are attended by pain in the back which radiates girdle-like towards the chest and abdomen. The pain is accentuated by turning in bed and by coughing and straining. As a rule, the discomfort lasts some weeks and clears up without deformity or disability. I have never observed any signs of spinal cord compression. Nor have I seen disabling deformities, even in cases treated by metrazol some six to eight years ago—patients in whom fractures were more common.

In rare instances fractures of other bones may occur. The literature mentions fracture of the femur and fracture of the humerus. I had one patient who sustained a bilateral fracture of the mandible.

These fracture complications are more likely to occur in stocky, younger males while the aged, feeble patients fortunately are spared. Perhaps the natural weakness of muscles in older persons, further enfeebled by weight loss, explains the rarity of fractures in such persons.

Such complications can be minimized, if not almost entirely prevented by the proper control of the patient and by the use of intocostrin (Bennett). Support to the jaw, hyperextension of the spine, and moderate holding of the extremities reduce the possibility of fractures. Then the additional use of intocostrin intravenously, $2 - 2\frac{1}{2}$ minutes before passage of the current, will soften the convulsion considerably. We employ two to four cc. of intocostrin – and, though this small dose does not eliminate the convulsive movements, it tends to lessen the severity sufficiently to save muscle pain. We start with a cautious dose, say $2 - 2\frac{1}{2}$ cc., and then increase with subsequent treatments as needed.

Utilizing the above precautions, we may state that traumatic complications are infrequent, and seldom, if ever, of a serious nature. Particularly when we compare the serious nature of the illness which we treat with the relative mildness of the potential traumatic complications, it is apparent that the odds are in favor of treatment.

Acute Toxic Delirious States

Among the complications which are sometimes encountered is an acute confusional reaction. This state develops in some three to five per cent of patients some time after the sixth treatment, as a delirious-like reaction. The patient, who had been improving with electrocoma therapy and was calm, cheerful, and grateful, quite abruptly becomes frightened and suspicious. One patient shrieked when the doctor approached her, fearing some hostile act, even though she had been friendly towards him on the previous day. She remained sleepless, sensitive to sounds and sights, suspicious and frightened for three days. Spontaneously and gradually she became calm and cooperative. Then she reached a stage of recovery, both from the original depression and from the confusional episode.

Another patient, also a woman, had been ill with a psychoneurotic depression of some two years' duration. Electrocoma therapy was instituted and she was given six treatments, with remarkable improvement. Twenty-four hours after the last treatment she began to ask odd questions, misidentified people, had visual hallucinations of peculiar activities going on outdoors. This delirious condition lasted about one week and then the patient became calm again. The mood improvement was moderate.

Such reactions, called organic syndromes by Kalinowsky, are temporary in duration and clear up spontaneously. As a rule, they do not interfere with recovery. Such reactions are more acute and resemble a toxic delirious state, rather than the common amnesia. Recently, since we have employed the Reiter-Wilcox-Friedman and motor techniques, this reaction is less likely to occur. Indeed, whereas in 1941 three of my first seventy patients developed this complication, I can hardly recall a single example in 1946, when we treated an even larger number of patients.

This reaction represents a sensitivity of the central nervous system to the current. It resembles the delirium of fever, of trauma, and of toxic substances. Fortunately, it does not require any special treatment and clears spontaneously.

THE POSSIBILITY OF DEATH

It is difficult to see how a brief convulsion lasting less than one minute could produce death! Yet, there have been reports of death occuring directly following or within some days after a course of electrocoma therapy. Undoubtedly some of these are but coincidences. When one considers the large number of patients who are receiving such treatments, the interval of weeks during which a course is given, and the age of patients, it is not unlikely that some of these are statistically destined to die in that interval. For instance, I was considering treating a woman of 63, but treatment was delayed by transportation difficulties. On the day the first treatment was scheduled, she developed a cerebral hemorrhage. Had the treatment been administered as scheduled and then the patient had become ill with a cerebral hemorrhage later, we would have concluded that the hemorrhage resulted from treatment. Actually, it would have been merely a coincidence. So, too, the deaths may be coincidental, since a brief convulsion lasting forty seconds can hardly injure bodily integrity to a fatal degree. Epileptics may go through a lifetime with severe couvulsions. Seldom is there a fatality.

In a study by Feldman and his co-workers, the small number of deaths occurring in connection with shock therapy were reviewed. Only three occurred in patients over sixty-five years of age. In several of the cases the cause of death was hardly related to the treatment proper.

More significant are the reports of thousands of patients treated without death. Kalinowsky reported 1500 cases treated safely. Holbrook gave 3,070 patients a total of 27,231 treatments without a fatality and with relatively few dislocations and fractures. Jackson states: "In properly selected cases fatalities should be almost nil. . . . . In Connecticut, not a single fatality had occurred until the middle of March, 1945, although many thousands of treatments had been given." Our series in Cleveland runs to several hundred patients without a death.

The use of intocostrin has added a possible cause of death. Several fatalities occurring in treatment may be attributed to this drug.

Tragic as this complication may be, it is rare indeed as compared to the frequency of death by suicide in nontreated patients. Every psychiatrist whose career covered the preshock and the present era, knows how rare suicide is among the treated as compared to the nontreated patients. As a concrete example, may I mention that during 1941 I treated seventy patients without a fatality, whereas among the lesser number who rejected this therapy because of fear or resistance of the family, there were several suicides.

Mode of Action of Electrocoma Therapy

If one were to simplify the nervous system into three levels, vital, emotional, and intellectual, then the passage of the electrical current through the brain affects all three instantaneously. Consciousness is obliterated, pulse is slowed, pallor or cyanosis develops, sweating may occur. When the convulsion ends, then quite promptly the vital functions of respiration and circulation return to normal. Intellectual functions return more slowly. But, in terms of clinical result, it is the mood which is chiefly affected by a course of electrocoma therapy. For, regardless of any changes in ideation, there is an early and often well sustained improvement in emotions. Depressed patients become cheerful and gay, even without knowing what they are happy about. Even schizophrenics become so cheerful that they neglect their private delusions to smile at the world of reality, for a time anyway.

Let us consider several possible modes of action of E.C.T.:

A. The psychoanalytic concept of satisfying the need for punishment.

Most depressed patients exhibit self-accusatory ideas, explained as a strong superego exacting its demands upon a guilty ego. The electrocoma treatment appears to be a form of punishment which, on the surface, exacts the penalty demanded by the superego, and thus frees the ego of its sense of guilt. However plausible this concept may appear, it is incorrect! For, when we used metrazol and employed a dose insufficient to produce a major reaction, the patients experienced the most horrible sensations of darkness, of dying. Such treatments certainly were the most disagreeable form of punishment for the ego and for the subconscious. Yet this failed to bring about recovery. On the contrary, patients became worse after such emotionally painful experiences. Likewise, some psychiatrists employed minor or petit mal reactions in their early electrical treatment programs. The results from petit mal reactions were poor even if they were "punishing techniques."

Then again, Dr. Guy Williams and I used nitrogen inhalation to induce states of coma in a series of schizophrenic persons. The anoxia led to unconsciousness, cyanosis, muscle tremors. Certainly this treatment was a threat to the ego and to deeper survival functions, a severe punishment to the ego. Yet, it did not alter the patient's mental processes to any appreciable degree. We subjected a series of some ten patients to such a course of nitrogen inhalation treatments thrice weekly for some two months, with a therapeutic result which was nil.

B. Electrocoma exerts a physiologic change in the brain.

Insulin coma and electrocoma produce a change which disturbs the brain wave patterns. Likewise, there is an altered metabolism within cells, a shift in the sodium-potassium balance, and an alteration in the cell membrane permeability. A convulsion alone can effect such alteration. What the exact chemical and electrolyte changes are cannot at this time be accurately described.

Therefore, we must content ourselves with a working hypothesis.

C. Electrocoma therapy may be effective through removal of inhibitory mechanisms or by stimulating inactive or dormant processes.

We know that severing frontothalamic fibers, as is done in lobotomy, removes tension and anxiety and leaves the patient more contented. Cutting these fibers serves to remove introspective fear of the future. Electrocoma therapy, likewise, tends to make the patient less self-conscious and more outgoing. Yet the value of electrocoma therapy cannot be merely the result of removal of inhibition because of the following observations:

1. Improvement (with electrocoma therapy) in mood may occur after one or two treatments. Patients state that they have slept more soundly, have relished the taste of food, have experienced a sense of well-being long before there is any significant dulling of intellectual processes. Likewise, in some patients, there is considerable clouding of mind without any appreciable alteration in mood.

2. Removal of intellectual processes does not necessarily lead to a change in mood. A recent clinical experience may shed light on this distinction. A man of sixty consulted me for a severe depression. As there was a history of a previous coronary attack, we postponed electrical treatment, with instructions to the family to watch him closely. Unfortunately, he attempted suicide by inhaling automobile exhaust gas. A rescue squad brought him to the hospital where he was revived. In the course of weeks he regained his vital functions but not his intellectual capacities. Indeed, he failed to recognize people, could read a letter without understanding or remembering what he read. He lost his grasp of events and of reasoning, though he had been a brilliant, well educated person. Despite his profound loss of memory and judgment, as a result of anoxemic brain damage – *the mood remained depressed*. He reiterated his suicidal threats.

3. Electrocoma is capable of subduing the exhilaration of the manic state. The dosage, as to number of treatments and the need to repeat them, is greater than that required for depressed patients. Yet manic patients do improve. Certainly, if electrocoma therapy worked through the process of removing inhibitory controls, one might expect manic patients to become worse, to become more

active. The fact of improvement of manics speaks against destruction of tissue or function as the basic mechanism of action.

D. My own working hypothesis is as follows: Mood is the dominant tone feeling which, though cyclic, tends to return to the base line of average normal. This tendency to return to equilibrium, a form of homeostasis, if you will, is inherent in all organisms. It is probably a property of all cell units as well as of some governing regions (diencephalon (?)). So, in normal persons, a depressed or elated mood will, after a few hours, a night's sleep, a short holiday, return to normal. Even in manic-depressive states, in which the mood deviation is more profound and enduring this tendency remains. For such patients usually improve spontaneously, even if the time interval be a year or more.

Electrocoma therapy accelerates this tendency to return to the average state! It achieves in several weeks what nature might accomplish in months or years. It works both in depressives and manics by a physical process which operates in the direction of the inherent recoverability of this disease. Thus, the passage of the current is not merely destructive, but directly beneficial. The passage of the current through the brain and the convulsion effect a physiological (chemical and electrical) change which proves to be both a stimulus to improved bodily function and a removal of self-attacking mechanisms. It tends to break up abnormally conditioned reflexes (Kessler and Gellhorn). The seat of this action may be in the pathways between cortex and thalamus, but this is merely a surmise. The observation of patients leads to the inference that electrocoma therapy is a positive physical treatment which speeds inherent recoverability – Hence, it is more effective in depressions than in schizophrenia.

The improvement in schizophrenias is difficult to explain. However, if we apply the same concept, it appears as though the electrocoma therapy corrects the mood abnormality promptly. This restoration of the mood towards normal may carry with it a change in ideation. If the illness be compounded of mood and intellectual mechanisms, a sustained improvement may result. If the basic disease, such as schizophrenia (hebephrenic type) be organic, little lasting improvement can be expected.

Whenever possible, psychotherapy should precede electrocoma treatment. Indeed, if psychotherapy proves successful, then one may not need to resort to the electrocoma method. However, if the patient fails to respond to psychotherapy and the symptoms become worse, then, of course, the shock methods are used. It should be clearly understood that electrocoma therapy is employed not to the exclusion of but often in conjunction with psychotherapy.

Treatment-Resistant Cases

Though most depressed patients recover, some are only temporarily benefited and others are not helped much. This small group, say about ten per cent, who do not show a significant improvement, may be termed treatment-resistant. Several such examples come to mind.

Mr. E. P. was a man in his fifties when he came down with a depression. In his family history is the item of his father's illness at sixty, with involutional melancholia, terminated by suicide. His past history was negative. He had been a highly intelligent man, happy in his home life, absorbed in many civic interests, and of average personality make-up. During the illness, he became fearful, sleepless; he lost confidence and thought of suicide. He was placed in a sanitarium for many months without benefit. Then a course of six electrocoma reactions was administered. The improvement was substantial, but temporary. Within weeks he became depressed again. Several additional courses, one of 15 treatments, were given, with slight change. Today, after several years of illness, he remains shy, has no confidence in meeting people, needs sedatives for sleep.

There is another patient, F. M., who was depressed to the point of several attempts at suicide. Once she was found unconscious in her automobile from the exhaust gas fumes. She recovered and then was given a series of some 12 electrocoma reactions. The improvement was temporary, and additional maintenance doses were given. She was able to be home, but lacked vigor, had no joy in anything. However, there were several disturbing situational factors such as economic problems difficult to remedy. While undergoing psychoanalysis she made another suicidal attempt with drugs. Therefore, a longer course of twenty electrocoma treatments was given. There were some days of brightness, but the deep, dark mood has persisted.

These are two examples of apparent failures of electrocoma therapy. Other cases could be cited. What is the meaning of these failures of electrocoma therapy in depressions?

Insufficient Treatment

Sometimes the fault is not the method, nor the patient, but the inadequacy of treatment. Certainly the percentage of recovery is much higher for those therapists who do not hesitate to employ longer courses and to follow them with secondary or maintenance doses.

For instance, N. M. was a severe case of involutional melancholia, who showed but temporary improvement with 16 treatments. Soon she relapsed and was given several additional reactions. These were repeated over a period of several months. All told, this patient was given 24 reactions. She became well and the recovery has been lasting. Had we advocated a routine of 12 or 15 reactions, as is the custom in certain clinics, her case would have been counted a failure. Adequate care meant recovery.

One may ask if the recovery was not coincidental and spontaneous. This possibility cannot be dismissed in one single instance. But experience has shown the consistent reaction in a high percentage of cases, so that the response to electrocoma therapy is almost as regular as to any specific drug or like therapeutic process.

Unresolved Situational Factors

There are some patients whose illness is caused or influenced by circumstances.

For instance, D. D. was a married man who became involved in an illicit love affair. Overwhelmed by a sense of guilt, he became depressed and made two suicidal attempts within one week. Electrocoma therapy was begun and its effect was remarkable. The patient became cheerful, forgot some of his problems, resumed normal living. But the attraction of the other woman seemed irresistible. His symptoms recurred. Another acute depression developed when this woman warned the patient that she was pregnant and that he might be the father.

Chronic Psychoneurotic States

There are psychoneurotic patients whose illness is deep set, constitutional, and chronic. They react to many situations with troubling somatic difficulties. Sometimes inner conflicts and external frustrations lead to depression. As a rule, such patients are not benefited to a significant degree by electrocoma therapy.

Sometimes a few reactions with electrocoma treatment are administered for the purpose of making the patient more outspoken and more amenable to psychotherapy. In such instances, we rely not upon electrocoma therapy, but upon psychotherapy.

If such a patient becomes severely depressed and a course of electrocoma therapy be administered, there may be some temporary betterment in mood, but the psychoneurotic symptoms will reappear. They may be so disabling as to represent serious illness. Such patients are likely to be resistant to electrocoma treatment and to other forms of therapy as well. This applies forcefully to the obsessional neuroses which may begin early in life and continue onwards over the years. If such a patient becomes depressed and receives electrocoma therapy, the improvement will not be basic. Frontal lobotomy has been carried out successfully in such cases.

Thus, there are a group of depressed patients who are not helped to an enduring degree. Perhaps we may know more about therapy for these resistant cases in the future.

Some cases appearing as depressed are concealed chronic schizophrenics – resistant to many therapies.

Psychotherapy as an Adjunct

It is our practice to interview *every* patient before *each* treatment and to discuss both immediate, practical problems and deeper conflicts. Then, after the course of electrocoma is completed, we make such suggestions as to residence and work and contacts as may be required in each case.

In many instances, the improvement in mood and the splendid change in well-being enable the recovered patient to cope with life's problems successfully. He can return to his customary environment and face those challenges which loomed insurmountable during the illness. Now he takes them in his stride.

Yet, there are many patients who are perplexed by everyday situations and who need counsel and guidance during the electrocoma program. Time should be arranged for analysis of problems concurrent with the treatment program. Later, as the patient improves, he may need help in the matter of physical difficulties, work, marital relations. During the weeks of follow-up observation, the physician has the opportunity to explain, remove fears, adjust the convalescent to life again. For electrocoma therapy and psychotherapy must be combined to achieve the greatest good.

Miscellaneous

THE CHANGING CLINICAL PICTURE DURING ELECTROCOMA THERAPY

In 1944 a patient was referred as a case of depression, after she had attempted suicide by slashing her throat. She had been given first aid, the wound sutured, and she was transfused. The physical state improved over a period of one week, so she was transferred to my service at the hospital. In the initial study she appeared downcast, weeping, sighing, "I want to die – I am a disgraced woman." Beyond these words of hopelessness, she would not converse. After a brief period of observation, electrocoma therapy was begun.

The immediate response to treatment was excellent. She relaxed, ate better, and participated in ward activities. She spoke of her economic and social problems, some of which were indeed serious. Then treatment was stopped and she was observed. Gradually she became quarrelsome, refused to take food, and accused the nurses of trying to harm her. Day by day the condition grew worse. She was fearful lest the bed be wired and became suspicious of spies surrounding the building. Thus, an almost typical paranoid state had seemingly developed in place of what was originally accepted as a depression. Indeed, when this condition first appeared, it resembled a toxic psychosis. Hence, we waited in the expectation of a spontaneous clearing up. But the paranoidal mechanisms grew worse as time wore on. Therefore, we decided upon additional treatments. We then gave ten treatments more and there was consistent improvement. The patient returned to her home, but later reports indicated that paranoidal ideas recurred.

How are we to understand this apparent transformation in the nature of the illness? Could the initial course of treatment have altered the fundamental nature of the symptoms? A better explanation, which fits this and other similar instances, is as follows: The patient had been basically paranoid and had then developed evidences of depression. These were so severe as to lead to suicidal attempts. The initial treatment removed the depressed state and revealed the underlying paranoid condition, as one may brush away a heavy layer of dust from furniture and then come upon deep scratches and defects.

Of course, it is possible that if our examination had been more extensive, or if the patient were more expressive, we might have uncovered her basic suspicions earlier. In such a case we would have planned a longer course of electrocoma therapy at the outset.

Such experiences suggest also another explanation for treatment resistance: the disease is schizophrenia and not a depression. The predominant surface manifestations are depressive, but deep within is a more serious, more chronic malady. Thus, we approach the case with a favorable prognosis only to encounter a tenacious illness which responds little, if at all, to our coma therapy.

The Absence of Epilepsy as a Complication

Earlier writers expressed the fear lest the use of convulsive therapy render the patient epileptic. I have not encountered this complication in any of my cases as yet. In over 130 patients treated by the electrical method during 1941 and 1942, not one has returned with a complaint of attacks of unconsciousness. We know that an average of 18 months may elapse between trauma and traumatic epilepsy. In my series, five to six years have elapsed and no epilepsy has resulted.

Combined Treatment

There are patients who show moderate or temporary improvement with electrocoma therapy. They may do better under insulin treatment. Thus, it is expedient to combine insulin and electrocoma, or follow one by the other. Secondly, a more prolonged treatment, so-called electronarcosis, has been introduced by Tietz and promises to benefit some patients who failed to respond to electrocoma therapy. There are some patients, particularly difficult schizophrenics, who may not improve under either electrocoma or insulin shock treatment. Such a patient was M. C., who remained in a catatonic state for many months despite the use of the shock methods. She would lie abed, refuse food, ignore her surroundings except at times to kick or bite an attendant. Recently a lobotomy was done, and the immediate results have been splendid. This patient is now pleasant, responds to questions in a friendly manner and carries out commands well.

Objections to Electrocoma Therapy

Despite the growing use of this procedure among an ever-widening circle of psychiatrists, there are some physicians who still oppose it. It may be of interest to consider the objections which are raised. There are some psychoanalysts who are prejudiced against a mechanical procedure. The very thought of passing an electric current through the brain seems to violate a sacred attitude. Such doctors will search avidly for any unfavorable clinical reports and may find an article which summarizes the failure of electrocoma in the treatment of chronic schizophrenia simplex, and use such data to refute the many favorable reports in the literature. The physician treats all organs of the body with respect, yet he does not hesitate to use drastic measures if experience proves their worth. Even lobotomy has helped a considerable number of patients.

Some psychiatrists are opposed to the method, because of a limited experience with an unfortunate selection of cases. For example, during several years of treatment, the great majority of patients responded favorably. There were, however, some failures several of whom were referred to the Probate Court for transfer to the State Hospital. A psychiatrist for the Probate Court missed the opportunity of seeing the recovered patients, but had contact only with failures. This limited contact led to the inference that E.C.T. was consistently unsuccessful.

There are other physicians whose experience has been limited to inadequate treatment or to accidental failures. I know a physician who, until 1945, believed electrocoma therapy to be unsuccessful. The basis for this belief was the fact that his patients were given brief courses, in which there were minor as well as major reactions. Naturally the therapeutic results were but fair. Then again, there may be a physician whose first case sustains a fracture or who has some other complication, and who thereafter shies away from the procedure.

These objections, namely a prior prejudice, contact with failures only, and unpleasant experiences, account for a certain opposition to the use of a method which has proved successful in the hands of those who use it properly.

Illustrative Case Histories

CASE I. *B. C. – Schizophrenia, with hebephrenic features – failure*

The patient is a young man of twenty-two, who had been a fairly healthy youth of average intelligence. After leaving high school, he took a job as a machinist and got along quite well. Yet he made few friends, did not date, but would putter around at a work bench in his basement. At times he would sit and daydream. After several years there was a decreased interest in his job, he became trembly and uneasy. He withdrew more and more from active participation and felt uncomfortable with others. Occasionally, he would whisper and chuckle to himself. His condition grew worse, so that he became passive and would spend considerable time at home. Some of his remarks were incoherent.

The initial examination revealed a healthy appearing, slender young man in the twenties. He sat in the examining room, a smile on his features. When spoken to, he mentioned that people looked at him oddly and would giggle to himself when discussing these matters. He was indifferent to current events and incidents in his home. When asked why he stayed abed, he remarked that he was very weak and tired, and promised that he would soon get going again. Though he was concerned about people's attitude towards him, he was not fearful, but rather smiled when he mentioned this subject. His dress was slovenly and his body showed considerable lack of care.

A course of electrocoma treatments was undertaken with a clear understanding on the part of the family that the prognosis was unfavorable. After four or five treatments, there was a surprising awakening of interest and energy. The patient was cheerful, took long walks, played baseball with his friends. Indeed, so remarkable was the activity of this patient that his family was positive he was well. However, our past experience with such initial improvement in schizophrenias caused us to caution the family against over-optimism. The treatment was continued, but somewhere around the tenth to the fifteenth treatment the patient became resistive, even more suspicious than he had been before. Additional treatments were given until a total of 25 was reached. At best, there was some moderate change in the physical condition and a slight increase in patient's activities. However, there was no fundamental change. He sits around the house, smiling and giggling for no reason, indifferent to people and to responsibilities.

CASE II. *W. P. – Acute schizophrenia – marked improvement*

The patient was a married woman in the middle twenties, whose health and personality record had been quite normal. She was happily married and went through her pregnancy without complications. Following the birth of her child early in 1945, she suspected that the hospital attendants were mistreating her. She became fearful and suspicious when she thought that people in the corridor were making unfavorable remarks about her. After she got home, she tried to take care of her child, but became fearful that he might be sick. Later she had an idea that perhaps he was dead. Her behavior became gradually worse.

At my initial examination in her home I found a pale woman with dry lips, restless and disturbed. "Everything around me has changed. Who are you? Your face is changing. Everything is changing." When the patient was a bit more calm, she stated that the radio talked about her and that the picture in the newspaper resembled her.

W. P. was placed in the hospital for observation. For several days she was overactive, sleepless; she tore her garments to shreds. "I am afraid they want to harm me; they want to poison me. Take me out of here." A course of electrocoma therapy was begun and she was given a series of 15 treatments. Her response was excellent, and she was permitted a trial home. However, her nervousness and preoccupation returned. She became worried about herself and about her baby. She could not manage her home. A series of ten ambulatory treatments was then administered. The response was excellent. Patient gained weight, became calm, took a wholesome interest in her family. Today, 18 months after the course was completed, she is in charge of her home, a happy, confident mother, a pleasant wife. She recalls the acute mental illness with clear insight.

CASE III. *R. I. – Schizophrenia, paranoid type – improvement*

R. I. was a young man of twenty-five, who had been sick at the age of nineteen and was helped by a course of insulin treatment. He was apparently well until early in 1941. At that time he became actively hallucinated and suspected that the house was full of traps. "I went into the bathroom and had the sensation of dropping through the floor. I made a slight gesture and I was right side up again, and suddenly I noticed a new light, a light that never existed before. I went to the store to get some pork chops and beef hearts. One of them looked peculiar and I had a feeling that there was some foulness in it." Patient also had olfactory hallucinations, remarking: "There are gas-like odors in the house. The food is changed." He sat in the home with a loaded pistol, apparently ready to defend himself against persecutors. When he was admitted to the hospital, he attributed all his difficulties to religion, stating: "I am an atheist. The religious people are against me; some of these religious people take mud and make it appear like food."

A course of electrical treatment was begun in April, 1941, and continued to June. Patient received some twenty treatments in all. He showed a remarkable improvement and was allowed to go home.

The follow-up in this instance has been through correspondence. This man is working steadily, is getting along very well at home. Indeed, subsequently I have treated several other members of the family for similar illnesses.

CASE IV. M. B. – *Schizo-affective disorder – remarkable improvement*

The patient was a married woman in the middle thirties, whom I examined in a mental hospital in February, 1941. The past history indicated that this patient was at one time a highly intelligent, energetic woman who was successful in her job as a sales person. She was married and apparently got along quite well. In 1936 she became nervous. The family stated that she was moody, sleepless, depressed, and worried about many physical conditions. In the course of time, she developed a strong impulse for killing and was placed in a psychopathic hospital. Later she developed suicidal ideas. The condition was so severe that M. B. remained as an inmate of several institutions over a five year period, until the time when I saw her.

In the initial examination I found a fairly well developed, talkative woman, who described voices that accused her of crimes which she had committed. She stated that she was being controlled by these voices. "They seem to read my thoughts even before I think them and they repeat these thoughts to me. Sometimes they make fun of me or make rhymes of what I am going to say. – "I am thinking of a chair and they say, 'Chair, comb your hair.' The voices accused me of being a Pied Piper."

This patient was placed in the hospital for observation and at one time wrote the following: "When you see my sister today, please tell her the truth regarding my condition. The confusion in my brain does not diminish. Medical skill can cure my body, but my soul is sick and only God can help me. I wish I had never been born. I know I can't live as I should with my thoughts in confusion. A long time ago I wrote and told her to send me to the hospital for the insane – I have nothing spiritual to guide me. Please let me die mercifully." Again and again she remarked that she would like to commit suicide and reiterated the phrase: "People are controlling me; they tell me what to do; they tell me to take my life."

A course of electrocoma therapy was begun in the spring of 1941. During the first few weeks there was little or no change. Even after the tenth treatment she would say: "My thoughts are being read; I hear the voices all the time. They only let up after the treatment, but then they come back again the next day." However, the patient looked somewhat improved physically. Gradually, between the tenth and twentieth treatment, she showed a phenomenal improvement.

In the summer of 1941 patient appeared vivacious, cheerful, and talkative. Her attention was focused upon the world around her and she denied hearing any voices. She had a sense of well-being and was making plans for the future.

I have kept in touch with this patient over a period which now approaches six years. During this entire time she enjoyed normal health.

This case was remarkable in that there were predominant schizophrenic features and a history of a long illness. From a statistical standpoint, the prognosis was unfavorable and the family was ready to commit her as a chronic, lifetime resident in a state institution. The immediate result of the treatment was splendid and the recovery has been relatively permanent.

CASE V. L. S. – *Depression, possibly reactive, but with features of involutional melancholia – successfully treated*

Mrs. L. S., a married woman of forty-five, had been healthy and free of nervous symptoms throughout her lifetime. There was a family history of depression involving two cousins.

In December, 1944, the patient became worried because her son was in service. She spent considerable time in a business against the advice of her boy, who wished her to remain at home. Then in January, 1945, she received a telegram that her son was missing in action. The mild nervousness of the previous few months became markedly worse. Patient could think only about her son. She was positive that he had died. She accused herself of having a guilty conscience. "My boy didn't want me to work, and now he is gone. If I had not worked, I could have spent more time writing to him; and now it is too late."

Subsequently she received news that her son was a prisoner of war and was safe, but she did not believe this statement. She thought it was a forgery.

During the initial examination, she was markedly depressed, tense, and agitated. "I can't sleep; I can't eat; I keep thinking about my boy. I know he is dead; he sends me letters, but how do I know that he has written them? It's all my fault - shameful, shameful."

The condition was looked upon as severe and immediate hospitalization was planned. However, a hospital bed was not available and patient was permitted to go home for several days. The family was warned about the possibility of suicide. On the following day she swallowed a bottle of Lysol and was rushed to a hospital for emergency care. Luckily, she vomited and escaped from this attempt with but a moderately severe chemical burn of the mouth and throat.

Patient was then admitted to the hospital and her depressive ideas were even more severe. She spoke in a husky voice: "It is not I alone, it is you and our whole race that are being dragged into this. Be careful, they are making notes, we are being watched." It seems as though a paranoid interpretation was superimposed upon the fundamental depression.

When the physical condition was improved, a course of electrocoma was started. Patient received a total of some 12 treatments. After the fifth, she remarked: "This is the first time that I am really alive. I must have said funny things to you when I thought this place was full of spies." When I mentioned her son, she replied: "When I see him, I will believe it." After several additional treatments, she was even more cheerful and stated: "I saw the post card and I know that my son is living."

This patient was discharged from the hospital and has been seen on occasion over the past twenty months. Her condition is excellent. Her boy did come back from the service and his return has added to her happiness.

CASE VI. *E. O. - Manic-depressive psychosis, depressive type, with frequent attacks; improvement*

Mrs. E. O. was a woman of forty-six who was referred to me in April, 1942, with a history of recurring attacks of depression over a period of years. The first had occurred in 1935, the second developed a year later. Patient stated that she has had attacks practically every year to 18 months. In 1936 she had consulted an analyst and was under his care for a period of three years. "At the time I felt that I was being helped, but my attacks started again."

The present illness had begun in December, 1941, and was continuous up to the time I saw this patient. "I feel miserable; I don't want to get up in the morning; I wish I could do something to end it all, but I lack the courage. I am a burden to my husband; I am of no use; I can't care for my home."

The symptoms were relatively mild, but in view of the persistence, we decided upon a course of treatment. After the third treatment, she was much better and was allowed to go home after four treatments. This patient remained well for 18 months and then had a recurrence.

In the fall of 1943 she was treated by a New York doctor when I was in service. In December, 1945, she had another attack, but once again four treatments brought about a prompt recovery. She enjoyed excellent health until December, 1946, when, as usual, another attack of depression occurred. This time she was given three treatments, with success.

This is an example of a rapidly cycling moderate depression. Prior to the present treatment program, the attacks lasted from four to six months. Now a series of four to six treatments in a period of a week or two have regularly brought about improvement. The improvement, of course, is limited to the attack only. Electrocoma therapy has been unable to alter the tendency to cycles.

CASE VII. *A. L. – Mixed manic-depressive psychosis – improvement*

Mrs. A. L. was a woman of twenty-nine, referred to me early in 1946 because of a history of overactive behavior which began shortly after the birth of her child. This patient developed a mixed manic-depressive psychosis. At times she would sit and weep, complaining of tiredness and weakness and inability to do things. More frequently, she was talkative, exhibiting flight of ideas, jumpy, moving about. The condition had grown worse during a period of observation and, therefore, a course of electrocoma therapy was begun. This patient received a series of 23 treatments over a period of two months. During this interval, she would show temporary improvement. However, when the treatments would be discontinued for a week or so, the manic behavior reappeared. The treatments were discontinued a year ago and the patient has been followed at intervals for psychotherapy. During the last visit she was seen to be well adjusted, taking care of her home capably, and free of any mood change.

Summary

Electrocoma therapy is being used by an ever widening circle of psychiatrists in the treatment of psychoses.

Psychoses, in which the major feature is depression, tend to respond to such therapy. Thus, the depressive phase of manic-depressive psychosis, involutional melancholia, schizophrenia loaded with affect, and sometimes manic states can be greatly benefited by such treatment. Certain types of psychoneuroses have also been helped by this method.

The course of treatment is individualized in accordance with the patient's condition, response, and type of illness. A compact series averages 6 to 12 treatments for depressions and twenty or more for schizophrenias. Subsequently, additional coma-convulsions may be needed, so-called maintenance doses.

Each treatment can be made more comfortable and safer by proper medication, attention during the convulsion, and post-treatment care. Sodium amytal helps to allay apprehension; intocostrin reduces the traumatic complications.

Electrocoma therapy can be administered in an ambulatory manner, provided there is a well qualified therapist and staff, and a careful selection of patients.

The family can help materially, especially in the handling of ambulatory patients, if they are acquainted with the program to be followed.

The therapeutic results of electrocoma therapy are gratifying. Viewed against the background of the status before such measures were used, we can see the striking improvement in the behavior of patients, the relief of suffering, the abbreviation of the hospital stay, the reduction in suicides, which can frequently be obtained by adequate therapy. The duration of improvement depends upon the inherent nature of the disease.

There are hazards to electrocoma such as temporary clouding of memory, traumatic complications, and the possibility of death. Fortunately, these hazards are few and are far less serious than the dangers of the disease. Indeed, many experienced therapists have treated large series of patients, numbering hundreds and thousands, without a fatality.

The mode of action of this treatment is a physiological alteration in the direction of recoverability. It is a kind of homeostasis, hastening equilibrium. It achieves no more than nature itself could accomplish, but it acts in a direct, positive, effective manner, saving time, suffering, possibly suicide.

There are a certain number of patients who fail to respond, who are treatment-resistant. Some failures represent inadequate therapy, others are caused by unsolved situational and psychoneurotic features. Then, too, there is a substantial percentage of schizophrenics who are not helped by any treatment.

My experience over a six year period permits the conclusion that at this time electrocoma, properly administered, is the most effective remedy available in a large number of psychoses. The method is being improved and modified, and it is hoped that the future will bring out techniques that are even safer and better than those we now have, or that preventive measures will make such methods unnecessary. Today, however, E.C.T. is a remarkably useful technique that has added immeasurably to the psychiatrist's ability to serve the mentally ill.

REFERENCES

Fetterman, J. L.: Electro-Coma Therapy of Psychoses. *Ann. Int. Med.*, 17:775 (Nov.) 1942.

Moriarty, J. D., and Weil, A. A.: Combined Convulsive Therapy and Psychotherapy of the Neuroses. *Arch. Neurol. & Psychiat.* 50:685 (Dec.) 1943.

Evans, V. L.: Convulsive Shock Therapy in Elderly Patients. Risks and Results. *Am. J. Psychiat.*, 99:531 (Jan.) 1943.

Kalinowsky, L. B.: Electric Convulsive Therapy, with Emphasis on Importance of Adequate Treatment. *Arch. Neurol & Psychiat.*, 50 652 (Dec.) 1943.

Neymann, C. A., Urse, V. G., Madden, J. J., and Countryman, M. A.: Electric Shock Therapy in the Treatment of Schizophrenia, Manic-Depressive Psychoses, and Chronic Alcoholism. *J. Nerv. & Ment. Dis.*, 98:618 (Dec.) 1943.

Evans, V. L.: Electroconvulsive Shock Therapy and Cardiovascular Disease. *Ann. Int. Med.*, 22:692 (May) 1945.

Friedman, E., and Wilcox, P. H.: Electrostimulated Convulsive Doses in Intact Humans by Means of Unidirectional Currents. *J. Nerv. & Ment. Dis.*, 96:56, 1942.

Liberson, W. T.: New Possibilities in Electric Convulsive Therapy "Brief Stimuli" Technique. *Institute of Living, Abstracts and Translations* 12:368, 1944.

Goldman, D.—Personal communication.

Perlson, J.: Psychologic Studies on a Patient Who Received Two Hundred and Forty-Eight Shock Treatments. *Arch. Neurol. & Psychiat.*, 54:409 (Nov.-Dec.) 1945.

Impastato, D. J., Bak, R., Frosch, J., and Wortis, S. B.: Modification of the Electrofit—1. Sodium Amytal. *Am. J. Psychiat.*, 100:358 (Nov.) 1943.

Bennett, A. E.: Preventing Traumatic Complications in Shock Therapy by Curare. *J.A.M.A.*, 114:322 (Jan. 27) 1940.

Bennett, A. E.: An Evaluation of the Shock Therapies. *Diseases of the Nervous System VI*, 20, Jan. 1945.

Myerson, A.: Experience with Electric Shock Therapy in Mental Disease. *New England J. Med.*, 224:1081, 1941.

Wender, L., Balser, B. H., Beres, D.: Extra-Mural Shock Therapy. *Am. J. Psychiat.*, 99:712, (Mar.) 1943.

Patry, F. L.: Abridged Technique in Ambulatory Electro-Shock Therapy. *Diseases of the Nervous System VI*, 18, Jan., 1945.

Fetterman, J. L.: Ambulatory Electro-Coma Therapy of Psychoses. *Diseases of the Nervous System VIII*, 5, Jan., 1947.

Feldman, F., Susselman, S., Lipetz, B., and Barrera, S. E.: Electric Shock Therapy of Elderly Patients. *Arch. Neurol. & Psychiat.*, 56:158 (Aug.) 1946.

Holbrook, C. S.: Five Years Experience with Electric Sleep (Electric Shock) Treatment. *New Orleans Med. & Surg. J.*, 99:147 (Oct.) 1946.

Jackson, A. H.: Electric Shock Therapy: Its Use in a General Hospital. *Conn. State M. J.*, 9:703 (Sept.) 1945.

Wilcox, P. H.: Electro-shock Therapy: A Review of Over 23,000 Treatments Using Unidirectional Currents. *Am. J. Psychiat.*, 104:100 (Aug.) 1947.

Colfer, H. F.: *Electrolytes of the Brain in Experimental Convulsions.* Paper read at meeting of Association for Research in Nervous and Mental Disease, New York, Dec., 1946.

Kessler, M., and Gellhorn, E.: The Effect of Electrically and Chemically Induced Convulsions on Conditioned Reflexes. *Am. J. Psychiat.*, 99:687, 1943.

Tietz, E. B., Thompson, G. N., van Harreveld, A., and Wiersma, C. A. G.: Electronarcosis, Its Application and Therapeutic Effect in Schizophrenia. *J. Nerv. & Ment. Dis.*, 103:144 (Feb.) 1946.

Kalinowsky, L. B., and Hoch, P. H.: *Shock Treatments and Other Somatic Procedures in Psychiatry.* Grune & Stratton, New York, 1946.

Katzenelbogen, S., Baur, A. K., and Coyne, A. R. M.: Electric Shock Therapy; Clinical, Biochemical and Morphologic Studies. *Arch. Neurol. & Psychiat.*, 52:323 (Oct.) 1944.

Kerman, E. F.: Electroshock Therapy. With Special Reference to Relapses and an Effort to Prevent Them. *J. Nerv. & Ment. Dis.*, 102:231 (Sept.) 1945.

Impastato, D. J., and Almansi, R. J.: A Study of over 2000 Cases of Electrofit-Treated Patients. *New York State J. Med.*, 43:2057, 1943.

Jessner, L., and Ryan, V. G.: *Shock Treatment in Psychiatry.* Grune & Stratton, New York, 1941.

Freeman, W., and Watts, J. W.: *Psychosurgery.* Thomas, Springfield, 1942.

Chapter VII

PSYCHOPATHIC PERSONALITY AND OTHER ABNORMALITIES

Psychopathic Personality

THERE is a disorder in which the patient himself does not complain of being sick so much as society suffers because of the patient's abnormalities. The swindler, the habitual criminal, the trouble maker among us, the Army's bad boy, is labeled "constitutional psychopath." He is the frequenter of courts and jails, the seaman for whom the brig was built, the soldier who spends time in the guardhouse, who goes A.W.O.L. again and again, whose nuisance value is so high that he is given a blue discharge (without honor) with relief and not regret on the part of those in charge. Such a person, briefly called the psychopath, is an individualist in an outfit whose success depends upon team play. He is extremely selfish in an endeavor that demands self-sacrifice; he seeks pleasure in a service that often exacts pain. He is unfortunate; or it is more truthful to say that we, his contacts, are unfortunate.

Man depends upon normal intelligence, normal physical qualities, and good emotional control to get along well. Lacking average intelligence, he is handicapped by mental defectiveness (low I.Q.); lacking normal muscles, he shows physical weakness; lacking proper emotional control, he manifests nervousness. Yet there is another quality that determines man's attainment. The human race is a relay race; each man is linked with his fellow. We depend upon each other as do members of a human chain crossing a river. The rules for getting along are the mores of the group. "From the cradle to the grave the human being, living in any particular society," writes Glueck, "is called upon by its mores, customs, and legal codes to achieve at least a certain minimal standard of conformity." The psychopath lacks the capacity for adaptation. He swims against the current of social effort. This difficulty, as will be explained later, is not due to a lack of intelligence or vigor but arises from a deficient moral sense.

This chapter deals largely with the problems that the psychopath presents rather than with the occasional instances of achievement which this deviation may produce. Myerson has stated: "Many of the most fruitful individuals the world has known could be labeled psychopathic. They have been riddled with psychopathic characteristics, but they have had what William James called 'a linkage with genius' and, consequently, they expressed, perhaps through their psychopathic traits, very high creative ability. One could thus speak of Edgar Allen Poe, Beaudelaire, Beethoven, Richard Wagner, and many others whose characteristics in general, aside from their genius, were psychopathic, but whose genius may have received a more intensive directive by this very conjunction."

Our concern, however, is with such types of psychopathy as the inadequate personality, nomadism, emotional instability, pathologic lying, criminalism, the sexual psychopathies, and paranoid personalities.

CONSTITUTIONAL INADEQUACY includes those who, either from lack of initiative, ambition, perseverance, or judgment, through shiftlessness, or tactlessness, or a planless existence, make a notorious failure of everything they attempt. Says Noyes, "They are improvident and shiftless ... they can neither work nor wait for deferred pleasure or reward ... the pleasure of the moment satisfies... .They are defective in sense of responsibility to themselves and society." Perhaps we can better understand the psychopath if we read the clinical record of L. L., age 25.

L. L. had a poor record in school, reaching the seventh grade at the age of 17. During these years he did not apply himself, was truant on many occasions, resting at home. He was a bed-wetter until the age of 16.

After he left school, L. L. took a job but did not keep it. His work record was sporadic. He quit his jobs because he was "tired and needed rest." This usually consisted of periods of loafing for several months. He did not hesitate to appeal to his parents for support, although he was physically robust and intellectually a low normal. During the last period of idleness, he "lived on Social Security," but visited members of his family for prolonged vacations.

In his early twenties he married. His wife soon left him and obtained a divorce on grounds of non-support. Then war was declared and L. L., inspired by patriotism (or shamed by his record), enlisted in the Navy. He made a poor adjustment, dropping out of drill and failing to do detail, complaining of pain in his back and head. He was discharged from the Navy within five months, the report stating, "There are no clinical findings of significance."

L. L. then enlisted in the Army Air Corps because, he said, "I'd be drafted anyway." In the Air Corps he failed again. "I was nervous all the time. The noise of the planes was too much for me, and the noise in the barracks was just as bad." Certificates from his officers stated, "Soldier was ineffectual, compensating for his inadequacy by complaint of dizziness and pain. He is reported to be untidy about his bunk area; he would rest on his bunk in his dirty coveralls; he would sleep with his coveralls on; he was not sociable and became silent and angry when a furlough request was not granted."

This soldier's record in the Army was one of complete failure—as it had been throughout his life. He lacked drive, was devoid of a sense of responsibility, completely inadequate to assume his position in life, civilian or military.

NOMADISM is inherent in some degree in all persons. It is so pronounced in certain races as to govern their mode of existence and social organization. In the pathologic nomad, the urge leads to a life as a hobo or tramp – he may beg, steal, trespass upon private property.

"The antisocial personality," according to Noyes, "shows a moral and ethical blunting, a lack of sympathy for his fellow men. As children, they are self-willed, play truant, commit petty thefts, are often cruel and untruthful...and as they grow older they show a brutal egoism, rarely feel remorse, are devoid of a sense of honor or of shame. Their offenses may constitute the whole register of crime–theft, embezzlement, forgery, robbery. Punishments are considered as expressions of injustice and have no deterrent effect."

T. M. illustrates features of emotional instability and antisocial behavior. Excerpts from his case record indicate that, as a child, he was a well youngster, free of serious injury or illness. He was raised in an average home. During his school days he did quite well until adolescence, when he became uncooperative and disobedient. He refused to continue school and took a job. He did not remain at it long, but instead joined some friends, "hitchhiking." At the age of 18 he was arrested for a minor theft and served 20 days in jail. He worked unsteadily and then "helped a friend steal a tire." Court records show a five-year suspended sentence.

This was followed by several arrests on "misconduct charges," and finally a sentence of 18 months in a state prison for forgery.

T. M. was drafted and became a soldier in the Army of the United States. Within two weeks he became ill of a venereal disease. When he recovered, he was assigned to the Engineers, where he applied himself during basic training. Once or twice he went on sick call, complaining of indigestion. He then went A.W.O.L. for 17 days. A court-martial sentenced him to two months' hard labor and forfeit of $18 per month pay. A portion of this confinement was remitted and he was released to duty.

Following this experience, T. M. was more diligent and went overseas with his outfit. Unfortunately, all he contributed was his presence, not performance. On several occasions he returned from leave, staggering and drowsy. He confessed to the use of reefers (marijuana) but promised to abstain. Yet he not only resumed smoking marijuana but he induced other soldiers to try it. Finally he was referred to the hospital by his company commander, with the note, "His behavior and unreliability in his company are having a deleterious effect on the other soldiers." From the time of this hospitalization for drug addiction, he lost time (and pay). At the overseas hospital, treatment was without avail. On the contrary, he initiated and was mixed up in several brawls in the ward.

T. M. was returned to the United States and hospitalized here. He complained of tiredness and indigestion. Although all tests were negative, he refused to do his share of ward detail, saying, "I am too weak. It will wear me down." He divided his time between staying abed or inciting fellow patients to trouble. Once a Christmas tree was knocked down, then a table was broken, a window broken – and T. M. was always nearby, always suspected but never caught.

When a ward officer spoke to him, he would insist, "I don't get any attention. I am a sick man and I am not getting the right medicine. The Army has done me wrong in three ways: My pay has been stopped, I can't get out to see a woman, and I am not getting proper medicine." Yet the record showed several months in the hospital, numerous examinations, guardhouse, and practically no service given to the Army.

A Board of Officers decided to separate T. M. from the service by Section VIII for "emotional instability" and to give him a blue discharge (without honor).

An example that has features of PATHOLOGIC LYING and

CRIMINALISM is supplied by an item in *Newsweek* (June 19, 1944): "Between April 13 and April 21, C. W., former member of the Flying Tigers in China, set himself a fast pace around the Army Air-Field at Santa Ana, California. Last week he faced the music, a court-martial on nine moral charges, including forcible rape, a charge of bigamy, and one of larceny - stealing a gold watch belonging to his first wife, who testified against him. C. W., who admitted he was married four times and had entered the Army fraudulently, was arrested after his alleged rape of a 17-year old dancer."

A current story that has gone the rounds may be retold to illustrate the impulsive criminal behavior of the psychopath as well as his moral callousness. This youth had been stealing and robbing and had served in all levels of institutions from reformatories to penitentiaries. On parole, he quarreled with his parents and was so aroused that he killed them. Tried in court for first-degree murder, he made an impassioned plea for clemency —on the grounds of being an orphan. A representative criminal in civilian life was John Dillinger.

A case in which early symptoms of psychopathy were present was recently brought to us for examintion:

E. M., a 12-year old girl, was brought by her mother, who complained that the child had been caught in numerous thefts in school, at home, and in a neighborhood store. She also showed violent temper, was lazy, hard to discipline, and fought with the two younger siblings. Furthermore, the mother found it impossible to get a truthful account from her about anything that had happened. The mother reported that these behavior deviations had begun seven months previously, during the mother's confinement in the hospital.

The patient began school at the age of five, was transferred from public to parochial school in the second grade, and repeated the second grade; now in the sixth grade, she barely manages to pass. The family consists of the parents, a brother 15 years old, and two sisters, five and two years. The father drinks heavily, becomes violent and fights with the mother. The children are all very much upset on these occasions and cry and scream. The mother, who accompanied the child, gave the impression of being somewhat dull and lacking in understanding of the seriousness of the child's problem. She spoke of being nervous herself.

During the interview E. M. was somewhat bewildered

but tried to be cooperative. She admitted thefts from the home and the neighborhood store, but denied having taken anything at school. She said she had been stealing money at home for two or three years, although the mother apparently had been unaware of what was happening. She also admitted that she found it hard to tell the truth, especially when it meant confessing her thefts.

The findings of the neurological examination were negative. The physical examination suggested glandular imbalance. On the Wechsler-Bellevue test of intelligence, E. M. obtained an I. Q. of 96, putting her in the "average" range in intelligence.

The picture as a whole is that of a child with constitutional psychopathic make-up, manifesting itself in stealing, lying, incorrigibility, temper tantrums, and general restlessness.

Another example is that of a young man who was accident-prone. He told his civilian friends that he had been injured in a plane crash and that he had parachuted from a remarkable altitude. This "story" was but a re-statement of the fact that ever since boyhood he had jumped from high places, usually on a dare. The young man had scars on his face, had sprained and fractured his ankle on several occasions, and had injured his back. The history revealed that in his childhood he was extremely jealous of an older and more stable brother, who did well in school and who won praise from his teachers and parents. The patient was impulsive, unstable, did not apply himself studiously. He sought for admiration by stunts. Thus it was that at about the age of ten he jumped from a two-story porch, fracturing his leg. A year or two later he dived from a high board into shallow water, sustaining further injuries. Again and again he would display his prowess as a jumper to win the plaudits of the crowd. In these jumps he sought for admiration, striving to outshine his successful brother, and there may have been the unconscious idea that when he was injured he was punishing his parents and the brother as well as himself.

His psychopathy was manifested also in other ways. He tried many jobs but seldom kept them. He had worked in one place for two months and then quit because he was "too tired." Later he worked at another job but decided he should go to college. He convinced his parents to buy him an automobile so that he could use it at school. After several weeks of apparent success, he left the school and drove off to California. The first intimation his parents had of his departure was a wire for funds. Impulsiveness, instability, lack of regard for his parents were prominent symptoms.

Case History of Common Type of Female Psychopath

V. M., a 16-year-old girl, was brought in by her parents following her second run-away from a girls' detention home (Blossom Hill). She was an attractive girl of average intelligence who had been sentenced to this home because of vagrancy and sexual promiscuity.

In her past history we learned that she was born in Cleveland, the younger by six years of two girls. There was a marked contrast between the two daughters, the older being well behaved, conscientious, and a model child. The patient was considered headstrong and obstinate as a child and she recalled frequent admonitions and comparisons with her sister. The parents attempted to maintain strict discipline and resorted to corporal means of punishment with little change in behavior. V. M. completed eight grades of school at the usual age and with no major disciplinary difficulty.

When 14 years of age, V. M. began staying out late, defying her parents more openly, lying, and finally about a year later (September, 1944) ran away from home to live with a man. Six months later she was picked up by the police because of the larceny of her "friend" and returned to her home. She completed a beauty operator's course and started to work, but a few months later (December, 1945) was arrested in a hotel room with a soldier and released to the detention home from which she ran away on two occasions.

The patient explained her behavior in the following manner: "It all began when my folks would tease me and bawl me out in front of my friends, and it got so they didn't believe anything I said. They believed me more when I was lying and I decided to go ahead and do the worst, as they thought it anyhow. But after that night that I first stayed with this man, I was afraid to go home so I just ran away. I was happier living with G. than at home. Nothing seemed to be important, least of all sex. I would stay with any fellow I liked at all."

"I hate this home; even before I ever went there I made up my mind to run away. People try to talk to me, to understand me I guess, but it doesn't seem to hit home. All I can think about is right now; the past is all over and I don't want to wait for the future. I don't feel I've done anything wrong, no one is helping me any. It seems there are two sides of me; I can get along all right with people and be honest, then something goes wrong, I get mad and go to the other side and don't give a darn about anything. I guess I would do most anything, lie or steal, if I thought I had to. It wouldn't bother me. I'd be careful about sleeping with men, though, because I've had enough to do with the police."

This patient exemplifies the gradual development of a psychopathic personality. When she was seen by us, she evidenced the lack of any kind of functioning conscience and disregard for the usual social mores and conventions. Her judgment was defective in that she was totally unable to forego immediate advantage for eventual benefit and obviously could not profit from experience. The fact that six months were added to her sentence for running away from the detention home did not deter her from a second attempt and from planning yet a third.

In our discussion thus far we have stressed the defect in the individual, with emphasis upon the innate or constitutional basis for this disturbance. The term, constitutional, is used broadly to include primarily inherent qualities, with the recognition that these may be molded by environment. Myerson states: "Environment acts as an evocative force; that is to say, the hereditary factors need an environmental evocation. Thus there are many boys who become criminal in an environment which easily favors that evocation, just as there are environments which are adverse, let us say, to the criminalistic tendencies which are probably dormant in most of us. The power of the environment in evoking constitutional factors has been very definitely discussed by such writers on heredity as H. S. Jennings. There are many experiments in genetics, by which change in the environment evokes different hereditary qualities, as in the classic experiments on the fruit-fly where warm moist laboratories produce different results than dry cold ones do. It is perfectly well known that certain parts of each city somehow or other evoke criminalistic conduct despite the character of the races that live there, and the Chicago sociologists have emphasized this a good deal."

In connection with the influence of environment in bringing to the surface psychopathic traits, we must recognize that the pressures around an individual may be significant. Myerson writes: "The general attitude seems to be that society and its demands are normal and that the individual is psychopathic. ... Society is psychopathic. It demands non-biological conduct, and there are many people who find it impossible to conform to these non-biological demands." The case history of V. M. is an example of a girl with strong sexual impulses, to which she reacted biologically. According to her attitude, the social pressures of law and custom were in error. She did not consider herself sinful, but that society was in the wrong.

Malamud summarizes the outstanding features of the psychopathic personality as psychopathic trends in the family history, a record of instability throughout the whole adjustment period, phases of worse behavior, some assets such as good initial adjustment to new situations. The demands of the Army, according to this writer, evoke accessory reactions. These include resentment against authority and regimentation, a tendency to blame others for one's own difficulties, and exaggerated swings of emotional stability as the final expression of dissatisfaction.

The actual grouping of the type of psychopathy varies with the major symptoms at any one time. A psychopath may conduct himself normally for a time, may express his illness by nomadism at one time and criminalism at another. The greater the stress, the more likely the development of new and distressing symptoms.

The diagnosis of a psychopath depends not merely upon the behavior at the moment, for it may be ideal, but upon the life story. For the psychopath, like the normal individual, may present his noblest side on certain occasions, especially to attain his goal. He may speak with the eloquence of an Anthony. Indeed, the psychopath, alert, smooth, unhampered by the restraint of truth, may seem interesting, convincing, entertaining. He may sell himself and his product until we, the victims, become painfully aware of the fraud. We may enjoy him as a Major Hoople, but usually in the Army his irresponsibility, his trouble-making practices make him unwanted.

SPECIAL PROBLEMS OF THE SEXUAL PSYCHOPATH

Deviations from normal sexuality have been interpreted by some as a form of psychoneurosis, by others as an endocrine imbalance. The Army includes them under the heading of sexual psychopathy because the difficulty is usually constitutional and the symptoms socially important. The sexual psychopath's deviations, like those of other psychopaths, anger society and invite punishment whereas such persons deserve sympathy and medical care.

In my practice I have seen homosexuals who were painfully aware of their problems and were struggling to correct them – often a losing struggle. As they related their stories, it was evident that early in life some of them had been different. A young man explained that, as a child, he played with girls rather than with boys, helping in the house, cleaning and sewing and decorating. In his earlier erotic dreams his sexual partner was another boy who was making love to him. In masturbation he fancied a man, strong and powerful, appearing in the nude. As he grew to adult life, he felt no desire to be with a woman, no thrill when dancing. He went on dates and liked girls to talk to—but never to make love to. However, the desire to be loved by a man was intense—a desire he fought consciously. He became fearful that he might fail to control his growing impulses, especially when one day, as he was addressing a class of men, it seemed as though all the individuals fused into one, and this one appeared as a huge penis. He became panicky, trembling, weak, and perspiring. He came for help to prevent trouble, presenting symptoms of anxiety. No outward expression of homosexuality had become manifest and hence the term, psychopathy, is not altogether correct.

Another case which illustrates this type of sexual deviation is that of P. L., who describes himself as a model boy, the only child of a widowed mother. "I was Mamma's boy and teacher's pet. I used to love to cut out dolls and design costumes. I remember I even played the role of a nun. I wanted to be a nun. I was taught to sew and cook and paint. I seemed to be afraid of boys – upset by them.

"My mother lived a chaotic life. She wanted to enter a convent but was forced into the business world. Then I came – an illegitimate child. I was something of an inconvenience at first but later I became a special charge. She wanted to take care of me – make me a perfect specimen. I was kept clean and neatly dressed and I stayed close to her. Then she 'remarried' – a large man who terrified me.

"When I was 12 years of age I began to masturbate and used to fantasy not *myself* but two men engaged in homosexual practices. As I grew older, all ideas of sex frightened me because I thought such ideas would offend my ideal of my mother. I took out girls – but never felt any thrill – never had any desire to caress or kiss them. But I felt an attraction to men – and I realized I was different. I tried to cultivate a feeling for women but it was no use – they left me cold. I became interested in a man. I loved to see him, to be with him, but I fought my impulses. I became disturbed, confused, weak."

This patient was a tall, normal appearing young adult, highly intelligent, struggling to contend with homosexual impulses. The cause of his deviation could be psychological, complete identification with his mother to whom he was unduly attached and who cultivated feminine traits in him. He feared his stepfather, could not compete with men. It was easier to be a woman than a man. Yet one cannot dismiss the significant, even if unseen, forces of glandular imbalance. Many male homosexuals exhibit a feminine type of body build, mannerisms of women, and accentuate this by dressing differently. So, too, female homosexuals may have masculine body build and dress mannishly. They show their deviations even though no environmental forces compel them in such directions.

It is remarkable that this patient has thus far combated his tendencies. There are other homosexuals, both male and female, who accept their deviations as something they cannot control or, in rare instances, as something to be proud of. They find partners with whom they fall in love, with whom they live in close association, or they depend upon casual "pickups" for sexual gratification. Some work together as members of a dance group or a band; others meet in certain neighborhoods of a large city. They indulge in various types of sexual practice, including mutual masturbation, oral or anal sexual experiences. Others are content to be in each other's presence like two Platonic lovers.

Many homosexuals are unhappy since they recognize the social ban imposed upon their "natural" impulses. Such individuals fear detection and punishment by society. Therefore they may seek subterfuges, as did one patient who used to admire male figures in physical culture magazines and who attended gymnasium regularly. He preferred wrestling, challenging powerful opponents from whose tactics he gained some sexual thrills. Others maintain rigid control until alcoholism weakens inhibitions and the two pals in a bar end up in a bedroom. Yet there is usually anxiety, doubt, and nervousness about such experiences. Many homosexuals either become ill nervously or are apprehended by civil authorities and punished. Some courts are more understanding and realize that homosexuality is an illness, not merely wickedness.

A useful classification of homosexuality is given in Myerson's section of the *Manual of Military Neuropsychiatry:* "There are three main groups of male homosexuals, and in a rough way the study of the hormone content of the urine corresponds with the clinical deviation.

"*First Group:* There is a homosexuality by cultural pressure, deprivation, or through the motive of financial gain. Thus, wherever the male is shut off from sexual relationship with the female, homosexuality springs up even in individuals who ordinarily would be heterosexual. Moreover, certain cultures and certain localities tend to emphasize homosexuality. The Greek culture, as exemplified by Plato's classical dialogue, placed homosexuality on a decidedly loftier and more ideal plane than the natural relationships of the sexes. . . .

"*Second Group:* This group is more biological in its origin. This is the type of homosexuality which is on the basis of endocrine disturbance. Such individuals are characterized by marked deficiency of either male or female hormones, or both, and the presence of the outward stigmata of endocrine disturbance, such as inferior genitalia, signs of pituitary disturbance, and less easily described but quite patent inferiority. . . .

"*Third Group:* This group we have called the true homosexuals. The true homosexual is one who from his earliest days on has been aroused sexually by males, and who either is without any sexual desire for the female or regards such relationship with loathing. . . ."

The homosexuality which results from the pressure of environment can be helped when the environment improves and the opportunities for more natural love relationships are made possible. Those whose deviation is the result of endocrine imbalance may be helped by sex hormones. I have seen two patients who have been definitely improved with male sex hormone (oreton) therapy. Psychoanalysis may be of some benefit to the other types. However, the results in general are not too promising for the true homosexuals.

Problems of the Psychopaths in Service

The success of an army depends upon leadership and team play. The teamwork of the smaller units, in the last analysis, depends upon the capacity of the smallest unit, the individual soldier, to cooperate. A dash of psychopathy is good seasoning for any soldier. It makes for spiciness, for acting with reckless abandon. It may account for certain deeds of valor, and one need not investigate if the "hero" was prompted by desire for exhibitionism or by a spirit of revenge against the enemy. His achievements are commendable. Indeed, if the play, *The Vagabond King*, be historically true, Francois Villon saved France from the Duke of Burgundy by a rabble army released from jails, to whom Villon appealed with the stirring song, "Oh, you sons of sin and sorrow, prepare yourselves for tomorrow."

Thus an element of psychopathy may be helpful. Picture the paratrooper swaggering down the streets of Columbus, Georgia, the jaunty walk, the pride in the distinctive uniform.

The psychopath may find success in the armed forces. Certain features of warfare activity – periods of rest and of violent activity, attacking the enemy as an outlet for aggressiveness – provide a tempo of life which is geared to his make-up. Thus a civilian who is bored and restless, who craves change, excitement and action, is thrilled with his uniform and his career as a paratrooper or in a submarine. He may exert just enough self-control to restrain impulses which might prove troublesome. His traits of character, impulsiveness, defiance, aggressiveness, may catapult him into the role of heroism. I have known of a soldier whose civilian record was one of instability and maladjustment and who was a problem of ineptness and discipline in his outfit. One day in combat he found himself aroused to a pitch of anger; he defied the order to retreat and went forward, bayonet in hand, hurling grenades. Unmindful of danger, he proceeded to attack, killing several Germans and taking prisoners. He was rewarded for his heroism and thereafter continued to exhibit feats of bravery.

Gillespie tells of a soldier who in civilian life was inadequate, unstable and anxious, who had been unable to hold any one job for more than a few months, but who "has, in the Services, succeeded, after a struggle, in being an efficient although not yet self-assured soldier."

Mira considers war conditions as likely to benefit rather than aggravate psychopathic personalities, since war provides a source of stimuli powerful enough to forget one's own conflicts.

Unfortunately, however, success is not the rule. If the psychopathy be more marked in the paratrooper whom we admired walking down the streets of Columbus, Georgia, we are likely to see a sadder picture hours later. We may witness the paratrooper staggering along, his hair disheveled, eyes bloodshot, clothes muddy, face bruised, being convoyed by an M. P. to the guardhouse.

The psychopath who fails is more common than the one who succeeds. Thus Harrison states that psychopaths constitute the third largest group of mental disabilities in the peacetime Navy, and in war they are the second largest. Patients with emotional instability are the most frequent, while the inadequate type comes second.

Mira described three forms of psychopathic reactions in the Spanish War. One type became nervously sick, worried and introverted in trying to repress his feelings of fear and disgust. This mood might explode in a "fit" or be dissipated. Another type developed an ever-growing resentment toward his leaders. The third, perhaps the most frequent and the most difficult to handle, expressed itself by an escape into alcoholism and drunkenness. (Alcoholism will be considered more extensively later in this chapter.)

"The psychopath," says Colonel Porter, "forms the largest class of mental deviates with which the Army has to deal... Some psychopathic individuals never succeed in being fitted into the military scheme. Their nuisance value is high. They take more of the time and energies of the company, non-commissioned officers, unit commanders and medical officers than their services deserve. However, there is frequently the feeling that the psychopath attempts to evade duty by artful design and by wilful insubordination. The temptation is strong to compel him to do military duty at whatever cost. Discipline, change of duties, personal counsel are sometimes successful in correcting the faults. However, under the exigencies of military service, it is more often necessary to discharge such a man because his nuisance value outweighs his virtues. Some aggressive psychopaths find an outlet for their antisocial feelings in action against the enemy and do well in combat organizations. The inadequate, passive types are not apt to do well because of their inability to make the personal adjustments necessary to comfortable group life. The sexual invert gets along well as long as he is discreet. If not, he becomes a social pariah to the other men and the very fact that he is a known homosexual reflects in his efficiency record, and antagonistic attitudes often precipitate mental crises of various kinds."

Many psychopaths try to get out of the Army, some by exaggeration of symptoms, others through persistent wasteful conduct, and a few even create symptoms or malinger. Porter mentions the item of bed-wetting as a symptom occurring in psychopathy and states, "One must remember that occasionally a soldier will attempt to float out of the Army in a sea of urine." So too, there are those who shuffle out with a gait disorder, and I know of one officer who vomited his way out. The problem of malingering will be taken up briefly later in this chapter.

The decision about discharging a psychopath depends not upon the diagnosis but upon the measure of his service to the Army. Some are a loss to the Service; the Army gains by their discharge. Others are capable individuals who, resolved to exercise self-control, may be salvaged.

It is my understanding that other armies treat psychopaths differently. In the German Army the criminal psychopath is confined to jail; the other types are retained in service. The majority are formed into a special battalion which is sent forward to receive the initial impact of the enemy. Interspersed with this special battalion are enough loyal, efficient soldiers to keep them from deserting. Yet my informant explained that many of the psychopaths of such battalions were among the first to desert and to surrender in the North African campaign. Mira stated that it was the practice in the Spanish Loyalist Army to retain psychopaths capable of making vocational adjustments but to discharge those with a severe and evident hereditary taint, whose reaction tendencies had made them unsuitable for social life and had required previous institutional care.

The Psychopath in Industry

The psychopath in ordinary life constitutes a problem to his family and to society as a whole. The psychopath, if and when he works, may become a problem in industry. He is likely to be unsteady and unreliable, taking time off for rest and recreation without consideration for his duty to his fellow workmen. Furthermore, he may be fault-finding, blaming others for any mistakes and feeling that he is mistreated. There is a tendency to accident proneness among psychopaths when they are depressed, impulsive, or emotionally disturbed. In such accidents, the psychopath unconsciously punishes others and thus gains a peculiar advantage. Following such an accident, it is not rare to have a prolonged period of disability, for the psychopath may have a neurotic tendency and the disability affords an opportunity for indulging in self-pity and inviting attention. The more aggressive types will become quarrelsome, arguing with personnel directors, dissatisfied with physicians, threatening lawsuits. Such was the conduct of V. G., whose case history is taken from my book, *The Mind of the Injured Man:*

> V. G., a young man in the early twenties, was injured in August, 1936, straining his neck muscles when he reached upwards. "I felt a snap in my neck, but I continued working. Later I had pain and was sent to a doctor. The doctor said it was something serious and placed me in the hospital."
> This patient was treated with a Thomas collar because of a suspected fracture, but in six weeks was permitted to be up and allowed to go to work. He worked for a few days and then gave up. For three years this man has been unemployed. He has the following complaints: "I have pain in the back of my neck; I can't find a comfortable position; I get nervous, can't sleep; sometimes I can't move my arms and legs." He expressed marked bitterness towards the doctor who treated him and towards the company. "They wanted me to go to work, but I was too sick. I think they gave me a job with an electrician so that I would be electrocuted. They want to kill me."
> The physical examination, including a complete neurologic study, was negative. The condition was at first thought to be a neurosis. This young man was seen several times later, after a summer outdoors. He looked swarthy and tanned and extremely healthy. He proudly announced that he had been drinking as much as two quarts a day. When asked about returning to work, he remarked, with a surly expression, "I'll get even with that manager. He'll know how I feel when he has his neck broken."
> Some weeks later he again appeared at my office, with a sarcastic smile, and began to upbraid the various medical

men he had seen. "A nerve specialist gave me some tablets. They were brown, but I was too smart for him. I opened up this tablet; the inside was white, nothing but flour. All the doctors ever give me is dope."

On his hand were several bruises, and when he was asked about these marks, he replied proudly, "I went to a clam bake the other day. I had good eats and drinks. When I drink, I like to fight. There was a beautiful girl in another party and I went over to 'make her.' There were 17 men in that party and you should have seen what I did to all of them. You know, it's easier for me to fight 17 than to fight one."

It is remarkable that this young man, whose physique would be a credit to any "physical culture" magazine, has so many complaints of weakness and pain. There is a notable inconsistency in the complaints about his helplessness and the braggadocio about his fighting prowess. He has a marked feeling of resentment towards the doctors who have seen him and the company that formerly employed him. His attitude is so irritable and resentful that it resembles the armed resentfulness of a paranoid. On several occasions, with flashing eyes, he expressed threats of homicide against the employment manager of the company for which he worked.

It is quite obvious that we are dealing with an abnormal personality which is undoubtedly inherent. The family physician stated that the family background was unstable and abnormal. V. G. had been a problem of discipline at home and at school. Later his work record was unstable – he changed jobs often for alleged mistreatment or because of "weakness." Then he sustained an injury upon which, like a paranoid, he projected all blame. He spends his time carousing about, apparently enjoying himself and, at the same time, fighting with symptoms and with legal aid, to be declared totally disabled so that he may receive $18.75 per week for the rest of his life.

A psychopath is often as much a troublemaker at work as when he is in the army. Sometimes he carries out a personal sabotage, again he may organize a rebellion. He fails to contribute his share to the common effort, casts blame upon others, invites accidents, or uses sickness as an escape and as a method of getting even. Industrial boards and courts should consider the constitutional psychopath when they meet certain claimants and litigants.

The Nature of the Psychopath

There is a little of the psychopath in all of us, which appears under favorable circumstances like dandelions on a lawn after a warm rain in spring. We may exhibit minor psychopathic traits for a time or show intense symptoms briefly. It is the intensity of the behavior deviation and, of course, its duration that characterize the psychopath. Fortunately there are not too many real psychopaths.

What is the cause of this condition? Although we recognize its manifestations, we are as yet ignorant of the cause. Some attribute this deviation to a faulty brain, others to failure in adjustment early in life. By definition, it is innate, constitutional. Gillespie says, "There are theoretically two senses in which the word 'constitution' can be applied to mental constitution: the congenital, probably inherited constitution, and the acquired – the latter being the result of persistent maladaptive reactions to experiences, so early encountered that the individual's mental development is ever afterward biased by them." Henderson suggests also that there is a disturbance in the energy endowment which accounts for periods of inadequacy, for explosive outbursts, and for impulsiveness. Certainly the early onset and its continuity favor an organic basis. This view is supported by the frequency of abnormal brain wave patterns among psychopaths. Indeed, Silverman reported 75 per cent of psychopaths as showing abnormal waves.

Noyes prefers to interpret the psychopathic personality as the product of psychic forces in conflict with environment: "As in all other human behavior, one must not unobservantly assume that the behavior of the psychopath, or the factors and steps that have gradually formed his character, may be explained on the basis of consciously rational motives. . The behavior may be reduced to an intrapsychic conflict, attempts to solve which are tried through adjustments that are socially inadequate or destructive. . . . Obstinacy, vindictiveness, or a disregard for ethical and social standards may represent efforts to compensate for the treatment received in childhood from a domineering and cruel parent. . . Society may represent to the criminal those persons in his childhood life toward whom he felt a hostility which he could not express."

It is my belief that the basic cause of psychopathy is an inborn defect, not necessarily visible in the brain cells but manifested by impaired social adjustment. Yet one cannot dismiss the influence of reactions to the environment, for life is more complicated than the laboratory and life does not separate tendency from contacts. Granting a constitutional impairment, the challenges, the impacts, the example and influence of people may determine the course of the behavior – lying, stealing, quarreling, nomadism. Just what is the nature of the defect?

It appears to me that the defect rests in a failure or a delay in the development of the faculty of inhibition. The infant, born helpless and dependent, still possesses the instinct to grasp, own, engulf any object in its environment. Its first movements are crude, weak, and clumsy. Growth of the brain and learning enable the infant to restrict its attention from every object to one specific article, to move one finger skillfully and not the entire hand clumsily. More important than learning coordinated muscle action is learning to live with the group. To acquire deftness and skill in walking, dancing, and skating, and in writing, painting, playing an instrument requires brain development. Even more development is needed to regard the wishes of others, to respect their views, to sympathize with their feelings, to perform one's duty in the face of obstacles, to postpone pleasure for the sake of the future, to set aside personal gratification for the good of the group. As we grow from infancy to adulthood, we acquire such capacity, which is largely the ability to identify ourselves with others and to inhibit our selfish desires or actions. A child whose brain has been damaged by injury or infection may become overactive, move about restlessly, lack control of muscle and actions; so the psychopath fails to acquire normal control.

Glueck undoubtedly interprets the problem in a similar way when he says, "The psychopath presents a certain playful childishness, an incapacity for removal or for identification of his emotions with those of his victims, an impulsiveness, a lack of planfulness, a reckless courage fluctuating with abject cowardice." The qualities of maturity, according to Glueck, bring great powers of reflection, inhibition, postponement of immediate desires for more legitimate later ones, the capacity of learning from experience. There is a delay in maturity of the psychopath.

Not all psychopaths are aggressive and criminal; some are inadequate, "weak sisters," pathetic. Others appear charming, talking smoothly, impressive and convincing; time, however, shows that their words were not backed up by worth.

Psychopathy does not always continue and maturity, though

delayed, may finally arrive. This explains the experience which Myerson has stressed: "Many people we call psychopaths recover; that is to say, in earlier years they show disorganization in the sexual, economic and conduct field which seems definitely psychopathic, but as time goes on they settle down and become conventional in their ways of life. . . . The reform process was slow in coming, but at twenty-five and thirty, the normal or at least conventional conduct became asserted and part of the habit of the individual."

Treatment of Psychopathy

From the military standpoint, selection at the Induction Station should exclude the serious psychopaths. Behavior records, records of arrests and sentences, should be made available to Selective Service, just as industrial and financial statements are obtained. For if such information is concealed, the psychopath can glibly describe himself as a model man and a loyal citizen. The following example of misguided patriotism on the part of a judge and concealment on the part of the soldier came to my notice.

B. F. had run away from home at the age of 14, lived as a vagabond for several years, had been arrested several times for vagrancy and for minor thefts, then drank frequently, had several fights, and finally stole a car. He had worked very little from the age of 16 to 22. When he was tried for auto theft, the judge studied the healthy physique of his "culprit" and remembered the Army's need for manpower. Waving an American flag and in a voice vibrant with patriotic zeal, he spoke, "Young man, you ought to be ashamed of yourself! I should send you to jail, but our country needs you. I'll give you one more chance. If you'll go over to the recruiting station and volunteer, I'll suspend the sentence."

The young man, faced with a long period of imprisonment, responded, "Your Honor, you've shown me my path to duty!"

He hurried across the street to the recruiting station, denied any health or social problems, "forgot" arrests, and was soon in uniform. Within six weeks as a soldier, he resumed his habits—drinking, going A.W.O.L., and finally developing serious nervous symptoms. Proper selection would have spared the Army the burden, first of training, secondly, of hospitalizing, and finally, of discharging a man whose record, if obtainable, would have excluded him. Fortunately, in many states, fairly adequate studies are made before a civilian becomes a soldier. Ebaugh has outlined a plan for collecting social service data on selectees in a state like Texas, comparable to procedures already used in other states. All states should consider it their responsibility to supply such data so as to save the Army (and thus themselves) the burden of hospitalization and later discharge.

As regards treatment, in the hope of making a useful citizen out of the psychopath, something can be done for him whose trouble is not too serious. Discipline will temporarily deter some psychopaths from repeating the misconduct or the crime. A change of duty towards one which requires more action puts the person in the limelight and may afford a useful outlet for the aggressive instincts. Then too, the mild psychopath in service may respond to the influence of the new group to which he is assigned, or he may be influenced by the authority and guidance of his officers. Such methods are worthy of trial even if they are not regularly rewarded by success.

Little can be done for the psychopath, though Schilder advocates analysis. Most physicians agree with Bleuler when he says, "The treatment of the psychopathies is not a very grateful task, for one cannot naturally change them; one must try to get along with them. It is important to create an interest, an aim for which the patients would strive, whereby definite traits of character, even if no virtues in themselves, such as vanity and pride, should often be made use of unreservedly, but should be developed within proper bounds. If the patient shows a helpless apathy toward useful occupation, he can perhaps be interested in sport, art, in some scientific hobby. At the same time, real work must never be neglected. In most cases it is impossible to educate the patients in the milieu in which they grew up; they must be taken elsewhere. The closed institution can in some regards accomplish more than the open one." Antisocial psychopaths who violate laws are confined to prison. Such confinement may not be ideal, but thus far psychiatry cannot offer society a more practical solution. There is also the hope that age, growing older, will reinforce the failing inhibitions, or, as Glueck states, "if the acts of delinquency began early in life, they were largely abandoned at a relatively early stage of manhood." Quoting once more from Myerson: "Even the so-called constitutional psychopath can learn finally that his conduct does not pay or, as I often put it, when the endocrines stop boiling, the forebrain gets a chance to work more in harmony with the better purposes of the individual."

The psychopath frequently exhibits symptoms of psychoneurotic or depressive types. Such symptoms can be improved by rational psychotherapy – discussion and reassurance. For an attempt to alter the deeper character formation, Schilder considers a deep analysis necessary – and hypnosis useless. Says Schilder, "Characters are the crystallizations of attempts at social adjustment, and we can speak of psychopathy when this attempt has not been very successful from the point of view of society. It is obvious that this pattern formation takes place at an early age, that constitutional characters and organic changes are of importance, and that the relation of father and mother is of decisive importance. The character formation of the psychopath offers great resistance against analysis."

As we embark upon an extensive program of rehabilitation for the veteran, we must not forget the psychopath. Whatever aid we give the veteran in the form of special financial assistance, retraining, treatment must take into account the soldier's pre-military record and his service to his country. We can never do too much to assist the conscientious soldier who fought in battle, who became ill while serving, or was wounded in combat. But we must beware the appeals of the psychopaths (especially the pathologic liars and swindlers). Such a one may have had a bad record throughout his life, yet blame the service for his "pitiable condition of nerves." He may strut on the street, his chest expanded with campaign ribbons (illegally gotten), while in his coat pocket is a blue discharge (without honor) deservedly given. This type of psychopath has contributed the least, complained the loudest, and will demand the most.

Lest the foregoing seem to malign the psychopath, it should be stated that the impulsiveness and individuality of some psychopaths become traits which are socially advantageous. Such persons may become colorful characters in the world of sport; they may leave the security of the group to become explorers and pioneers, daredevils to venture into risky endeavors. Indeed, one may mention the remark of Bleuler, "Psychopaths and insane, such as Mohammed, Luther, Loyola, Rousseau, Pestallozzi,

Napoleon, and Robert Meyer, have influenced the course of our civilization in a fateful and beneficent manner."

Malingering

Malingering is the falsifying of sickness for a purpose. The alleged patient claims symptoms that are nonexistent, acts ill, or inflicts damage upon his person to obtain compensation or to escape unpleasant situations. Norris subdivides malingering into four groups: (1) invention of symptoms, (2) exaggeration or fraudulent magnification, (3) perseveration – or false continuation of previous symptoms, and (4) transference, or attributing to one cause symptoms that arise from another source. Norris states, "Soldiers and other service men may seek to evade the dangers and hardships of war, or even the dull routine of barrack life by inventing or exploiting illness ... e.g., self-inflicted gunshot wounds, or poisoning by cordite or by picric acid. Costedat, quoted by Norris, called attention to the existence of establishments near military camps or barracks in which an unscrupulous chemist or other person was prepared, for a small payment, to induce an abscess by the subcutaneous injection of an irritating substance.

In my experience, clear-cut malingering is uncommon. Emphasis upon symptoms – the group labeled exaggeration by Norris – is relatively common. When the situation is tough, the soldier who has sustained an injury or developed an illness may cling to his symptoms tenaciously. Fear, anxiety, interest, all contribute to this overemphasis so that this tendency hardly deserves an odious label which appropriately belongs to conscious purpose, planning, perpetration, deceit. Malingering is insincere, dishonest... exaggeration is too near normal, and may be normal.

CASE HISTORY OF MALINGERING IN SERVICE

B. M., recently inducted into service, attempted to simulate mental symptoms. During drill he was seen to stand in a blank manner, to stare long into space. Even in barracks at night he sat alone, mumbling. Several days later he refused all food, ignored those who approached or addressed him. He was therefore hospitalized and studied on a neuropsychiatric ward.

When he finally answered questions, he stated that God was warning him not to eat, that some calamity would overtake America. Indeed, on the next day he held on tightly to the wall because he could feel the building rocking. Sadly he awaited his doom, listening to voices and mumbling a reply.

While the medical staff pondered over this problem, light came to them in the form of a visitor, an agent from the F. B. I. He inquired about B. M. and casually dropped the hint that the name of B. M. had been found on the records of a "fraudulent" school which was teaching men to act insane. The doctors tried intravenous amytal as a "truth drug" and the patient became loquacious and honest. "Yes," he said, "I went to that fellow and he told me how to act and what to say. It wasn't my fault. My mother made me do it. She said she would die if I was sent across. So she took me there. I was told to act this way at the Induction Station, but I didn't have the nerve to start it then. But in the Army it got kinda tough and at night I was lonesome. So I began to sort of hear the voices which I was taught. Then I realized I could get out of the Army and go back home if I kept on hearing the voices."

This is an example of malingering in a soldier whose past record was psychopathic. He had done poorly at school. He worked irregularly, leaving job after job because of alleged weakness and unfavorable working conditions. He spent much time "loafing," left home many times, and quarreled often with his father. Many a time his mother's intervention saved him from violence at the hands of his father. For our patient was unstable, sensitive to the least rebuke, slow to serve, quick to suspect. Whenever an unpleasant duty presented itself, he "played sick," left town, or cleverly proved that the job ought not to be done.

Brussel and Hitch consider that almost every malingerer has a psychopathic personality. His effort in avoiding responsibility, his lack of remorse, his troublemaking are psychopathic traits. However, some malingerers do not have a past record of psychopathy, but their feigning of illness is planned definitely to meet or solve a specific situation. Myerson calls attention to the observation that malingering increases by leaps and bounds as one passes from the Induction Station to the camp or training center, and to the combat zone. The relation of situation to malingering is even more apparent in a statement by a Russian psychiatrist, Ossipov:

"Malingering in its pure form appears usually in times of great social upheaval when punishments for crimes are very severe or when the situation is such that one's life is threatened.

In such periods large numbers of people develop defense reactions by means of which they hope to escape punishment or death. Thus there were quite a few cases of malingering in the U. S. S. R. during the civil war... In the days before the revolution there was malingering to avoid military service; at the present time one hardly finds this."

Myerson mentions the frequency with which amnesia is claimed in wartime, in contrast to its rarity in civilian practice. "In most cases," he says, "the loss of memory has been a cover and an escape for delinquency or some way to cut the Gordian knot of a tangled situation in which the individual has become enmeshed, and since one does not punish a sick man, he simulates a sickness difficult to disprove, to wit, amnesia."

My personal experience is in agreement with the above statement. There come to mind three instances of amnesia, one civilian and two in the armed forces. The first case is that of a woman who bruised her own forehead with a brick, slumped to the ground, and was picked up and brought to a hospital. She acted in a blank manner for several days, until the hospital physician, puzzled by her behavior, made plans to commit her to a mental hospital. Some time later, when questioned critically, she explained to me that this "acting ill" was a technique she had used to get out of tense, threatening situations:

CASE HISTORY OF MALINGERING IN CIVILIAN LIFE

Mrs. R. B. was referred by her physician, Dr. Marcus, because of the history of a head injury, with such symptoms as headaches, dizziness, and forgetfulness. She had been brought to the emergency room of a Cleveland hospital after she had been found in a stuporous state, lying at the curb on the street. The police emergency had brought her to the hospital in this "unconscious" condition. The examination by the physician in the accident room revealed bruises over the forehead. Obviously there was a suspicion of a concussion, and this patient was admitted to the hospital and observed carefully. X-rays of the head were made, blood pressure was taken regularly, and even a spinal puncture was done because of the suspicion of a serious head injury. The skull x-rays were negative, the puncture showed no blood, and there were apparently no positive neurologic signs other than the stupor and blankness. This patient remained in a coma-like state for 96 hours and then became alert gradually. On the fifth day she was able to respond to questions. She improved rapidly and was allowed to go home, diagnosed as a case of concussion.

It was two weeks after this episode that this woman was referred to me for examination. As is the usual procedure with head injury cases, a detailed inquiry was started and the patient was asked to explain precisely and minutely how she was hurt. Her replies were vague and evasive; the more obscure she became, the more definite were the questions put before her. Such a detailed investigation was made not because I suspected malingering, but in the hope of guiding an individual whose memory might have been affected, to recall more accurately how she was hurt. The patient lowered her head, tears came into her eyes, and she sobbed: "I guess you have caught me, so I had better tell you my whole story. My childhood was very unhappy, largely because of a stern stepfather. Whatever went wrong at home brought punishment. I was blamed and often severely beaten if I ever did anything out of the way. Even if my report card was poor, I would be disciplined and often punished. I loved to read and I remember the story of a little girl who was found unconscious and taken to a hospital. Her picture was in the paper and it showed her surrounded by toys and the article described how the whole town was interested in identifying this lovely girl who could not remember her name.

"Several days after I read this story I did something naughty in school and the teacher gave me a note to give to my parents. You may imagine how terrified I was and how faint and weak I became as I walked slowly home carrying in my purse the note which surely would bring the painful beatings by my father. As I walked, feeling trembly and weak, the thought flashed through my mind, 'What if I were found unconscious, wouldn't it be nicer to be in the hospital and given the things I would like?' And almost immediately my legs gave way under me and I slipped to the ground unconscious. People hurried and shook me and I half heard them, but I made no effort to awaken. I acted 'dead' and I can remember the crowd forming and the ambulance coming. It was quite thrilling to be lifted into the ambulance and taken to the hospital. The doctor came and talked to me, but, though I half heard him, I acted blank and did not answer. When my mother and father came, they stood sadly by the bedside, their faces becoming wrinkled and worried when the doctor spoke of a serious coma and perhaps sleeping sickness.

"My parents stayed at the bedside; they brought me candy and flowers and toys. Inwardly, I felt happy when my father and mother told me of how sorry they were for the treatment they had given me and how kind they would be if only I would get well. I kept on acting this way for several days and then one morning I woke up alert and happy. Deep in my mind I felt that I had won a victory, for I had escaped a beating; for the first time in my life, my stepfather was sympathetic and talked sweetly to me.

"Three or four times in my life I have resorted to the same escape. When I felt sure that I might get a beating, or later when I was threatened with a serious situation which I could not solve, I would automatically sink into unconsciousness.

"Recently things were going very badly at home, my husband was quarrelsome, creditors were pressing us, and I just could not face my responsibilities. I was working to help out financially, but my job was very unpleasant. I had consulted an attorney about a divorce, and the thought of going to court upset me terribly. One evening, worn and weary from the day's unpleasant work, dragging myself home to a place where there would be quarreling and bickering, I so longed for a rest or for freedom. How nice it would be to have someone take care of me, someone be kind to me. Just then I remembered that I wasn't far from a hospital and so I could not resist the impulse to go behind a building, pick up a large brick, and scrape it against my forehead. And then when the street seemed empty, I walked to the curb and allowed myself to slump, face forward, on the pavement. Once again, people gathered about me and an ambulance was called; I was rushed to the hospital. I acted as though I was in coma for several days, but when the doctors talked about sending me to the psychopathic ward of City Hospital, I awoke."

In the Army I recall several examples of amnesia "put on" to assist the person in a troubled period. W. E. became bored with Army routine, got lonesome for his wife, dreamt of hunting in the woods in the fall. The longing to be free, to visit his family, to hunt, became irresistible. One day he left his post and arrived home, stating that he was on leave. He was happy to be with his wife and was thrilled with a sense of boyish irresponsibility as he tramped the woods, a rifle on his shoulder. For two weeks he enjoyed this freedom. Then came fear that he would be apprehended and court-martialed. He left his family to return to camp. En route, he was confused, lost, and decided to state that he didn't know what he was doing. "I must have wandered away without knowing where I was going. I must have been in a daze. Suddenly I woke up . . . and then I realized I was A.W.O.L."

At first W. E. reiterated the story of utter blankness, of not knowing who he was, where he had been, of automatic behavior. He was given an injection of sodium amytal intravenously and was encouraged to review in detail every step of his departure and of his two weeks' vacation. He succeeded in accurately recalling his activity (which real amnesia cases cannot do) and finally told the real facts about his going.

Another example is that of a pretty WAC, who was A.W.O.L. several days upon her return from a furlough. She was found wandering in the street and did not recall her name, her home or her destination. The complete cloud lifted several days later. She responded to the friendly questioning of the examiner with a statement of what had occurred. "I was miserable in the WAC. It wasn't what I expected. One day I got a wire that my mother was ill and I asked for a furlough. There was a stopover at the railway station of several hours, so I started to walk. A man met me and we had a few beers . . . anything to "forget" my troubles. I liked him and we spent several days together. It was grand not to have to get up for drill, not to obey orders, and so I stayed. Then I became afraid I'd be picked up by the M.P. So I acted dazed and blank and turned in at this hospital." Although this case has many features of hysteria, it exemplifies the conscious acting of illness for a purpose.

There are many gradations of malingering from the school boy who plays sick so that he can stay home on a day of examinations to the person who acts crippled after an accident so as to obtain a large settlement. We consider the former type as normal and smilingly accept it. The latter is a form of dishonesty which we condemn. Yet deceit by sickness to obtain material gain is far less common than swindling, selling fraudulent securities, and other thieving techniques of cunning psychopaths who would rather spend days scheming to outwit their fellow men than work for a few hours to obtain the same material gains. Such faking of illness is antisocial and harmful even though some authors consider malingering as unconsciously motivated, however material the obvious goal may be. Allowing this point of view, the practical attitude still demands the detection and proper disposition of the malingerer.

There is no simple formula for detection; it requires alert attention, careful study, plus individual techniques for specific problems. The experienced physician suspects fraud when the patient's story doesn't ring true. Myerson says, "For the detection of the malingerer, psychiatrists must possess and manifest the wisdom of the serpent and the guilelessness of the dove."

Ossipov presents some useful points in detecting those who feign a psychosis: "Every malingerer is an actor who portrays an illness as he understands it . . . A carefully conducted interview often reveals malingering, especially if the malingerer is caught contradicting himself. In imitating the behavior of a psychotic patient, the malingerer goes to extremes . . . When someone shakes hands with him, he uses the left hand instead of the right. Another malingerer when going to sleep puts on his glasses and lights his pipe." Ossipov mentions the example of one criminal who for more than a year was in a state of stupor and then burst out laughing when his attorney made a comical remark about him during the trial. Then and there he stated that he was tired of acting and confessed the crime.

To detect malingering may be simple or proves a challenge for a diagnostic Solomon. A critical history can reveal inconsistencies; the examination shows bizarre behavior which does not fit common patterns. Special mental tests may disclose conscious efforts to deceive (Minnesota Multiphasic). Sodium amytal may dissolve the conscious wariness or reduce the resistance of the patient. Technical procedures (electroencephalograms in cases of alleged blindness, the tuning fork pressure test (Fetterman) for alleged pain, the dynamometer for hand-weakness) have a field of usefulness. Detection is important, for malingering must be discouraged.

ALCOHOLISM

Alcoholism may be defined as the irresistible tendency to drink to an unhealthy degree physically or socially. It is a fairly common condition which often begins innocently but may end tragically. At the outset, the pathological drinker does not appear any different from the everyday, normal, social drinker. But in the course of years, the abnormality is recognized when a man spends a week's pay in an overnight round of bars and reels home unsteadily, or when a wife conceals a bottle of liquor from her husband and consumes it stealthily alone, neglecting all her duties.

In its pathological form alcoholism may lead to one or several neuropsychiatric conditions:
1. Impairment of personality
2. Neurologic disturbances, tremors, unsteady gait, polyneuritis, epilepsy (so-called whisky fits)
3. Delirium tremens
4. Alcoholic hallucinosis
5. Korsakoff's syndrome

PERSONALITY CHANGES—CHARACTER DEFECTS

Often there is an underlying defect to account for chronic alcoholism, for it isn't the alcohol that pursues the man, it is the need in the man that craves for and finds the alcohol. There are those who consider alcoholism a psychoneurosis – a form of insecurity and maladjustment which seeks for an escape in drinking. Others believe that states of depression lead to the use of alcohol as a means of getting a lift. Then there are some persons who are latent homosexuals and who find in the camaraderie and the socialization of the bar a legitimate expression of forbidden instincts.

Such deviations of personality may be responsible for the chronic tendency to drink. But the result of repeated drinking produces additional changes, both primary and secondary. The person loses interest in the higher ideals of life, fails to plan or work towards success, and just drifts along. He tends to neglect his job or his duties socially. He makes excuses, lies in order to get away to drink. Then he goes through periods of remorse with self-blame for his inability to keep his promise not to drink heavily any more. Or the person may become quarrelsome, projecting blame upon others for their admonitions or inhibitions.

Says Mrs. L. D.: "This drinking is my husband's fault, not mine. It's because he says I can't drink any more that I do it - for spite, just to prove to him that I am not a baby and that he can't boss me." Thus spoke a woman of 35 who began to drink socially in her early twenties. Later she consumed more liquor: "I'd have six or seven highballs in an evening, sometimes doubleheaders - and I'd wash them down with beer."

At the age of thirty she married and in the following years had two children. Yet, though she had a fine husband, two young children, and a nice home, the drinking continued: "I'd get bored with everything - tired of keeping house, so I drank. As soon as my husband went to work, I'd hurry to the liquor store to get a quart - and I'd drink most of it during the day. Of course I didn't keep my house in order and sometimes I'd neglect the children."

This patient was placed in a hospital but resented her husband's efforts to help her. At first she dismissed the subject of her drinking as entirely due to her husband's bossiness. Later, when she felt free, she told the above story of her drinking.

The outstanding symptoms included a lack of a sense of duty, neglect of her responsibilities, frequent lying to her husband - symptoms which suggest psychopathic personality.

It seems as though the use of alcohol has subtracted something from the already defective personality and results in a weakening of character. The patient fails in his duties and resorts to self-blame occasionally: "Oh, what a louse I am to go drinking again when I should be doing my work." More often, however, he will conceal and lie about drinking or continue to project blame upon others.

In the course of years, there is a weakening of resolve and ambition, like a shore that is washed away by the waves. At first the individual has been able to maintain a certain integrity and to keep his job. Later, however, he confesses to his failure, stays away from home. He is disowned by the family, divorced by his wife, and ultimately may end up as a resident in some wayfarers' lodge. This is the path which certain severe alcoholics descend.

M. F. was brought to the hospital in a disheveled state, clothes tattered, face unshaven, lips dry - a strong odor of alcohol on his breath. He pleaded that he be treated because he was nervous and sleepless. He gave the following history:

"I was an only child of a strict father and a gentle mother. She died when I was several months old and I was raised by an indulgent grandmother. In my grammar school days I was happy because my grandparents were so nice – and I enjoyed school. Then my father remarried and I lived with him and a stepmother.

"Life changed for me. I was no longer the center of attention but was spanked for everything. I tried to make myself conspicuous to get attention but only got into trouble.

"I had difficulty in high school and then started college. I was shy and unhappy so I began to drink. I seemed so clumsy and bashful and I felt better when I drank. My school work was neglected and I was dropped from college.

"One night when I was in a bar and had a few drinks, I met a girl and persuaded her to drink with me. I felt so courageous that I convinced her to spend the night with me. In the morning when I was sober I got scared. I was afraid that the girl's family would hurt me because she might become pregnant, so we got married.

"I tried to work but when I got tired or sick at heart, I drank. I lost job after job and my wife divorced me. Then I didn't work for a long time. I was too shy to apply for a job.

"For the past ten years I have been drinking heavily. I work long enough to get some money, then I go on a drunk. I know I never grew up – I can't control myself – I am the same adolescent as I was 15 years ago."

This patient is a highly intelligent, well read, and interesting adult in the middle thirties with a history of alcoholism of some 15 years' duration. He presented no evidence of neurologic or psychotic disorder. His life record is that of a complete failure, disowned by his father, self-derogatory, yet pleasant and witty when he is sober. He has been to many hospitals and doctors and has made many resolutions. Yet the need and the habit are so intense that he contrives somehow to get drunk again. He states: "I drink because it bolsters me when I feel inferior or lonesome – I am a weakling or I would help myself."

This patient was kept in the hospital for several weeks, given a program of activity and psychotherapy. He improved sufficiently to leave the hospital and obtain a job. For several months he maintained this good record – then slipped again.

Neurological Disturbances

Some patients maintain fairly adequate personality adjustments, but the pathology of alcoholism appears in the form of neurological symptoms. Tremors and unsteady gait are quite common in alcoholics. Occasionally, however, one sees a patient who develops burning pains in the arms and legs, with numbness, tingling, and weakness. In the more severe cases there is definite atrophy of the muscles, especially in the lower extremities.

An example of this type of disorder is that of M. E., a man of high intelligence who began to drink heavily when he was a student in college. He did not finish his college course, but did some part-time writing. He could not earn a livelihood because of his drinking, using up a generous inheritance over a period of years. This man drank heavily, up to two quarts daily, for many years. In the course of time he developed numbness and tingling in his legs and drank more to overcome this distress. Finally he reached the point where he could not walk.

I saw this patient at the University Hospitals, lying uncomfortably in bed, in great distress because of the burning in his legs. His personality was still cheerful and he was very much interested in cultural subjects and world events. His arms were thin, weak, and tremulous. The lower extremities were markedly atrophied, the reflexes were gone, there was loss of sensation, especially over the feet. The skin over the hands and feet was scaly.

In addition to this evidence of polyneuritis, the patient had an enlarged liver and vomited blood as a result of varicose veins in the esophagus.

M. E. was treated with vitamins, both orally and by injection, and showed a remarkable improvement. In the course of months he regained his ability to walk and was relatively free of pain.

There are other neurological conditions which are far less common than polyneuritis. I have seen patients with degenerative processes in the spinal cord and several patients who had convulsions after heavy drinking bouts, so-called whisky fits.

Delirium Tremens

More frequent than peripheral nerve disturbances are acute disorders of mental functioning characterized by marked delirium along with intense tremors of the hands, so-called delirium tremens. In the Army this is probably the commonest form of delirium. In civilian life such cases are not rare. Several examples of this form of delirium are included in Chapter VIII on Toxic Psychoses. Such patients were troubled by visual hallucinations in which they see small objects, dark in color, moving about. These patients, as a rule, are restless, wakeful, frightened, trying to escape from the dangers of their hallucinated objects. Crawling mice, tiny insects in bed, rather than pink elephants, are the animals which threaten them.

Alcoholic Hallucinosis

There are some alcoholics who develop a serious disturbance

characterized by hearing voices. Unlike delirium tremens, in which the hallucinations are visual, the major symptoms in this form are auditory. The patient hears the voice of someone he knows or of strangers. In some instances the voices are sharp and clear, warning, threatening, accusing. Such a patient will hear one person or a group of people reviling him with foul names, accusing him of all kinds of sins. The subject may be repeated again and again or may change. Sometimes the voices are not sharp and clear, but there are sounds which are buzzing, blowing.

Along with the hallucinations, the patients are troubled by the feeling that they may be punished, that others are threatening to do them harm. Thus there are delusions of persecution. Despite these hallucinations and delusions, many of the patients can make a reasonably good adjustment to reality situations.

I recall a man whom I saw at the Neuropsychiatric Clinic of Lakeside Hospital from 1923 until some time in 1940. He had been a heavy drinker and yet maintained a good work record as a laborer for a paving company. He was a bachelor who lived alone, having no other interests than drink and work.

Some time in 1923 he first heard voices who accused him of all manner of perverted sex activities. He was particularly incensed when they accused him of sex relations with animals. Yet he did nothing about these hallucinations except to spit continuously. He often would spit into his palms in a very dramatic fashion, stating: "I am spitting on them and trying to clean myself from their damned insults."

In some instances the alcoholic hallucinosis is undoubtedly a form of schizophrenia. However, the disease runs a long course and deterioration is not common.

Korsakoff's Syndrome

This is an organic disorder occurring with alcoholism. It is a combination of impairment of memory, sometimes clouding of consciousness, neuritis and, above all, delusions of persecution. In some instances the cases are acute and severe. In others the course is milder and more chronic. Quite commonly the patient becomes impotent and accuses his wife of unfaithfulness as the cause of his impotence. The memory is considerably impaired and judgment affected. There is often a disturbance of speech to the point that the symptoms resemble paresis. At times Korsakoff's psychosis follows an acute illness such as delirium tremens.

The neurological and mental symptoms with alcoholism thus take on many forms depending upon some peculiar vulnerability of the individual. The most common in my experience are those involving character impairment rather than medical problems. Frequently there are mixed forms in which personality changes, tremors, neuritis, and medical disorders are present.

Treatment of Alcoholism

The treatment of alcoholism is a challenging problem for which there is yet no satisfactory solution. The immediate medical symptoms of neuritis and even of delirium can be removed to a large degree by intravenous vitamins, chlorides and glucose. This should be followed by an adequate diet plus such additional vitamins, orally or by injection, as may be required in the individual case. The patient, M. E., who had a severe form of neuropathy, responded favorably to such medicinal measures along with psychotherapy. Indeed, he remained quite well for several years.

A program of psychotherapy, including the items covered in Chapter III, may benefit certain alcoholics. We aim to learn what the alcohol stands for in the present life of the patient—is it an escape from an intolerable situation, a compensation for fears of inferiority? We may find that the alcoholism is a repetitive effort to overcome deeply buried inner conflicts. Such patients may possibly be helped by a thorough-going psychoanalysis. Unfortunately, most patients do not cooperate for a sustained period of time and frequently resort to alcohol again and again. A practical form of group psychotherapy which has proved distinctly valuable is Alcoholics Anonymous. This organization accepts the alcoholic and attempts to elevate his ego; it provides an opportunity for the patient to identify himself with certain outstanding individuals who have recovered. He is given the opportunity for socialization and for restoring his ego confidence. It lessens lonesomeness, strengthens the ego structure—and thus has helped some to resist the tendency to drink.

The alcoholic, who presents a picture of an enfeebled physical state and a profound weakening of ego, can hardly rehabilitate himself at home. His own statements, his promises and the scoldings by his family prove futile. Hospitalization is necessary. Such a transfer to a hospital may break the link of the tragic chain of events, protects the patient from his accustomed resort to the "remedial use of alcohol." At the hospital the patient can receive adequate dietary and vitamin regimes plus psychotherapy. When the patient has improved in the hospital, he should then be followed closely by the doctor in the hope that rehabilitation can be accomplished.

Addiction

Closely allied to chronic alcoholism is addiction to drugs. Some patients not only are chronic alcoholics but alternate with the use of large amounts of medication. An example of the alternation of drugs and alcohol is as follows:

Mrs. W. T. had been an unstable nervous woman who began to take chloral because of sleeplessness. She was seen in 1942 with symptoms of weight loss, tremors, and weakness. Drug addiction to chloral was diagnosed. She responded well to psychotherapy. Two years later a sister died and patient became nervous again. At this time she began to drink heavily. When the subject of her drinking was mentioned, she denied the use of alcohol and attributed her nervousness to her husband. "He mistreats me, he runs around; there is nothing wrong with me; he needs a psychiatrist. - I do take a beer now and then."

The usual addiction is to drugs and often to one drug alone, such as opium and its derivatives, barbiturates, chloral, paraldehyde. As a rule addiction is a serious and tragic symptom of psychoneurosis.

Brief Case History of a Patient Addicted to Barbiturates

W. B., a woman of 35, was brought to my office complaining of nervousness. She was a pale, emaciated woman who talked thickly and walked unsteadily. She denied the use of drugs at first but later gave the following data:

"I was one of many children, tall, thin, and awkward. I did splendidly in school - yes, I won a scholarship. But my family was poor and so I had to work. I was quite shy and nervous and seldom went out on dates. Some of my teeth were extracted so that I had to wear a plate even before I was 16. I was unhappy because I had no boy friends.

"Then when I was 19, a man paid attention to me and took me on dates. It was nice to have someone pay me compliments and I fell in love with him. One night we had intercourse – and I became pregnant. When I told him, he confessed that he was married. Ashamed and heartbroken, I had to tell my parents – and how sick at heart I felt because I was to have an illegitimate baby. I thought of running away, of committing suicide. I couldn't eat or sleep. Doctors gave me sleeping medicine. When the baby was born, I wanted it – I loved it, but my family forced me to give it up. My nerves got worse. I couldn't sleep unless I took more and more medicine.

Since then I have had many operations (some were definitely insisted upon by the nervous need of the patient for self-punishment). The insomnia persisted and so also the use of drugs.

"I can't sleep unless I take medicine. I use two to three capsules of sodium amytal (gr. six to gr. nine). I have taken as many as eight capsules of nembutal. Once I felt so hopeless that I took twenty phenobarbital tablets – I just didn't want to go on. I must have such medicine or I won't get any peace. I must have it to get over my nervousness."

At the present time this patient is slow, neglects her responsibilities, was unreliable in regard to her history. For example, she had concealed this story from her family and her previous physicians.

Originally the sedative drugs served a psychological need. Now they are taken even though there is no apparent cause. They have been maintained as a habit. There is no longer the obvious need for escape that there was ten years ago. Yet this patient persists in taking a steadily increasing amount of sedatives – offering some pretext to account for a "conditioned reflex."

Addicts obtain some relief, an escape, by the drugs they take. Anxiety is lessened, fear allayed, temporary security or forgetfulness obtained. Such an escape, be it in alcohol or in opium, is more serious than the common escape of nervous symptoms. For the use of drugs or alcohol dulls the mind, lessens the will to get well, reduces the physical status. The alcoholic patient develops avitaminosis, the drug addict suffers from impaired digestion. Both may develop delirium. For instance, the patient who ran through the hallways of University Hospitals (Chapter VIII, p. 250) was a professional man who had taken excessive amounts of bromides. Whenever he was upset or nervous or fearful, he would reach for more bromides (and other drugs). He had lost his appetite and was undernourished. Delirium followed the emaciation and the overuse of drugs.

Alcoholism and addiction thus constitute a serious problem for the person himself and for society. There is the matter of obtaining the item - relatively easy for alcohol and difficult for drugs. There is the cost - often a sacrifice. There is the tendency toward chronic and habitual use, for the person who needs such escapes in the face of one situation will encounter repeated situations of like degree to justify his need for alcohol or drugs.

It should be our policy to give such drugs cautiously - trying to remedy the cause rather than to encourage resort to possible habit-forming methods. The reliance upon alcohol, now glamorized as a social attribute, carries a potential danger for those whose neurosis may lead to dependence upon it. Intensive psychotherapy should be undertaken as early as possible in any patient showing addiction.

REFERENCES

Glueck, S.: Discussion in: Banay, R. S.: Immaturity and Crime. *Am. J. Psychiat.*, 100:170, 1943.

Noyes, A. P.: *Modern Clinical Psychiatry*, 2nd edition. Saunders, Philadelphia, 1939.

Malamud, W.: Psychopathic Personalities. *Manual of Military Neuropsychiatry*, p. 160. Edited by Solomon, H. C., and Yakovlev, P. I., Saunders, Philadelphia, 1944.

Gillespie, R. D.: *The Psychological Effects of War on Citizen and Soldier.* Norton, New York, 1942.

Mira, E.: *Psychiatry in War.* Norton, New York, 1943.

Harrison, F. M.: Psychiatry in the Navy. *War Medicine*, 3:113, 1943.

Porter, W. C.: What Has Psychiatry Learned During the Present War? *Am. J. Psychiat.*, 99:850, 1943.

Fetterman, J. L.: *The Mind of the Injured Man.* Industrial Medicine Book Company, Chicago, 1943.

Henderson, D. K.: *Psychopathic States.* Norton, New York, 1939.

Silverman, D.: The Electroencephalogram of Criminals. *Arch. Neurol. & Psychiat.*, 52:38, 1944.

Ebaugh, F. G.: Major Psychiatric Considerations in a Service Command. *Am. J. Psychiat.*, 100:28, 1943.

Schilder, P.: *Psychotherapy.* Norton, New York, 1938.

Bleuler, E.: *Textbook of Psychiatry.* Macmillan, New York, 1924.

Norris, D. C.: Malingering. From *Rehabilitation of the War Injured.*, p. 123. Ed. by Doherty, W. B., and Dagobert, D. R.; Philosophical Library, Inc., New York City.

Brussel, J. A., and Hitch, K. S.: The Military Malingerer. *Mil. Surg.* 93:33, 1943.

Myerson, A.: Malingering. *Manual of Military Neuropsychiatry*, p. 189.

Edited by Solomon, H. C., and Yakovlev, P. I., Saunders, Philadelphia, 1944.

Ossipov, V. P.: Malingering: The Simulation of Psychosis. *Bull. of Menninger Clinic*, 8:39, 1944.

Fetterman, J. L.: Two Clinical Tests Valuable in War Medicine and Medicolegal Practice. *War Medicine*, 3:155, 1943.

Strecker, E. A.: Alcohol and Alcoholism. *Manual of Military Neuropsychiatry*, p. 180. Edited by Solomon, H. C., and Yakovlev, P. I., Saunders, Philadelphia, 1944.

Strauss, M. B.: Multiple Neuritis—Differentiation of Nutritional Polyneuritis from Other Multiple Neuritides. Chapter XII in *Nutritional Deficiency in Nervous and Mental Disease*, A. Research Nerv. Ment. Dis., Williams & Wilkins, Baltimore, 1943.

Bowman, K. M., and Wortis, H.: Psychiatric Syndromes Caused by Nutritional Deficiency. Chapter XV in *Nutritional Deficiency in Nervous and Mental Disease*, A. Research Nerv. Ment. Dis., Williams & Wilkins, Baltimore, 1943.

Curran, F. J.: The Effects of Barbiturates and Bromides on Mental and Emotional Processes. Chapter VIII in *The Inter-Relationship of Mind and Body*, A. Research Nerv. Ment. Dis., Williams & Wilkins, Baltimore, 1939.

Myerson, A.: Sexual Deviates. *Manual of Military Neuropsychiatry* p. 185. Edited by Solomon, H. C., and Yakovlev, P. I., Saunders, Philadelphia, 1944.

Caldwell, J. M.: Neurotic Components in Psychopathic Behavior, *J. Nerv. & Ment. Dis.*, 99:134, 1944.

Karpman, B.: Moral Agenesis, *Psychiatric Quart.*, 21:361, 1947.

Chapter VIII

TOXIC AND ORGANIC PSYCHOSES

AN interesting group of cases are those which show mental symptoms in relation to a recognizable disturbance in the brain. The pathologic process in the brain may be a transitory edema or inflammatory reaction, or it may be a chronic, progressive compression by a growing brain tumor. This group includes cases in which the brain is affected by injury, infection, deficiency, excessive use of drugs, inhalation of poisonous gases, tumors, and a large variety of vascular and metabolic disorders.

A comprehensive classification would cover many individual diseases, among them alcoholic psychoses, the psychoses with febrile disease, the drug psychoses. Then there are the psychoses with tumor, with vascular disease, with metabolic disorders. We may simplify the subject by subdividing this large group into two, the acute or toxic psychoses whose major feature is that of delirium, and the chronic organic psychoses, the cardinal evidence of which is deterioration of brain functions. This chapter will deal with examples of mental illness which occur during the course of, or closely connected with, medical disorders. Apparently similar mental states may result from dissimilar causes since a like reaction may follow a variety of insults. The toxemia of pneumonia, the edema from trauma, the chemical changes of deficiency may produce like symptoms in the form of delirium.

Deliria

In a state of delirium consciousness is clouded, attention is shallow and fleeting, memory defective, while inner emotions, unchecked by critical awareness, express themselves too freely. A part of an object is taken as a complete experience and is interpreted in line with drives and fears. A white object thus is misinterpreted as a ghost who is pursuing the individual to punish him for his wrongdoing. An alcoholic patient heard a sound in the hallway which he interpreted as footsteps. As he had read about a torso murderer, he was seized by the horrible fear that this murderer was coming to destroy him. And so, to escape such destruction, the alcoholic leaped through the window. In the state of delirium, whether it be in connection with alcohol, fever, drugs, or anoxemia of the brain, certain basic functions are disturbed.

Clear thinking and sound judgment depend upon the integration of all functions. They are served by correct reports from the special senses. They rely upon appropriate correlation of such stimuli with past experience. They are dependent also upon the correct evaluation of time and the fitting in of the present experience in its logical time sequence. Normal thought and action require the ability to be critical of oneself and to distinguish fantasy from fact. Sudden damage to the brain, whether it comes from trauma, anoxemia, or deficiency, disrupts such functions. If the damage be sudden and extensive, the patient may become unconscious. But if the process be more gradual and some brain areas more affected than others, there occurs a dysfunction which we may call delirium.

In the total picture of delirium the following figures stand out:

A. Disturbances in Special Senses and in Peripheral Nerves

There is likely to be a hypersensitivity to stimuli so that hearing becomes more acute and the patient is aware of even the slightest sound. He may become sensitive to light. More often there is an actual hallucination of sound and sights and perhaps odors. Rosett attributes hallucinations to the released functions of areas in the brain which have been damaged. Perhaps too, the damage to the peripheral nerve endings causes burning and tingling and crawling. In the clouded mental state the patient may actually look for tiny objects such as insects which are causing these peculiar sensations. The clouded state causes him to misidentify scenes, for attention is fleeting, inner fears are predominant, and suggestibility may be heightened.

B. Disturbances in Memory

In states of delirium recent memory is markedly affected. In part, this is due to the inability to concentrate upon any one impression but, in addition, there is an inability to retain what one hears or sees. A patient may be told the date or the place where he is, but he will quickly forget this information.

C. Disorientation

Because of the clouded state and disturbed memory, there is usually an inability to orient oneself in relation to the environment. The patient thus is frequently unable to recognize the persons or objects in his surroundings and cannot clearly place himself in the time relationship of things. The patient may be greeted by his doctor, can see the charming nurses in their starched white uniforms and every indication of a hospital in his surroundings and yet say he is in church or working in a factory. He may be instructed to look out of the window and see that it is late in the afternoon and the green buds and new leaves give every evidence of springtime, yet he may not recognize the true significance of what he sees. Thus delirious patients are disoriented as to time, place and person.

D. Delusions and Confabulations

As the patient lacks the ability to appraise himself and his situation critically, fantasies take precedence over facts. Experiences or even reading imbedded in the memory may come to the surface as though they have actually occurred this very day. The patient may report activities such as dancing or working on the farm or sailing, though he may have been confined to bed for days with fever or a fractured leg. Such reports of experiences, or confabulations, are common in delirium. Indeed, past and present, experience and reading, reality and imagery are jumbled and sometimes fused. It seems as though the orderliness of normal thinking has been disarranged.

E. Bewilderment and Confusion

Not all mental functions are damaged, so that the patient may have partial realization of his surroundings. He tries to fit together the actuality which he recognizes with the hallucinated, disoriented world around him. The jumble of his imagery and falsification of memory clash with his actual sense impressions. The patient is bewildered, dazed, he can't understand.

F. Fear Reactions

Failing to comprehend the world around him and bombarded by stimuli, many of which are terrorizing, the delirious patient is often in a troubled state of fear. He is in the dark as far as his surroundings go and, like a child who is fearful of the dark, he is uneasy. An approaching friend seems to threaten him. The reflex hammer of the doctor causes him to pull away as though it were a tomahawk.

Other symptoms, in addition, are related to the clouding of consciousness. Sense impressions lack clarity, concentration cannot be maintained. There is drowsiness alternating with restlessness, there is fatigability. It may be remarked that the consciousness of the delirious patient fluctuates. It changes like the sun on a cloudy day, peering brightly for a few moments when the clouds pass by, and then completely darkened and hidden from view.

The mental processes of delirious patients are active but are confused. Delusions springing from inner, perhaps repressed sources, come to the fore. A well educated woman who was married to a tailor announced that she was the wife of a doctor, during her period of delirium following typhoid: "I have had a good education, I belong in the upper classes. My husband is a doctor; he is a great man." Indeed she misidentified the visiting physician and referred to him as her husband. She attempted to prove her scholastic attainment by reciting lines of poetry in a loud voice.

Woven out of memory and desire, combining past, present, and future, statements are offered which represent achievements. For example, a sergeant who had been injured in a jeep accident stated that he had just come in from sailing on the lake. Despite the fact that he had been in the hospital for weeks, he insisted firmly that he had just been out with some friends in their sailboat. Another patient, a woman who had delirium tremens, stated: "I just came home from a lovely party. It was gorgeous. There were so many important people and I was among them. I was very popular." She described the dress she wore and the people she met—though her dry lips, trembly hands, and rapid pulse were part of a serious, acute illness. When it is pointed out to the delirious patient that he has been sick in bed for a day or for weeks and that he could not possibly have had the adventures that he tells of, he will good-naturedly agree with this. However, he will emphatically repeat what he believes to be his experience.

I recall quite vividly a colored patient who was ill with pneumonia. He became restless and sleepless and insisted that he "leave this place" so that he could join his friends. He could hear them calling him. Some time later he announced: "I've got to go back to that dice game. I have won a good deal of money and boy, now I'm going to get that pretty girl I love."

Let us review in a general way some of the chief findings common in delirious patients. The appearance of the patient reflects some underlying physical illness. The patient usually is restless, confused, mumbling. He is whispering a reply to an hallucinated voice or even angrily talking back to some accuser. Perhaps he is picking little objects from his clothes or trying to hide away from his enemies.

The stream of talk is usually incoherent and irrelevant. His remarks may have no relationship to immediate surroundings. The mood is apt to be anxious or sad. Very often patients are fearful, dreading danger. The patient's mind is preoccupied with delusions and hallucinations. These are shifting, changing from hour to hour. Hallucinations are common. The sensorium is clouded; there is disorientation for time and place; judgment is affected and insight lost.

The physical and neurological manifestations in delirium are important. As a rule, the patient looks acutely ill. He may show signs of fever such as flushing, rapid pulse, dry lips. He may be drowsy for a period of hours and then awaken suddenly, startled by what he believes to be the approach of danger. There are physical weakness, tremors, with abnormality of reflexes – depending upon the underlying cause.

Types of Delirium

The diagnosis of delirium is usually a medical problem in which mental symptoms occupy the foreground. Practically any infection of the nervous system, acute febrile disease, deprivation of vitamins, anoxemia may produce such delirious states. A thorough examination is required to determine the basic cause of delirium. A few of the more common types are as follows:

A. Delirium with Febrile Illness

Influenza, pneumonia, typhoid, malaria are sometimes responsible for acute delirious mental states. I have also seen patients with subacute bacterial endocarditis and with rheumatic fever who showed similar disturbances.

The case history of Mrs. M. S. is briefly as follows: She had taken sick, with a temperature of 101° and headaches. During the night, she became restless, fearing danger in her home. The condition grew worse, she became sleepless, refused food, and talked in an incoherent manner. She seemed to be looking for objects in bed. During the initial examination at her home, she cooperated quite well but was confused about time and place. It seemed to her that her thoughts and actions were being controlled by others. She would remark: "The people want me to do this. They exercise a domination over me."

This patient was hospitalized, during which time she refused all food, spitting out anything that was offered to her. Tube feeding became necessary. She became disoriented for time and place. She believed that the hospital room was the interior of a church. She "recognized" it as a famous church in Italy where she had once traveled. She misidentified persons, referring to me as her husband. About ten days after onset, the temperature was 103, the pulse 130. The patient continued to be restless, talked on and on: "You are Howard (husband's name). No, you are Dr. S. (family doctor). You are Dr. S. Freud. You are tall, dark, and handsome." She would repeat these phrases again and again (perseveration).

The nature of the illness for which she had been treated before I was called was flu. She was later given large doses of sulfadiazine with a good result.

As the fever came down and the physical condition improved, there was a gradual improvement in the mental state. Patient took some food and became better oriented. However, some two weeks after onset, she still talked oddly: "I am an Indian chief; I do the polka barrel dance." She jumped out of bed and went through some dance steps to illustrate her remarks. The condition lasted some three or four weeks and there was a complete recovery.

This patient had had no previous mental symptoms. She has been seen occasionally for a period of four years following this illness and has remained mentally well.

B. Delirium from Alchoholism: Delirium Tremens

One of the commonest forms of delirium is that which occurs with alcoholism. Recent work indicates that the cause is not so much the alcohol as the vitamin deficiency. Such a mental illness may begin gradually, with restlessness and sleeplessness. Then the patient becomes tremulous, uneasy. Some hallucinations develop. These are often visual and the patient may see tiny objects moving. Auditory hallucinations are not uncommon; voices are likely to be accusatory. In the acute illness, the patient may misidentify what is happening and act in accordance with his interpretation.

For example Mrs. G. U. was admitted to the Lakeside Hospital for some surgical condition. During the night she became terribly alarmed, thought that she was outdoors, and pictured a series of small coal cars moving around her.

Another patient was rather amused by his hallucinations: "When I was in bed, I saw a little figure coming through the doorway. He was a tiny little man. In fact I called him Tom Thumb. He danced into the room and jumped into my bed. I tried to catch him, but he always eluded my grasp." This patient also "saw" outside his window a group of little people milling about. Then there seemed to be fighting, as though two gangs were attacking each other. He became frightened by the scene that he had witnessed and was about to call the police. These two hallucinations, the experience with Tom Thumb and witnessing the little people fighting, were the most colorful experiences during several days of sleeplessness, tremors, fever, and confusion. With proper treatment, he recovered quickly.

There was another individual, a responsible business man, who had been drinking heavily. He came home one night staggering, his hands trembling, his voice unsteady. He complained to his wife that the house was moving. As he looked out of the window, it seemed to him that he was on a globe actually revolving, and that in the distance he could see another world which was passing by him. When he was questioned about this unusual hallucination, he later explained that he had been to the World's Fair and had seen the panorama on a moving car. The hallucination was a fragmentary reproduction of this experience.

One of the most dramatic cases of alcoholic delirium is that of the patient whose case history was previously mentioned. This patient had been drinking a quart or two of liquor a day for a matter of months. He came home tired and exhausted. After a short rest, he tried to read the newspaper. He was attracted by the headline and the news story of a torso murderer. The story had described the dismembered torso which was found near the lake in the City of Cleveland, and told of several suspects who were being questioned by the police. As he read this story, his eyes became blurry and he went off into a fitful sleep. He awakened startled. "I heard footsteps in the hallway; I'm positive they were footsteps coming nearer to my door. Who could it be? ... It must be the torso murderer and I'm to be his next victim." As the footsteps grew louder, the patient's terror increased and then, at the moment when he thought the "murderer" was about to open the door, this patient dashed towards the window and leaped out. In this jump he fractured several bones and sustained severe bruises and contusions.

C. Delirium from Drugs

Drugs are also responsible for a certain number of delirious states. Two cases come to mind. A professional man had been quite nervous and hypochondriacal. To get relief from his anxiety, he began to take tablets. In the course of time he needed more and more medication to obtain rest. His fear of disease grew and he was hospitalized at the University Hospitals. On the first night he was found running in his pajamas through the hallway, and at this stage I was called in consultation. The patient was pale, trembly, and in an obvious state of alarm: "I can't stay here another minute. This room is moving around. My doctors are nothing more than murderers. They are planning to have an operation done on me. They think I have a tumor in the back of my brain, a most unusual tumor, and they would like this specimen to show in the Museum of Pathology. They are going to kill me. Please be careful. If you try to befriend me, they may get you.... Be careful as you walk in my room. I think there is a trap door under this carpet and both of us may find ourselves in the museum." The delusional ideas of this patient were predominantly fearful and they took on the interesting form linked with pathology.

The physical and neurological examinations showed diminished reflexes and some tremors, but did not reveal the cause for the delirium. However, a blood specimen for blood bromides showed a tremendous increase to 350 mg. Discontinuance of bromides, salt medication, and hydrotherapy brought about improvement.

At the Lawson General Hospital I was called to see a WAC who had been sick for several weeks with pain in the back and sleeplessness. Medication had been started and she had been taking bromides for several weeks. Quite abruptly she became noisy and cried out: "I can hear them outdoors; they are going to operate on me. They think I have a baby in my stomach and they want to keep me in the service. I would rather have the baby." This patient was fearful and clung to me, stating: "You are my rabbi, you will protect me from this. Things are awful here. The food tastes different; I am sure they put urine in my water. I hear people talking about me outside. I believe it's my husband who is out there. I'm sure it is. He wants to visit me, but they won't let him. Please protect me."

This patient's delusional ideas revolved about the subject of a baby as she had been married for years and was childless. Apparently she wanted to get out of the service and perhaps believed that pregnancy would achieve this for her. She had hallucinations of smell and of sound. There was marked mis-identification of sound and she interpreted all activity around her as hostile efforts to destroy her. She was particularly terrified lest she be operated on without an anesthetic. She continued in a tense, watchful state, restless, sleepless, and alarmed for about ten days. Then she became calmer but was still uneasy and suspicious. Gradually her physical state improved and all mental processes were free of abnormality. The blood bromide level had been 400 mg.

Treatment of Delirium

The major steps include the removal or treatment of the cause, sedation, replacement methods, feeding, and miscellaneous procedures. The cause of each delirium is different and careful diagnostic methods are necessary to determine the nature of the delirious process. The history is particularly important. A careful physical and neurologic study and such laboratory procedures as spinal fluid tests and blood examinations are necessary. The cause should be removed or treated with such specific measures as are available.

Obviously in those patients whose delirium is related to alcoholism or drugs, it is important to discontinue them. If there is infection, say syphilis, specific measures are used. For the delirium of other fevers the sulfa drugs and penicillin may prove beneficial. It is not always possible to remove or treat the cause effectively, but all patients require sedation. The patient is in a state of fear and restlessness because of the ceaseless bombardment of disturbing stimuli. He can be protected from his bombardment and given relaxation and sleep by the use of hydrotherapy and drugs.

The two hydrotherapeutic methods in vogue for the treatment of delirium are the wet pack and the continuous tub. It is the experience of those who have treated acutely ill mental patients that a wet pack properly administered may enable the disturbed patient to fall into a needed slumber. So too a warm tub used for hours will bring relaxation to an otherwise overactive, disturbed patient.

In addition to hydrotherapy, medicinal agents will dull the patient's alertness and provide rest. The most commonly used drug is paraldehyde, which may be given by various routes, orally, rectally, intramuscularly, or intravenously. It can be given orally either "straight" or in ice water, orange juice, or milk. The rectal dose may be administered in olive oil, glycerin, or in a 4 per cent starch solution. The dose should be started with a small amount of the drug, but increased until an adequate amount has been given. As a rule, paraldehyde is fairly safe and effective. When given intravenously, of course small doses are used with caution.

The barbiturates are likewise effective drugs in the delirious states. My own favorite is sodium amytal in doses of 3 to 6 grs. orally. However, if the patient refuses oral medication, the same drug may be injected intramuscularly or even intravenously. Other barbiturates are valuable as is hyoscine hydrobromide, gr. 1/100, combined with morphine, gr. ¼. In the milder states of delirium, bromides and chloral may be used.

Along with sedation, there is need for supporting measures and replacement therapy. The foremost therapeutic method, as recently established by Strecker and Rivers, is the intravenous administration of a combination of glucose, insulin, and thiamin chloride. These authors advise the combined administration of 100 cc. of fifty per cent glucose, fifty units of insulin, and 120 mg. of thiamin chloride. Such a dose may be repeated every three hours if necessary, care being taken that sufficient sugar is given to the patient orally. If the patient is not taking sugar by mouth, the dose of insulin is reduced. My own experience is in line with the favorable results obtained by these authors, particularly in alcoholic deliria, but also in other delirious states.

In addition to this intravenous technique, it is important that the patient be given as much liquid and food as he can possibly take. If the patient refuses food, then tube feeding becomes necessary. The tube feeding which I have used consists of three eggs, an ounce of cod liver oil, two ounces of olive oil, one cup of fruit juice, eight ounces of cream and two ounces of sugar in one quart of milk. This combination has a caloric value of over 2,000 calories. Sodium chloride, Brewer's yeast, and drugs may be added to this mixture.

In addition to the above methods of treating deliria, it is necessary that the patient be protected and that he receive adequate nursing care. In some disturbed patients shock therapy has been tried, not as a cure of the delirium but in the hope of converting a combative patient into a cooperative individual.

Course and Prognosis of Delirious States

As a rule, a toxic psychosis is an acute illness which tends toward recovery. The course of the mental symptoms is dependent upon the continuation and severity of the underlying cause and also upon treatment. The professional man who developed a bromide psychosis improved in some two weeks after the bromides were stopped. The woman whose mental symptoms came during an attack of influenza became well in several weeks. Alcoholic deliria in previous times generally cleared up in several weeks, although a certain percentage of patients, particularly those in poor physical states, died. During recent years the early use of effective treatment has cut short the duration of the illness and has reduced the mortality. Today, a patient with delirium tremens may become calm in 24 to 72 hours – and the death rate has been reduced to a minimum.

In some cases a toxic psychosis resembles schizophrenia and, though it clears up, subsequent mental symptoms appear years later. For example, W. T., age 18, was brought to Deaconess Hospital because of a bronchopneumonia. After about seven days of fever, he became restless and tried to run out of the hospital. "I see horrible faces on the wall; they are leering at me; they want to get me – yes, I can hear them talking about me; they want to kidnap me." For some days he remained in a state of alarm. Then, as the temperature returned to normal, his mental state improved. He slept quietly and was freed of the terror of his hallucinations.

He made a splendid recovery and was apparently well. The brevity of the illness, its symptoms, and its occurrence during a febrile illness indicated a toxic psychosis. However, two years later, during apparent well-being, he noticed men at work "spying" upon him. Indeed he was being followed by certain persons in the streetcar. Automobiles would cruise on the street near his home and park facing it. He became fearful lest they try to kidnap him or bomb his home. So he stopped going to work and concealed himself. A psychiatric study revealed the features of a schizophrenia. Apparently the mental symptoms which appeared during fever represented a vulnerability - a reaction type.

Thus what begins as a toxic psychosis may be a phase of a later, more serious illness. Yet, by far the greater number of acute deliria run a relatively brief course toward recovery.

The Organic Reaction Types

The organic reaction types, a term first used by Bonhoeffer for the mental symptoms occurring in arteriosclerotic brain disease, are similar to the deliria because there is organic brain pathology. However, the course of the disease is progressive rather than reversible as with the deliria. The organic reaction types, as was mentioned at the beginning of this chapter, include particularly the psychoses with cerebral arteriosclerosis, with metabolic diseases, with tumor, etc.

The clinical picture will be determined by the personality of the patient, the rate and extent of the causative agent. There will be certain specific features depending upon the underlying disease processes. Henderson and Gillespie, in describing the psychoses with cerebral arteriosclerosis, state: "The onset may be apoplectiform. The patient has the realization of being less efficient than before. He tires more easily, he shows less initiative, the comprehension is duller, there is a failure of memory. Emotional instability is an early symptom, with tearfulness or explosive anger.... There is a progressive narrowing of interest. The power of comprehension becomes less elastic and thought becomes sluggish. The person sticks to an idea obstinately and dislikes departure from the beaten path of daily routine. There is failure of memory especially for recent events. The memory defect becomes more diffuse and gaps are filled in by fabrications. Patches of amnesia increase till there are losses extending into childhood. On the basis of memory defect, suspicions and ideas of persecution develop. Attention is poorly sustained, disorientation involving time and place and person develop."

I have seen a considerable number of cases of organic reaction types who have shown the above features. The outstanding difficulty is the impairment of memory. The patient is unable to give proper attention to stimuli and the full meaning of any act is not realized. Bleuler mentions a paretic who walked out of the window to get a cigarette butt, unmindful of the danger of this step. The same author tells briefly of a senile patient who stole a barrel of wine from in front of a wine shop in broad daylight and asked two policemen to help him roll it home when he became too tired. Bleuler states that there is a restriction of thought to a specific cluster of ideas - "Physically speaking, it is like an attempt to get one's bearings through a keyhole." This exposes the patient to committing great stupidities. Such patients cannot distinguish the specific from the general, cannot shift quickly from one subject to another. There is a tendency to repeat again one performance or one phrase (perseveration).

I recall a patient who lost his ability to work and would lie around the house. When reprimanded by his wife, he would become quarrelsome. He talked in a garrulous way. He had periods of blankness, twilight states.

There was a man in the seventies who lost the sense of time and could not distinguish day from night. He became suspicious of his family and thought that they as well as strangers were plotting to rob him. He would awaken at 2:00 or 3:00 a.m., wander out of the house, and go to the bank, fearing lest the contents of his safe deposit box might be stolen. When this man was placed in the hospital, he had complete loss of memory. Even when he was visited by members of his family, he could not recall this visit. Though he had been retired for several years, he would urgently request that he be allowed to go to his office to transact important business waiting for him. At times his condition improved and he would recognize his daughter and grandson and carry on a fairly lucid conversation.

Another patient is a woman in the seventies who gradually lost interest in people and events of the day and would sit blankly looking out of the window or staring at the newspaper. Though she scanned the newspaper for hours, she could not recall one single item of what she had read and of course had no concept of the meaning of news events. Her husband had been dead for years, yet she would often remark: "My husband is unfaithful. He hasn't been home for days. I'll bet he is running around with pixies. He should be in hell for the way he has been carrying on." This patient would become extremely aroused and violent if her husband's name was mentioned. She still believed he was alive and explained his absence by the fact that he was keeping several girl friends in expensive apartments.

This patient had no idea of time or place, lost the ability to calculate. For the most part she was calm, but when she was questioned, she would become embittered and insult the examiner. In the course of time she lost all sense of propriety and even emptied her bladder in a public restaurant.

There are many specific varieties of organic reaction types, for these may occur with any medical disease. Those which occur in syphilis will be discussed in a separate chapter.

A rather dramatic case in my experience was that of a young man of 17 who had been suffering from diabetes. He was treated with protamine zinc insulin and one day became unconscious. He was brought to the hospital in this state of unconsciousness and remained comatose for several days. Gradually he emerged from this state and in the course of a week became aware of his surroundings. When he recovered physically, he had lost the ability to read and write and had forgotten simple acts. For instance, when I offered him a cigarette, he reached for it and brought the cigarette to his lips. I then showed him a box of matches but he did not know what to do with them. I lit one for him and offered it to him. Instead of lighting the cigarette with the burning match, he was about to bring the match to his lips and I barely stopped him. He had also lost his sense of propriety, urinating and defecating in his room.

The case appeared to be a serious and almost hopeless dementia due to encephalopathy. However, in the course of months he improved considerably. When he was seen in another hospital about six months after the acute illness, he gave the impression of being a schizophrenic because of certain delusional statements and incoherent remarks. His condition continued to improve so that about a year after the catastrophe he was able to take his place socially and even to do routine work.

I have seen several cases of psychoses with thyroid disease, several with pernicious anemia, and of course other cases with brain tumor.

The treatment for the organic reaction types must be individualized according to the specific problem involved. In the more chronic varieties, a protected environment such as a hospital, with good nursing care, is necessary.

REFERENCES

Rosett, J.: *The Mechanism of Thought, Imagery and Hallucination.* Columbia University Press, New York, 1940.

Strecker, E. A., and Rivers, T. D.: Preliminary Report on Adjuvant Treatment of Toxic States. *Pennsylvania M. J.*, 45:601, 1942.

Bonhoeffer, K.: *Die Symptomatischen Psychosen im Gefolge von Akuten Infektionen und Inneren Erkrankungen.* Leipzig: F. Deuticke, 1910.

Henderson, D. K., and Gillespie, R. D.: *A Textbook of Psychiatry.* Oxford University Press, London, 1930.

Bleuler, E.: *Textbook of Psychiatry.* Macmillan, New York, 1934.

Strecker, E. A., and Ebaugh, F. G.: *Practical Clinical Psychiatry.* 5th edition. Blakiston, 1940.

Chapter IX

NEUROSYPHILIS

WHEN Columbus and his sailors returned from their voyage of exploration, syphilis made its European debut as an infectious disease, and from the early 1500's onward the shadow of this disease has followed invading armies and darkened the footsteps of illicit love. In its earlier history, syphilis is reported as a disease of high mortality and striking cutaneous manifestations. Indeed, until recently the cutaneous and osseous manifestations were so striking that chief attention was paid to them. In recent decades the disease has become less virulent and the involvement of the nervous system has become more commonly recognized. It is with this phase of the disease, neurosyphilis, that we will for the most part deal in this chapter.

The campaign which was started by Surgeon General of the United States Public Health Service Thomas Parran in 1936 and which has been carried on for many years has contributed to a better understanding of this disease and even to a reduction in its spread. Likewise, the employment of the serologic tests for syphilis by the Selective Service, their common use in premarital and prenatal examinations, and their extensive use in routine examinations have made possible an earlier recognition and treatment. Consequently the incidence of serious complications will be reduced.

Life Story of This Disease

Diseases, like persons, have a life story. To understand a disease properly, we should not stop at a study of one phase, however striking or dramatic it may seem, but trace the illness from its inception to its disappearance or to the tragic end of the patient. This running account, this trajectory of the disease over a period of time, I have called the chrono-kinetic approach (chronos – time; kinetic – movement). What is the chrono-kinetic course of syphilis?

The initial stage is the chancre, a red, round, hard sore on the genitals or other exposed parts of the patient. This chancre develops some two weeks after neglected exposure. Within the chancre are numerous spiral organisms, the spirochetes of syphilis, which have found in their host an ideal environment in which to live, multiply and spread. Within six weeks of the appearance of the chancre, the patient may become ill with slight fever, headache, and a rash. At this point, the secondary stage, the skin is spotted with small reddish spots and in some cases there are sores in the mouth as well. The lymph nodes in the groins and neck and armpits are enlarged and tender. It is during this stage that swarms of spirochetes are streaming in the circulation, lodging in the patches of the mouth, in the skin rash, and even in the meninges, for the spinal fluid during the secondary stage commonly shows evidence of irritation or involvement.

This phase of syphilis, at times quite striking in its manifestations, gradually subsides. The rash fades, the patches heal, the changes in the spinal fluid tend to clear and the malaise is replaced by well-being. The patient feels comfortable and thus believes that he is well again. Some do remain symptom-free for life, but the majority are merely lulled into a feeling of false security, from which they are awakened months or years later by the sudden or gradual development of symptoms.

As a rule, the secondary stage is followed by a period of dormancy on the part of the organisms; at least most patients are untroubled by symptoms. Yet this stage is not one of utter inactivity for the organisms. Indeed, the spirochetes which have lodged in the skin, in the lining of a bone, or those which have nested in the aorta or in the brain may in a year or two set up an active disease. Thus a thick, nodular sore may appear on the skin (a gumma); the tissues around the bone may swell (periostitis); or the damage to the lining of the brain may incite an acute meningitis.

As we focus attention upon the invasion of the nervous system, we see that the spirochetes may attack the nervous tissue proper, its linings, the blood vessels, or combinations of these structures. The extent of involvement and its rapidity vary from patient to patient. In some instances the active disease damages the brain with the speed of a consuming flame; in others it causes a slow change like a smoldering fire.

An example of an acute syphilitic brain involvement is that cited by Sezary. A man of forty developed an extensive rash one month following the chancre. Forty-five days later, this patient suffered an acute hemiplegia and died very soon after this incident. The autopsy revealed thrombosis of the left Sylvian artery, which vessel was involved in an extensive arteritis. The histologic study of the brain and cord showed spirochetes in the parenchyma and a meningeal cellular reaction.

Such a rapid and overwhelming termination in the early stages of the disease is indeed rare, for as a rule there is an average lapse of 10 years between the initial chancre and symptoms of tabes, while a longer period of time frequently elapses before paresis begins.

Although the patient may be free of obvious symptoms, yet it is possible that the organisms are not entirely inactive; they may be mobilizing for an attack or may be infiltrating and weakening the blood vessels or cells of the brain, like fifth columnists. The person affected may be no more aware of such infiltration than a nation is of its fifth columnists, when suddenly he is attacked with headache, a convulsion, an acute mental disorder, or hemorrhage and death.

A. B. was an apparently well man who reported to work as usual. He was seen busily engaged in the night shift at one time, but an hour later was found dead – sprawled on the ground. Because of the circumstances attending this sudden death, there was a suspicion of accidental electrocution. However, careful studies showed no source for an electric shock.

A complete autopsy revealed pathologic changes localized to the brain. The cause of death was an extensive subarachnoid hemorrhage. Histologic studies, done by Dr. Francis Bayless of the Institute of Pathology, Western Reserve University, and substantiated by Dr. Joseph H. Globus of New York, revealed a widespread meningeal exudate and severe arteritis. The vessels showed intimal proliferation, with occlusion of small branches as well as exudate in the adventitia and the meninges. Dr. Globus and Dr. Bayless interpreted these changes as due to syphilis and having existed for months or years. Six months after the autopsy we obtained a history that this patient had had a 4 plus Kahn test, twice confirmed, in 1934. Apparently the initial clinical symptom was an extensive subarachnoid hemorrhage. The first clinical evidence was the exitus of the patient. Like a neglected battery, which may run down slowly and then stop "dead" suddenly, so the pathologic changes in the nervous system may progress silently until a sudden catastrophe announces the clinical stage of the disease.

However, it is more common for the symptoms to develop gradually. In tabes, for example, there may be numbness in one leg, gradually spreading to the other in the course of months. Then come shooting pains, which dart like lightning down the legs. Months later the individual may exhibit difficulty in walking at night and later ataxia in the daytime. Thus years may elapse from the onset of the initial symptoms until the case is fully developed. This same slow development applies to paresis also, a disease which customarily starts insidiously and progresses irregularly, even with periods of clinical improvement, followed by relapses.

Groups of Symptoms—Classification

The type of symptoms depends upon several factors: the area of the nervous system involved, the rapidity of the attack, and, as always, the person affected. So variable are the possible regions and combinations that many different symptom groupings or syndromes are possible. A classification in use in the United States Army is the following:

CLASSIFICATION OF NEUROSYPHILIS

(Abstract from Circular Letter 74, Surgeon General's Office)

Asymptomatic: Early or late cases free of symptoms and signs whose spinal fluid shows abnormalities.
Acute syphilitic meningitis: Low grade meningeal involvement, with or without cranial nerve involvement, occurring within the first two years.
Diffuse meningovascular: A catch-basket category to include all patients with neurosyphilis who do not fit into other categories.
Tabes dorsalis: The typical history and such findings as Argyll-Robertson pupils, areflexia in the knee jerks and ankle jerks and sensory loss involving posterior columns.
Taboparesis: To be used for patients showing psychiatric signs of paresis complicated by evidence of posterior column involvement.
Psychosis with syphilitic meningo-encephalitis (general paresis): Limited to cases of psychosis with neurologic signs and "paretic formula" in spinal fluid.

Miscellaneous: Optic atrophy. Gumma. Psychosis with neurosyphilis.

We will take up in some detail tabes dorsalis, paresis and meningovascular syphilis, and mention one case of optic atrophy.

Common Clinical Syndromes of Neurosyphilis

Tabes Dorsalis

This is a form of syphilis in which the disease has affected chiefly the posterior columns of the spinal cord, the nerves which connect the spinal cord with the lower extremities, and the tissues surrounding these nerves. The major pathologic changes occur in the posterior columns of the spinal cord, but there are similar processes in the dorsal root ganglia and in the posterior roots. Of course, involvement in the brain, brain stem, cranial nerves, and other peripheral nerves may also occur. Such pathologic processes lead to a growing series of physical symptoms and disabilities.

The patient suffers from shooting pains in the legs and develops loss of position and vibratory sense and of power in the legs. As a rule shooting pains are the earliest manifestation. They are likely to occur at night, may involve one leg first, then spread to the other, and become persistent and excruciating. Patients describe them as darting, striking in one spot, then in a different region and then in the other leg. So intense are they and so persistent that patients must resort to strong medication. Some require repeated injections of large doses of morphine. Once present, such pains may recur intermittently during several decades. As the disease progresses, unsteadiness and weakness develop. Thus the patient's gait becomes weak and unsteady, known as ataxia of locomotion.

The legs tend to become flabby and insecure. The patient has difficulty in walking, particularly upon an uneven surface and when in the dark. The disease has damaged the sense of muscle position. Consequently the tabetic cannot feel the position of his feet and legs and must watch carefully or he will fall. The loss of position and the muscle weakness combine to produce a faltering, stumbling gait.

Sometimes in the early stages, though more commonly in the advanced period of tabes, the patient experiences difficulty with bladder control. There may be delay in starting the stream of urine or the urine may dribble away involuntarily. Some patients are unaware that the bladder is full or cannot completely empty it. This is a troublesome symptom which invites infection and is socially shameful. Patients who have bladder symptoms are apt to be sufferers from impotence or difficulty with penile erection.

Other symptoms include girdle pains, a sensation of encirclement, tight and uncomfortable; or the more serious condition of gastric crises. In this condition the patient suffers from attacks of severe abdominal pain and vomiting. As the name "crisis" implies, these bouts are so violently distressing that the patient is unable to obtain relief from the long period of vomiting and pain. Quite in contrast to this symptom is that of a swollen but painless deformity of joints, known as Charcot's joint. The knee and ankle are most often involved but in rare instances the spine, the elbow, and the foot joints may be affected by this curious swelling. It seems as though injury leads to an unhealthy overgrowth of tissue in and around a joint—which becomes excessively loose and insecure.

Though the major defects occur in the lower extremities, yet the brain stem and even the brain may also be affected. Inequality of the pupils is common; weakness of extraocular muscles or eyelids may occur. Occasionally there is a progressive involvement of the optic nerve, leading to optic atrophy and sometimes to blindness. Thus tabes is usually a serious disease, capable of a variety of manifestations as is illustrated in the following case histories:

> P. S., a man of 42, developed sharp pains in both legs. He would be awakened from sleep by darting, intense pains, "500 times as violent as a toothache." Then he became uncertain in walking at night and finally could not walk steadily. Examination revealed the telltale pupils, absent reflexes and loss of sensation - all suggestive of tabes. This clinical diagnosis was confirmed by a positive Wassermann test on the blood and the spinal fluid. P. S. recalled that he had a chancre at the age of 20, for which he received a few intravenous injections. He believed himself "cured" - yet the disease was dormant for twenty years, only to become active again as a serious form of syphilis at the age of forty.
>
> A similar tragic experience was that of S. B. In his early twenties, as a private in the Army, he pursued the ladies without care or caution. Then in his more mature thirties he became a serious soldier and was promoted several times

until he became a master sergeant. One day, after drilling, he developed a swollen knee. The swelling grew larger and larger. Although the knee joint was painless, he suffered sharp, "lancinating" pains in both legs at night. Examination showed the bone and joint changes of a Charcot joint as well as other abnormalities. Thus at 38 this sergeant became useless to the Army and potentially a cripple because of syphilis contracted 15 years previously.

A typical case of tabes dorsalis is that of R. E., who was referred to my office because of difficulty in walking. He had a chancre at the age of 23, treated by a few injections until the sore disappeared. At the age of 40 he developed some weakness in one leg and a slight limp. At first this trouble was noticed only at night, but later it grew worse. He was then bothered by fleeting pains in the legs, of moderate degree. Later came difficulty in voiding. Finally this patient fell and fractured one ankle, which did not heal but instead the ankle and foot became more swollen and weaker.

The neurological findings of significance were small pupils which did not react to light, absent knee and ankle tendon reflexes, marked impairment of position and vibration sensibility in both legs – and radiographic evidence of a Charcot's joint of the left ankle.

The blood Wassermann was 4 plus. A lumbar puncture revealed the spinal fluid Wassermann to be 3 plus, with a cell count of 24, protein 55 mg./per cent, and a colloidal gold curve of 22321000.

Treatment with induced malaria and tryparsamide arrested the progress of the disease.

¶ Although the classical case has many of the features menioned, some patients exhibit only one symptom–a part of the picture. For instance, R. O. showed recurrent severe attacks of gastric crisis; another patient was troubled by urinary incontinence; a third had a Charcot spine – the other symptoms wanting. Again, tabes may be merged with paresis, so that the patient shows a combination of brain and cord symptoms. Numerous variations are possible.

Paresis—Dementia Paralytica

A more common form of neurosyphilis is paresis, known popularly as softening of the brain and in medical books as dementia paralytica. It may develop so slowly and secretly, symptom by symptom, that its grave import is not recognized until too late.

First there are headaches, then nervousness, sleeplessness, then forgetfulness – certainly everyday symptoms, innocent in themselves. In the course of time come failing interest, neglect of person and duties, and expansive plans despite weakening judgment. The patient neglects his attire, his home, his business, yet seems buoyed up by an unusual and unwarranted spirit of success. At this stage there may be twitchings around the mouth, tremors, slurring and indistinct speech, unsteady gait, and sometimes attacks of unconsciousness. If the progress of the disease is not checked, then in the course of months or years attention to reality dwindles, memory is lost and judgment becomes impaired. Peculiar ideas, undue cheerfulness in the face of poverty, expansive feelings of wealth and power amounting to delusions of grandeur may appear. While these mental symptoms grow, the patient may have peculiar attacks of automatic behavior or convulsions. Physical difficulties, such as tremors, weakness and even paralysis set in. Ultimately in its last stages we see an emaciated patient, too helpless to walk, speaking in a slurred, indistinct manner about his great wealth, obvious delusions of grandeur. Let us look at several clinical examples:

D. W., age 37, was referred in 1933 by his physician, Dr. S. Kamellin. In the spring of 1933 the patient had had one convulsion, as a result of which he was taken to the emergency room of a local hospital. Here a blood test was made, revealing a 4 plus Wassermann.

On the basis of several positive blood tests and irregular pupils, this patient was given a course of neoarsphenamine. Under routine treatment, D. W. was free of convulsions but began to show slight changes in personality. The family reported that whereas he had formerly been friendly and gracious, he had now become quick, irritable, and quarrelsome. These disagreeable traits occurred occasionally, yet they were signficant. The patient was hospitalized and the spinal fluid examined. The cell count was 11, globulin 4 plus, Wassermann 4 plus in all volumes, and the gum mastic curve 5554310000. At the time of the examination this patient was keen, had good memory, showed no speech defect and no hallucinations or delusions. The one convulsion and episodes of slight personality change might be looked upon as pre-paretic. This patient was inoculated with malaria and allowed to have eight paroxysms. Later, he was given a course of tryparsamide and bismuth. For almost five years he has remained clinically well.

This case history is significant in calling attention to (1) the importance of a convulsion as the warning signal of the early vascular change which occurs in paresis, (2) the progression of the disease during routine chemotherapy, and (3) the prompt and, it is hoped, permanent response to fever therapy.

Let us look briefly at another example. A sergeant was sent to the local general hospital because of paralysis and attacks. During lucid intervals he smiled happily, saying, "I am no sergeant. I am an officer; I'm a major." When asked about orders, he replied, "I don't need them, I issued them myself."

Although he had numerous attacks, was paralyzed and unable to walk, yet he was optimistic, spoke cheerily of good health, and was proud of his promotion (a delusion). In the intervals between his attacks he was able to recall, "Yes, I had trouble before, when I was a young soldier on duty overseas. It was double plus syphilis and I got some shots for it." The blood and spinal fluid tests were positive.

It is noteworthy that in his delusion the sergeant imagined himself a major – rather than as Napoleon or Croesus. To be a major was the ultimate goal of his wishes.

There was L. I., who at the age of 35 considered himself a failure as a clerk. So he became an insurance salesman, trying hard but with little success to sell policies. Thus months passed by, during which he showed apathy, made few contacts, avoided friends and family. Quite suddenly he became overconfident, busied himself and called on all sorts of prospects. Indeed, he would awaken people from their sleep at all hours during the night to talk insurance to them. So odd and disturbing was his conduct in the hotel at which he resided that its manager referred him to a physician. While waiting in the doctor's reception room, he busied himself with a column of figures which filled a page.

"What are these numbers?" he was asked.

"They are my profits on my insurance sales. I get $250 whenever I sell a certain policy. I can sell such a policy in half an hour, and that means 48 sales a day. I won't take time off for sleep. You see, I don't have to sleep. Multiply this figure by seven and you have my weekly earnings; now multiply this number by 52 and that's my annual income. Now add my bonuses and interest and multiply this by thirty and I'm a millionaire."

Although the last figure ran into millions, L. I. was

shabbily dressed, had not eaten for some time, and was far behind in the payment of his rent. The physical examination revealed unequal pupils, facial twitching and increased reflexes on one side. His speech was dysarthric, memory for recent events impaired and judgment severely affected. He could not repeat test phrases, could not recall items of current interest. Curiously, his calculations were correct, but not the significance of what he calculated. The blood Wassermann was 4 plus. The spinal fluid cell count was 32, protein 69 mg. per cent, and the gum mastic 555421-0000.

In other cases the symptoms of paresis may appear abruptly and the disease run an acute course. C. W. flew planes from the United States to North Africa. His route began in Florida, passed through Natal, Ascension Island, and terminated in Dakar. His earlier health record was excellent, save for some "difficulty" in his early twenties. Now, at 38, he was strong, well liked, and an expert pilot in the ferry command. He had completed a dozen or more trips.

As he flew his plane eastward on his last journey, C. W. was unusually gay. "It's a great world," he sang. "My rich aunt in Oklahoma is going to leave me $30,000,000."

During the periods of relief by his co-pilot, he talked loudly and became chummy with other members of the crew. As a matter of fact, he offered to loan the navigator $50,000. Landing safely in Dakar, his high spirits continued. Then his friends found him buying several "diamonds" from an Arab street merchant, spending most of his cash for this purpose.

"Boy", he exclaimed, "I got a swell bargain! Six diamonds for $100 cash now and $100 more on my next trip! I sure fooled that Arab; he's never going to collect the rest from me."

"How do you know the diamonds are genuine?" he was asked.

"I tested them," he boasted. "I struck one with a hammer and it proved hard; diamonds are hard."

Upon the return journey, C. W. continued the story of his expected wealth and the sum grew with the distance of travel.

"It's $40,000,000 I am getting and I expect to share some of it with you guys," he announced. When his co-pilot received this astounding information with doubt and anxiety, C. W. could not understand it. When the co-pilot asked him to rest, he assured him that his body was perfect, that he didn't need to rest. Then he added that he could fly the plane without gas, which he tried to prove by doing some fancy maneuvers in the sky.

"Funny," he said later, "no one seemed to believe me. Even when I offered them a million each they weren't happy, but looked at each other in such a puzzled way. It made me laugh how they begged me to rest and how worried they looked when I refused. I was the boss and I showed them."

When the plane landed in Brazil by a miracle, C. W. was examined by a physician, forced into another plane and brought to Florida. Upon examination he was talkative, eyes gleaming, exuberant with statements of wealth and power. "I am now one of the richest men in the world," he said. "I'll give you $5,000,000 to start a hospital. My eyes are jewels, diamonds, emeralds", etc., etc.

These delusions of grandeur and the accompanying exuberance were found to be the result of syphilis of the brain.

The mental symptoms of paresis need not always appear as grandiose delusions. Indeed, in some cases the patient is depressed, blaming himself for misdeeds and becoming suicidal. Thus one patient, normally a worrisome, serious-minded person, began to brood about "mistakes." She lost interest in her household duties and feared she would be punished. Harassed by such fears, she made a suicidal attempt. The examination showed a sad woman, sitting with drooping posture. The pupils were miotic and the tendon reflexes unequal. There were forgetfulness, slurring speech, and positive spinal fluid findings. Malarial treatment followed by tryparsamide was curative.

Another patient, who was always uneasy and distrustful, became unduly suspicious. She believed that the neighbors were spying on her so that they could burglarize her home. She spent hours peering behind drawn blinds to watch their movements. Her mental symptoms resembled a paranoid psychosis, but she exhibited evidence of far advanced paresis.

A clerk who had been meek and studious took out his savings and purchased a Cadillac car and raced through the neighborhood. He announced to his family that he would go out West and be a racer, enter the movies. He became over-active, jumpy, showed flight of ideas; he resented his brother's counsel and became combative. He looked like a typical manic. The blood and spinal fluid tests furnished the clue to the diagnosis–paresis.

Thus the underlying personality traits will influence the type of symptoms which occur in paresis, whose delusions may express inhibited fears and wishes.

The tempo of the disease is also extremely variable. The onset may be insidious and slow or abrupt and stormy. The course may be rapid – like galloping consumption. Then again the disease may advance slowly, show remissions for months and years, only to flare up again later.

A woman in the forties, who had been a calm and efficient person, suddenly became talkative, sleepless, and incoherent. She was placed in a nursing home for a rest. The symptoms subsided and she returned home. For two years she was apparently well and could manage her household satisfactorily. However, this was only a two years' remission. She became slovenly, neglected her duties, made serious blunders such as burning her husband's valuable papers. She was then examined carefully and found to have loss of memory and judgment, unequal fixed pupils, abnormal reflexes, a positive Wassermann reaction of the blood, and positive spinal fluid findings. Induced malaria was then given for fever therapy but it was too late to repair the damage which had been done.

Whether continuous or interrupted, the disease tends to follow a downward course, the patient ending up "sans eyes, sans ears, sans everything"– a pitiable, emaciated, mentally impoverished person, yet offering to share his fabulous wealth with you. Hence paresis is recognized as one of the most serious of all maladies– accounting for some 10% of admissions to certain State hospitals.

MENINGOVASCULAR TYPES

These represent symptom groups which result from syphilitic change in blood vessels and in the meninges. Depending upon the vessel involved, particular symptoms develop. One patient has symptoms of a cerebral hemorrhage, with paralysis of the right arm and leg and loss of speech; another loses the use of both legs, gradually or suddenly; a third develops pain in the arm and then a dulled sensation in it.

We may glance briefly at several examples.

(a) R. S., a man of 39, worked steadily for a steel mill, when quite suddenly he felt a burning in his legs and he dropped to the ground. He was brought to the Warren City Hospital, his legs paralyzed, and unable to void. I saw this man in consultation with the late Dr. C. W. Thomas and found unequal, fixed pupils, loss of reflexes in the lower extremities, and loss of pain and temperature sense below the umbilicus. The condition was one of thrombosis of the ventromedian artery, a form of meningovascular syphilis. It was successfully treated with antisyphilitic therapy.

(b) In St. Louis in 1936 I saw a colored woman who suddenly developed weakness in all four extremities and in movements of her tongue. The spinal fluid Wassermann was positive and the cell count increased. Her condition was due to a vascular lesion in the lower medulla.

(c) Y. Z., a man in the late fifties, had been troubled by episodes of headaches over a period of years. These were intense, kept him awake during the night, and did not respond to the usual medication. Finally, an episode of headache was attended by a period of speech disturbance. The patient could not express himself well. The laboratory examination showed a 4 plus blood Wassermann. The spinal fluid showed a pressure of 250 mm. of water, a cell count of 300, globulin 3 plus, Wassermann 3 plus, and a slightly altered colloidal gold curve. The diagnosis was obviously syphilitic meningovascular disease. Because of a previous coronary attack, it was deemed unsafe to use malaria. Treatment with tryparsamide, mapharsen and bismuth resulted in a relief of symptoms.

(d) A case of optic atrophy will be discussed in the part dealing with treatment.

Causes of Symptoms

The spirochete finds in the central nervous system a favorable tissue for its growth. It nests in tiny blood vessels, stirring up a reaction of swelling and inflammation which may reach the degree of blocking the lumen completely (endarteritis obliterans). By its presence or its toxins it leads to an inflammation of the meninges and a thickening which strangle blood vessels and nerves, reducing the blood supply to such nerves and to the spinal cord. In paresis, swarms of spirochetes occupy the brain tissue itself, annihilating ganglion cells, stirring up reactions of glial tissues, occluding its blood vessels. Thus, unchecked, the normal pattern of cells in the gray matter is disorganized, the brain shrinks. It is this irritation and brain damage which lead to headaches, confusion, spells of unconsciousness. Then the alertness and judgment fail; there are released freedom of emotional display and delusions of grandeur. Sometimes these represent the person's hitherto unattained strivings and dreams for wealth and power.

He believes these goals attained: "I am Napoleon." "I am wealthy." "I have more wives than King Solomon." The damaged brain deprives the patient of the power to distinguish wish from reality.

The pathology in the brain produces loss of alertness, defects in recent memory, slurred speech, and defective judgment. As the ganglion cells are further destroyed, tremors, paralysis, or convulsions set in. Likewise, emaciation may occur, possibly because of damage to vital metabolic centers. Paresis is a disease of widespread pathology and protean manifestations.

The Diagnosis of Syphilis of the Central Nervous System

There are several ways in which one can diagnose syphilis: (1) history, (2) physical findings, and (3) laboratory tests. Where it is possible to obtain a reliable and complete history of infection it would be easily suspected. However, such a history may be lacking or unavailable. In thirty per cent of patients there was no recognizable initial sore or chancre. Likewise, even if present, it may be so brief, so transitory that it is forgotten. Also the early symptoms may be so common that they are not significant. However, if a patient had syphilis and obtained some (inadequate) treatment and then later showed serious nervous symptoms, we must think seriously of neurosyphilis. Even if the history is negative, we cannot be lulled into a feeling of security, for some do not know and others will not tell.

The physical findings are more important. First are the eye signs. For the poet, the eyes are the windows of the soul; for the doctor they are a door to a diagnosis. Pupils, tiny and pinpoint, which do not react to light, are usually telltale evidence of a spirochetal scar in the brain stem. A combination of eye signs, twitching of the muscles of the face, and abnormal tendon reflexes are often present in paresis. Eye signs, absent knee reflexes, and unsteady posture are a threesome of tabes.

The combination of a positive history and physical findings is quite convincing, but usually we await confirmation by positive laboratory tests.

The blood serology tests (Wassermann, Kline, Hinton) are highly specific. They confirm the clinical evidence; they reveal that the patient has been infected with spirochetes even if the disease is inactive. Even more valuable is a test of the spinal fluid; a count of the number of cells, the amount of protein, and the Wassermann or other serologic test, when positive, afford corroborative evidence of syphilis and of its type.

In a classical case of paresis the cell count will be elevated from 10 to 100 cells; the protein will be increased, 50 to 200 mg. per 100 cc.; the Wassermann positive in all volumes; and the gum mastic curve 5554432100. In tabes the cell count may be increased, the protein moderately increased, and the gum mastic curve 1233221000. In meningovascular syphilis and in any type of treated neurosyphilis, the spinal fluid findings may vary considerably and be less characteristic. In all diagnoses, of course, the laboratory data must be correlated with the clinical findings.

The ideal time to treat syphilis of the nervous system is in its early states – even before symptoms appear. It is too late to diagnose and treat paresis in the Napoleonic stage; then it is usually Waterloo for the patient. To prevent paresis the diagnosis must be made on the early spinal fluid findings. Thus physicians must perform tests of the spinal fluid routinely in all cases of syphilis. To rely upon the assurance of a negative blood test alone after a series of treatments is to neglect the most sensitive index, to fail to "stop, look, and listen." An early L.P. may prevent a late G. P.

The Treatment of Syphilis

The spectre of the spirochete casts its shadow over all illicit intercourse. This is a warning which means avoid exposure. But if you are exposed to a spirochete, do not rely upon hope and trust, but upon chemicals. Methods are now available which will protect a high percentage of those exposed, if used early enough. Prevention and early recognition of syphilis are extremely important. We must prevent the spectre of the spirochete from invading the soma and haunting the soul of man. Public health measures include the isolation during the contagious stage of those patients likely to spread the disease.

PSYCHOTHERAPY OF THE PATIENT WITH SYPHILIS: I have seen patients who have just received the sad news that their sore, or rash, or other symptoms were caused by this disease. They described an overwhelming self-loathing, a sense of horror passing through them when the doctor, with an accusing glance and pointed finger, announced the verdict –"You have syphilis!" "I couldn't sleep, I couldn't eat. I was afraid to touch any person; I hesitated to take a fork or spoon in my hand. I was afraid to go to work because it seemed that people knew of my shame. I wanted to run away. I wanted to die – to think that I had this loathesome disease and might now pass it to my family. I looked at my skin and could picture upon my face those horrible sores I had once seen in a movie."

Such are the tragic thoughts that have been expressed by certain patients who had been frankly, sometimes brutally told of the diagnosis. In some instances, harsh, frightening frankness may be necessary. For example, a callous person with lesions that are potentially contagious, who is indifferent to the dangers to others and who neglects treatment, should be "shocked" into cooperation. But such an approach is not necessary in most instances and is unwise where the syphilis involves the nervous system, was contracted years previously, and is not contagious. It is better to present the matter in a more kindly, more hopeful manner.

To a patient with neurosyphilis I would say: "Your symptoms come from an infection which you acquired many years ago. Sometimes we don't know when it came. But we are sure you have it. If you get treatment, we are reasonably sure it isn't contagious. You can continue living at home and attend to your job. You must get your treatments faithfully, however. There is a good chance that you can be helped. We have some remarkable methods of fighting this disease. There is hope for you!"

Such an introduction to his malady, followed later by further explanations in response to the patient's questions, does not take away self-respect and does not shatter the personality. Yet, gentle as it sounds, the fact of the syphilis is clearly impressed, and at the same time the hope with treatment. Both elements, need and hope, keep the patient faithful in following the course prescribed by the doctor.

TREATMENT OF THE EARLY CASE OF SYPHILIS: The danger of contagion which is present in the stage of chancre and in lesions of the skin and mucous membranes must be guarded against. Isolation in some cases, caution in others, and early treatment in all patients is the rule.

The "Guides to Therapy for Medical Officers" (T.M. 8-210, C 1, May 6, 1943) suggests the following program: "Arsenoxide (mapharsen) will be used as the standard arsenical. Emphasis should also be placed on the completion by each patient of the full schedule of treatment in the time called for, regardless of early serologic reversal. It cannot be too strongly emphasized that the regularity of treatment schedule, without long or short time variations or lapses, is critically important to both infection, control and cure."

The recommended plan covers 26 weeks: Oxophenarsine hydrochloride is given twice weekly during the first ten weeks, plus bismuth subsalicylate, intramuscularly, once weekly for five weeks. Then the patient is given a six weeks' rest period from arsenic but receives weekly doses of bismuth. In the last ten weeks he again receives oxophenarsine hydrochloride twice weekly. Thus the entire course consists of the injections of oxophenarsine hydrochloride, each approximately sixty mg., for a total of 2400 mg., and ten injections of bismuth, each of 0.2 grams of bismuth subsalicylate.

Recently penicillin has been tried for the treatment of early syphilis. It promises to be a valuable addition to our methods, but with this drug also there is no certain cure. Leifer reported excellent results in the treatment of early syphilis, using sixty intramuscular injections of 20,000 units of penicillin in saline solution at three-hour intervals, day and night, for seven and one-half-days. The Committee on Medical Research and the United States Public Health Service recently summarized their studies on the use of penicillin in early syphilis. They advocated a longer course, 3.6 million units (90 injections of 40,000 units each given every two hours or sixty injections of 60,000 units every three hours) for seronegative and 5.4 million units for seropositive primary and early secondary cases. They suggest the combination of arsenic and bismuth with penicillin. Careful follow-up of all cases for relapses is necessary.

TREATMENT OF NEUROSYPHILIS: Whereas neoarsphenamine and oxophenarsine hydrochloride have been effective in the treatment of early syphilis, involvement of the nervous system is a resistant problem. Either the type of spirochete is different, or has been altered by time, or is protected by the tissues in which it lodges. The arsenic which is more effective is a pentavalent form (neosalvarsan and oxophenarsine hydrochloride are trivalent), tryparsamide. This drug is valuable in paresis, although it must be used cautiously because of possible damage to the optic nerves.

When chemical methods are impotent to halt the progress of the disease, as is true in most cases of tabes and paresis, fever treatment is needed. Thanks to the discovery of Wagner von Jauregg, many an early paretic, formerly doomed to deteriorate with dementia and paralysis, can now be rescued. Employing the proper diagnostic and treatment methods, a physician can now maintain or restore to health patients with early forms of tabes and of paresis.

Von Jauregg demonstrated that fever has a healing influence on paresis. Either the organisms are destroyed, or their growth discouraged, or some change is produced in the "soil" so that further damage by the disease is halted and a certain amount of healing takes place. Many methods for producing fever were tried by Von Jauregg but of these malaria was most effective. To this day malaria is still considered most valuable, although in many clinics artificial fever methods are being employed more and more. Fever-producing boxes, such as the inductotherm, can be regulated and operated safely.

The patient must receive an effective amount of fever: 150 hours over 100° Fahrenheit or fifty hours over 104° Fahrenheit. This is arranged in a series of treatments in a fever cabinet or by a series of paroxysms with malaria. The malarial method, which has been widely used for over twenty years, begins with an inoculation of the patient with the blood of one already undergoing treatment. Some days after the inoculation the patient begins to chill, and then goes through regular periods of chills and fever. As a rule he is permitted to have ten to fourteen paroxysms. (See J. E. Moore: *Modern Treatment of Syphilis*, 3rd Edition.)

The success of fever therapy cannot be attained without risk. The growth of the malaria, even though artificial, dissolves erythrocytes, and the fever, either from malaria or electrically produced, brings about a rapid pulse and a fall in blood pressure. If proper caution, with good nursing and medical care, is used, the hazards can be reduced to a minimum. My motto has always been: A live patient with a few spirochetes is better than a dead one with all spirochetes killed. Thus treatment should be interrupted or stopped entirely if there are any signs of imminent danger. Quinine is used to terminate the malarial fever.

The fever treatment is supplemented by chemotherapy. Some

physicians give oxophenarsine hydrochloride simultaneously with the fever cabinet treatment.

Penicillin is used with the fever therapy. It has been my custom to administer 4,000,000 units of penicillin, in doses of 30,000 units intramuscularly every three hours. These injections are given before, during, and after fever therapy. Reports indicate that penicillin alone is helpful and that the combined use of penicillin and fever therapy is even more effective.

One of the most striking examples of improvement which I have ever obtained in neurosyphilis is that of S. M., who was developing blindness from syphilitic optic atrophy. This patient was referred to me by Drs. W. E. and A. B. Bruner, who had found blindness in one eye and beginning loss of vision in the other eye. S. M. was admitted to the University Hospitals. The neurologic examination showed Argyll-Robertson pupils; blindness in the left eye, the disc of which was white; and impaired vision in the right eye, whose disc was pale. He could read only the headlines of a newspaper. The pupils were unequal and did not react to light. The laboratory findings included a positive Kline test of the blood, a positive Wassermann in the spinal fluid, and a gum mastic curve of 332210000.

S. M. was inoculated with tertian malaria and penicillin was started immediately. He was given 10 paroxysms and 4,000,000 units of penicillin. The progressive loss of vision in the right eye was halted and the vision in this eye gradually returned to normal. There was no change in the eye which was already totally blind.

Stokes and Steiger reported upon the effectiveness of penicillin in neurosyphilis, advocating a dose of 4.8 million units of penicillin sodium intramuscularly. O'Leary and his co-workers are less enthusiastic, stating that penicillin alone is not capable of controlling the parenchymatous forms of neurosyphilis. "However, in cases of the meningeal forms of the disease . . . the results thus far are encouraging." Both authors stress the value of penicillin in relieving the lightning pains of tabes. Reynolds, Mohr, and Moore have treated 41 paretic patients, 24 with penicillin alone and 17 with penicillin and malarial therapy. These authors conclude: "The effectiveness of concurrent penicillin-malaria therapy is such as to make it, for the present at least, the treatment of choice for patients with dementia paralytica."

Previously it was my practice to use fever therapy and follow this with tryparsamide, one injection (one gram to three grams) weekly for 50 to 100 doses. For the past year I have used the combination of malaria and penicillin in all cases of active neurosyphilis. Higher doses of penicillin of 6 to 10 million are advocated.

The results in the main were dependent upon the stage of the disease and the type of patient. Patients with early forms of meningoencephalitis (paresis) were improved. Late cases and those with tabes were far less favorable. "If it were done when 'tis done, 'twere well it were done early."

Problems of Rehabilitation

Following a course of fever treatment, the patient needs physical rebuilding with iron, nutritious food, and graduated exercise. Most patients respond promptly, with renewed energy and reawakened interest. In special instances, such as patients with locomotor ataxia, walking exercises, walking with the aid of cane and with constant attention to the ground may help to improve the security and coordination of the gait. Paretics who have lost memory and judgment may but slowly regain such functions. Some remain handicapped; many show remarkable improvement. C. W., the Ferry Pilot whose paresis was acute, should respond favorably to treatment.

The employment problem of the patient with syphilis is serious. Certainly an employer whose physician finds evidence of neurosyphilis would be justified in hesitating to employ such a person. Yet many treated patients succeed in obtaining employment and making good. Where an employer does hire such a person, any risk from the disease should be the employee's.

The matter of re-employment or continued employment is different. R. E. was a delivery man who had worked faithfully for a large company for some 18 years. Although he was walking oddly for some months, no one paid any attention to his peculiar gait. He fell at work and injured his ankle. Recovery was delayed. Definite signs of tabes appeared requiring fever therapy. He improved after treatment, although he retained some unsteadiness of walking. When the physician's statement explaining R. E.'s absence from work was submitted to the employer, he refused to re-employ him on the ground that company rules excluded the employment of persons with syphilis. It was pointed out that R. E. was healthier after the disease was recognized and treated than before. Also he had seniority based upon 18 years of service. His employer generously gave him a trial and this patient made good. Walking with care and watching his step, he had no more falls and performed his job satisfactorily and faithfully. A tragedy was averted when the employer set aside regulation and followed reason and a regard for the individual.

P. M. acted queerly at his work on the machine bench. Later he talked in a peculiar manner and made blunders at work. A careful examination showed an early form of paresis. Fever treatment was instituted after which the patient came regularly for tryparsamide injections. The response to treatment was remarkable. However, when P. M. was ready to return to work, the employment manager objected to rehiring him. The company physician was friendly to the man and the firm was desperately in need of men. P. M. had been capable and experienced, and so he was given a "trial" – subject to discharge at the least sign of failure. Instead of failing, P. M. showed more attention and interest than before. During the rush of war work which his firm had in 1939 to 1942, P. M. proved one of the most loyal and capable workers – indeed, he was promoted to the position of foreman.

Again and again I have seen individuals make good, despite a statistical shadow which follows them. In syphilis, as in other diseases, it is the specific situation of the single patient and not the group that must be considered.

The newer drugs used in treatment, and the earlier recognition of neurosyphilis by routine spinal fluid studies give much hope in a disease previously considered grave. The routine blood tests in many clinics, and premarital and prenatal examinations make it possible to discover syphilis before it has done irreparable damage. With a continuous educational program for prevention and improved methods of treatment, the ravages of syphilis should be reduced to a minimum.

REFERENCES

Parran, T., Jr.: The Eradication of Syphilis as a Practical Public Health Objective. *J. A. M. A.* 97:73, 1931.
Sezary, A.: *La Syphilis du Systeme Nerveux*. Masson et Cie, Paris, 1938.
Leifer, W.: The Treatment of Early Syphilis with Penicillin. *J. A. M. A.*, 129:1247, 1945.
Moore, J. E.: *The Modern Treatment of Syphilis*, 3rd edition. Thomas, Springfield, 1945.

Stokes, J. H., and Steiger, H. P.: Penicillin Alone in Neurosyphilis. *J. A. M. A.*, 131:1, 1946.

O'Leary, P. A., Brunsting, L. A., Ockuly, O.: Penicillin in the Treatment of Neurosyphilis. *J. A. M. A.*, 130:698, 1946.

Reynolds, F. W., Mohr, C. F., and Moore, J. E.: Penicillin in the Treatment of Neurosyphilis. *J. A. M. A.*, 131:1255, 1946.

Moore, M., and Merritt, H. H.: Role of Syphilis of the Nervous System in the Production of Mental Disease. A survey of the various forms of neurosyphilis occurring at Boston Psychopathic Hosp. from 1912–1934. *J. A. M. A.*, 107:1292, 1936.

Fetterman, J. L.: Early Forms of Neurosyphilis. *Ohio State M. J.*, 36:35, 1940.

Merritt, H. H., Adams, R. D., and Solomon, H. C.: *Neurosyphilis.* Oxford University Press, New York, 1946.

Dattner, B.: *Management of Neurosyphilis*, Grune and Stratton, New York, 1944.

Chapter X

EPILEPSY

THE essence of epilepsy is the recurrence of attacks of diminution or loss of consciousness with the release of convulsive movements or other abnormal reactions. The detailed symptoms which may occur under the heading of epilepsy are numerous. Some are primary, the attacks proper. Others are secondary and consist of the physical, social, and industrial complications that result from the seizures.

The Primary Symptoms of Epilepsy

The primary symptoms of epilepsy are the attacks, which may be listed under the headings of grand mal, petit mal, psychomotor, Jacksonian, and special varieties. Although certain patients exhibit one type of attack only, the majority have an assortment of attacks. If we study the life story of an epileptic patient, it is not rare to find that the initial disturbances were brief petit mal spells, but that at a later time grand mal attacks developed. Likewise, a patient whose seizures are predominantly Jacksonian also shows generalized, typical grand mal seizures.

A. Grand Mal Attacks

These are the dramatic features described through the ages and vividly portrayed in pictures and in words. Lucretius, in 95 B. C., wrote of an epileptic seizure:

"Oft too some wretch, before our startled sight,
Struck as with lightning, by some keen disease
Drops sudden:—by the dread attack o'erpowered
He foams, he groans, he trembles, and he faints;
Now rigid, now convulsed, his laboring lungs
Heave quick, and quivers each exhausted limb,
Spread through the frame, so deep and dire disease
Perturbs his spirit: as the briny main
Foams through each wave beneath the tempest's ire.
But when, at length, the morbid cause declines,
And the fermenting humors from the heart
Flow back—with staggering foot the man first treads.
Led gradual on to intellect and strength."

As an aid to a better understanding of the convulsive attack, it has been my custom to divide the seizure into three periods. I designate these periods as pre-crisis, crisis, and post-crisis. (Crisis is the French designation for the epileptic seizure.) The term, pre-crisis, applies to the period of warning, of uncomfortable symptoms that precede the loss of consciousness. It includes the hours or minutes of changed feelings which each patient recognizes as foreboding trouble. Some describe a heightened awareness, "being alerted" for trouble. Others feel dull and uncomfortable. In most patients, there is no long stage, but odd sensations which last but moments. One patient describes blurred vision, another speaks of a humming sound in his head, a third is troubled by palpitation or abdominal distress, a fourth becomes aware of weakness or trembling in one limb. In rare instances there is a feeling of bliss welcomed by the patient (Dostoevski). Such sensations, recurring rather consistently before each attack of loss of consciousness, are in the nature of a warning. Patients seek to protect themselves in the face of such warning. Some try clenching their fists or start rapid action to "overpower the spell." Others seek a safe position to await the attack. At times there is no warning whatsoever and the initial manifestation is the loss of consciousness.

The crisis, as has been vividly described again and again, consists of a loss of consciousness, often accompanied by a cry, and a sudden fall. The patient may pitch forward, slump to the ground, or fall in any other direction. At first the patient is rigid, with jaws clenched, arms extended, legs outstretched. Then he begins to shake violently, the head striking the ground, the arms thrust repeatedly outward, the legs jerking up and down, the jaws opening and closing, chest muscles set so that the features become cyanotic and a bubbly foam appears in the mouth. After about a minute's convulsing movements, the shaking slows, the muscles gradually relax, and the patient can then resume breathing. Gradually his color returns to normal and he may fall off into slumber. During the attack proper, there is commonly injury from the fall, and, in some attacks, involuntary emptying of the bladder.

The third stage of the attack, or post-crisis, is the period of a return to consciousness. Some patients wake up rather briskly when the convulsion is ended; others fall into a deep sleep which lasts for minutes or hours. The majority are stuporous for minutes and then gradually open their eyes to blurred, confused surroundings. The patient does not know what has happened, does not understand how he got to be on the ground, objects and people seem blurred in one indistinct image. In the course of minutes, he notices that his head aches and that his muscles are sore, and gradually becomes cognizant that he has had an attack. Objects then grow more distinct and he is able to recognize individuals. Step by step consciousness returns and, in the course of time, the mind is fully clear. As a rule, there is no recollection whatsoever of the attack proper.

Of course the three stages vary in different patients and in the same patient from one attack to the other, yet the pattern is recognizable to the patient and to the observer.

B. Petit Mal

Petit mal, or little sickness, designates the brief spells which epileptics have. In the petit mal spell, there is usually a brief diminution rather than a complete loss of consciousness. The patient stops whatever he has been doing, stares vacantly, makes peculiar movements with his lips and tongue, may twitch or shake; another patient changes color and is troubled by epigastric and other visceral symptoms. In some individuals there is merely an involuntary thrust of the arm or a kick of the leg. Any object that is held in the hand is flung; the leg may bump into a chair or table. If this occurs while the patient is eating, the spoon is dropped or thrown. The episode, as a rule, is so brief that within moments the patient can resume quite normally the task that he was doing before this occurred.

Lennox subdivided petit mal spells under three headings: (1) pykno-epilepsy, (2) myoclonic epilepsy, and (3) akinetic epilepsy. The first designation is applied to the very brief periods of blankness lasting from five to 30 seconds. During the temporary "blackouts," which occur very frequently, there may be a little twitching and some automatic behaviour. In the myoclonic variety, there is obvious muscle contraction without detectable loss of consciousness. The akinetic type consists of a sudden loss of postural control, with nodding of the head or a sudden fall. Without any warning and without coincident muscular jerk, the patient collapses.

A petit mal is essentially a lapse in consciousness during which other release phenomena may appear. The staring, the twitching, rarely incontinence, the automatic movements are some of the release phenomena.

C. Jacksonian Attacks

A specific kind of seizure, first described by Hughlings Jackson, has certain characteristic features. The attack begins in one region of the body in the form of muscle contractions such as twitching or spasm, or with sensory disturbance such as numbness, tingling, or burning. The contraction of the odd movement spreads from the original site, say the right foot, upwards to involve the entire right leg, the right arm, and face. So too the odd sensation marches upward and radiates over the entire side of the body. Often the sensory disturbance is quickly followed by contraction which spreads over the same half of the body. As a rule, the patient remains conscious during the initial phase of such an attack and sometimes throughout the entire experience. However, he may be conscious during the beginning moments of the contraction or paresthesia and then lose consciousness as he goes through a generalized convulsive seizure.

Jacksonian attacks signify a focal lesion in the brain. The region of the body in which the symptoms begin corresponds to the area in the brain which controls its function. Thus, if the initial symptom be a contraction of the right big toe, the location of the lesion is in the paracentral lobule of the left hemisphere. If the initial symptom be a burning sensation in the left hand, the lesion is likely to be in the right postcentral hand area.

A patient who is subject to Jacksonian attacks may also have generalized convulsions. As a rule, if the symptoms continue over a period of years, they do not remain as pure Jacksonian seizures, but are likely to include generalized attacks as well as the focal ones. Quite commonly such attacks denote an organic pathologic process in the brain and require a careful search for such a lesion.

D. Other Special Types of Attacks

There are spells characterized chiefly by peculiar mental states, by odd behavior, and particularly by continued automatic action. The term, psychomotor equivalent, has been used to describe such spells. A common experience such as that reported by one of my patients is as follows: He will be walking along Euclid Avenue and notice the store windows at East Ninth Street and that a clock on the corner reads 11:30. He may then continue walking a matter of a mile and suddenly notice that it is 12:00. He has been entirely unaware of sights seen or sounds heard, and has no recollection whatsoever of what he has done. His behavior was purely automatic.

During such automatic states, the patient may carry out simple routine performance or he may execute some unusual and perhaps dangerous act. An example of the latter kind is that of a soldier who, while on guard duty, shot his gun, killing a soldier who was a total stranger to him in a tent quite a distance away. A careful study of the case showed no motive whatsoever for this act. The history revealed that the patient had for some years been having occasional lapses, with drooping of his head and sagging of his arms. He described certain periods of automatic behavior. An investigation, using sodium amytal intravenously, did not reveal any recollection of the event of the killing. An electroencephalographic study showed slow brain waves such as are seen in psychomotor equivalents. On the basis of such findings, this soldier was discharged with a diagnosis of epilepsy, rather than court-martialed for criminal behavior.

There are other interesting types of spells which are associated with lesions in the temporal lobe. The patient may go into a more prolonged trance, a sort of dream state in which he lives through, in imagery, a scene which seems very familiar to him. During each of these spells, the same scene is relived. It has all the aspects of familiarity and recognition.

For example, a young woman stated that, during the period when she would look blank, she found herself in an oriental bazaar in a city like Bagdad, looking at beautiful tapestries and precious stones. The scene was familiar as though she had been in such a place frequently during her childhood, yet she had lived in the City of Cleveland all her life. Such experiences, called déjà vu, are thought to be related to lesions in the temporal lobe.

Another interesting type of experience of epileptic patients is known as an uncinate gyrus fit. The patient becomes aware of a faint or pungent odor in the room. This is an hallucination because there is no external, real cause for such an odor. The patient may mention the smell of burning onions and actually look for the source of this burning, when quite suddenly he may lose consciousness and fall to the ground in a convulsion. Such attacks are related to lesions on the medial aspect of the temporal lobe where there is a center for the sense of smell. Recently I saw a patient who had two kinds of attacks, the psychomotor equivalents in which she would wander away and be lost, and several episodes of smelling some strange, pungent odors. Both the symptoms pointed to a lesion in the temporal lobe. The examination showed a difference in the reflexes on the two sides and early choked disc. An exploratory operation was carried out, revealing a tumor deep in the temporal lobe.

Secondary Symptoms of Epilepsy

If we view the basic symptom, namely loss of consciousness, as the primary symptom of this disease, let us take up two groups of symptoms which can be considered secondary. We shall include here first the complications that occur from attacks and secondly the psychological, social, and industrial problems that arise because of seizures.

A. Trauma

Patients who lose consciousness, fall, and whose muscles contract violently are apt to injure themselves. Thus, a bitten tongue or an abrasion of the lip and cheek is fairly common as the result of a major attack. In the fall itself patients have burned, cut, and injured themselves to some degree. Then too, the violent muscular contraction may cause a fracture of the spine. Some years ago Dr. Eugene Freedman at University Hospitals x-rayed routinely the thoracic spines of some fifty epileptic patients. We were amazed to find that in six of them there had been compression fractures. These fractures were minimal in degree, without deformity, troublesome pain, or other disturbing symptoms. They were silent fractures at the time of the examination, although the history revealed that the patients had back pain following a severe attack some time in the past.

More serious injuries occur if an epileptic has an attack while driving a car. I recall one or two patients who had such tragic experiences, wrecking their machines and sustaining severe bodily injury.

Another complication of attacks is a period of mental confusion following the seizure. Practically all patients have loss of memory for the attack itself; occasionally, however, the attack is followed by a prolonged period either of sleep or of actual clouding of consciousness. Indeed in some cases a patient may be clouded or confused for many days. I recall several patients who were confused to the point of irrational behavior which lasted several days and then cleared up. There are also some instances of psychoses of a chronic type which may occur in connection with epilepsy. For example, F. S. is a young woman of 18 who has had attacks for many years. Then she developed a loss of interest in school, neglected her duties at home, spent considerable time in daydreaming. She now presents the features of a psychosis which certainly resembles schizophrenia. Such instances are indeed rare in private practice.

B. Psychological Symptoms of Epilepsy

Since time immemorial the epileptic has been looked upon as "possessed" by some demon or evil spirit, a person who is eccentric and peculiar. In ancient times epileptics might be considered as especially favored by the gods or more often as outcasts. The patients with severe epileptic seizures and some mental disturbance were frequently housed in colonies. Thus the sufferer from epilepsy had a sense of degradation, a feeling of being unwanted. In more recent times the epileptic child who had seizures in the classroom was often excused or expelled from school and not permitted to return. The epileptic adult who had attacks was fired from his job and not rehired.

Patients frequently labor under the fear of being detected, perhaps dread the next attack because it may mean humiliation, heartbreak, and loss of a job. Some disorders confer a certain prestige, as one may realize when he visits a patient recovering from an appendix operation, but the sufferer from epilepsy feels stigmatized and is somehow conscious of social shame. This sense of having something undesirable and the fear of unemployment represent two major psychological handicaps of the epileptic.

Unemployment itself is a definite complication. During the 1930's following the depression, many an epileptic who was so unfortunate as to have an attack at work, found himself minus a job. No one would rehire him if he admitted the nature of his illness.

Another fear is that of "loss of mind." It had been the false belief that patients subject to this malady showed deterioration. Quite commonly the epileptic or his family would ask me how long it would be before the patient would lose his mind.

Recent observations tend to disprove the age-old belief that epileptics as a class deteriorate. Some years ago M. R. Barnes and I started a serial study of the intelligence of epileptic patients and found no serious change over a period of some five years. Several of these patients have been checked in 1946 by E. J. Wilson and the I. Q. level is approximately the same as it was 20 years ago when the initial tests were made. Paskind reported that many of his private patients, housewives, clerks, teachers, professional men and women, were capable of maintaining their jobs and their positions in society despite years of epilepsy. So too Lennox has observed a similiar encouraging situation. Of course certain epileptics are feebleminded to begin with or lose intellectual capacity as the result of a progressive organic brain disorder such as hydrocephalus.

Causes of Epilepsy

Any interference with the function of the brain may induce a convulsive attack. Yet there is a certain susceptibility which may explain the continued tendency towards attacks, the chronic nature of epilepsy. The exact nature of such susceptibility is not known, though the abnormalities commonly found in brain wave studies point to some latent electrical disturbance in the brain as reflecting this susceptibility. In addition to the tendency, a second factor is a brain lesion such as the swelling and scar formation from trauma, infection, vascular disease, tumor, etc. A correlated factor is a sudden alteration in the blood supply or in the sugar metabolism of the brain. Thus, an abrupt cerebral anemia which occurs in Stokes-Adams and in the carotid sinus syndrome may lead to loss of consciousness and convulsions. Although all three factors may be interwoven as a cause of attacks, nevertheless one etiologic agent, sufficiently severe, can precipitate a convulsive seizure.

Some years ago Cobb listed many possible specific disturbances in the brain, ranging from embryologic defect to senile degeneration, and including chemical changes and the results of drugs. He listed several common denominators such as anoxemia and impaired circulation.

Penfield subdivided the causes of epilepsy into two major groups, those with a demonstrable cerebral lesion and those without such a lesion. In the former group are included tumors of the brain, scars which have arisen from injury or infection and a variety of gross defects, some congenital and others acquired. The second group, according to Penfield, includes cases caused by abnormal chemical or circulatory disturbances plus those which are called idiopathic (occurring without obvious cause).

It is my custom to subdivide epilepsy into two classes: idiopathic and symptomatic. The idiopathic, by far the more common, usually begins early in life, particularly in the pre-puberty and puberty periods, and may continue onwards. There is no recognizable local or physiologic cause for the attacks. The symptomatic variety may commence at any period in life and one is able to discover a specific cause for the attacks. Within the second category are cases of head injury, brain tumor, and syphilis.

History-Taking in Epilepsy

In order to appraise the nature of the attacks and particularly to learn something of the personality of the patient who has them, a detailed history-taking is significant. An outline which I have used in my office is the following:

I DESCRIPTION OF ATTACKS
    (A)—Major
        Pre-crisis: Odd sensations, changes in mood and feeling, motor manifestations or somatic symptoms.
        Crisis: A description of the manifestations as experienced by the patient and/or reported by observers.
        Type of fall, turning of head, frothing, motor phenomena, incontinence.
        Post-crisis: Confusion and amnesia, headache, muscle soreness, effects of injury (sore lips, cheek, or tongue).
    (B)—Minor
        Subjective experiences and objective observations referred to as Petit Mal, or by various designations. Lapse, dazed period, blackout, faint feeling, little one, spell, twitching.
    (C)—Miscellaneous
        Deja Vu phenomena, olfactory hallucinations, acts performed during periods of hypoconsciousness (psychomotor equivalent, automatism, fugue).

II CLINICAL COURSE
- (A)—Time relationships: Date of onset, time of occurrence, and frequency of attacks.
- (B)—Diagnostic studies and results.
- (C)—Therapy received and response to therapy.
- (D)—Sequence of events as to attacks, social and industrial experiences, educational advancement and personality growth.

III PAST HISTORY
- (A)—Birth and development: Symptoms of cerebral trauma or congenital defect; blue baby, convulsions, vomiting; retarded development.
- (B)—Childhood illnesses and injuries: Evidence of involvement of the brain during an illness or from trauma (unconsciousness, spasms).
- (C)—The past occurrence of "spells" which appeared during a short period of time.

IV FAMILY HISTORY
- (A)—History of the occurrence of sick headaches, fainting spells, spasms, convulsions, or mental illness.

The next step, of course, is a complete examination with a detailed neurological study. Practical laboratory tests include an x-ray of the skull, a blood Wassermann, and usually a spinal fluid examination. Of outstanding importance is an electroencephalogram or brain wave study. This new method is of particular value in the epileptic patient. It helps to distinguish the epileptic spell from other attacks and may serve to localize a focal lesion. If the history of the attacks, the physical findings, or the brain wave studies show evidence of a probable focal lesion, then a pneumoencephalogram should be done. The injection of air or another gas into the spinal canal will provide a clear visualization of the ventricles and the subarachnoid pathways as an aid to the diagnosis of a focal lesion such as a brain tumor.

The Electroencephalogram in Epilepsy

(Contributed by F. A. Gibbs)

"Since almost any chemical disturbance in a tissue will give rise to small electrical disturbances it is not surprising that the brain produces electricity. The record of the electrical activity of the brain is called the electroencephalogram, E.E.D., or brain waves for short, but the long word is not so hard to say either: "Electro" for electric, "encephalo" for brain, and "gram" for writing; electroencephalogram. It can be recorded by fastening electrodes to the scalp and connecting them to an amplifier and

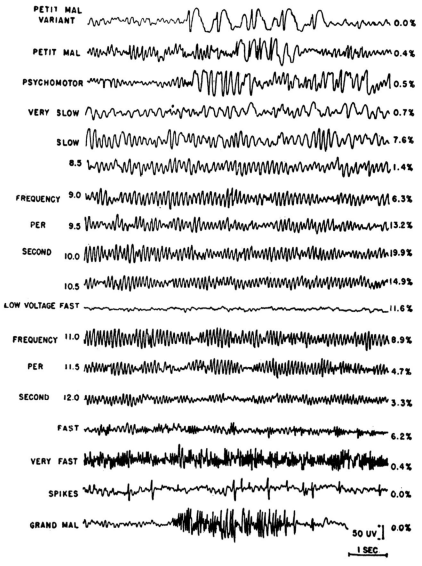

ink writing meter. The instrument which records the electroencephalogram is called an electroencephalograph.

"The extraordinary thing about the electrical activity of the brain is that it is definitely rhythmic. In adults the waves that are recorded have a frequency of about ten cycles per second. In infants they are much slower; around two to four cycles per second. Newborn infants, while awake, show nothing that can be clearly identified as an electroencephalogram. It is only at the third month that rhythmic electrical activity becomes clearly evident in the waking state. The next important and extraordinary fact about the electrical activity of the brain is that it changes with disturbances of consciousness, particularly those that occur in epilepsy and related organic brain disorders. It shows no alterations in schizophrenia, manic-depressive psychoses, neurosis, hysteria or a great variety of psychiatric disorders. It cannot read thoughts or test intelligence.

"Of all the diagnostic studies that can be used in epilepsy electroencephalography is the most informative. As has been stated, the normal cortical rate in the adult is about ten per second. If this speeds up to thirty or forty waves per second a person is likely to lose consciousness and go into a convulsion. If it slows down to three or four waves per second a person is likely to become stuporous or lapse into coma. In about 85% of epileptics an electroencephalogram taken atrrandom shows abnormal waves. The 15% of persons whose electroencephalograms are normal on routine examination, but who have a history of epileptic seizures if studied at the time of the seizure or repeatedly on other occasions, will show electroencephalographic abnormality. A normal electroencephalogram is like a negative Wassermann, presumptive but not positive evidence of normality.

"A different type of wave appears in association with each of the three major types of epileptic seizure. An alternate 3-per-second wave-and-spike pattern or dome and dart, as it has been called, is associated with typical petit mal seizures. Grand mal seizures or tonic-clonic convulsions are associated with fast activity which begins at a low voltage but increases in voltage as the disturbance proceeds, while at the same time becoming slower in frequency. A psychic equivalent or psychomotor attack is associated with flat top 4-6 per second waves. Characteristic samples of each of these patterns are shown in the classification chart. Such discharges appear not only at the time of a seizure but also between seizures. At times no clinical manifestations occur with a brain wave discharge such as ordinarily accompanies a clinical seizure. In such a case the discharge is called a sub-clinical seizure discharge. The detection of sub-clinical discharges in the absence of any clinical history of epilepsy is suggestive of epilepsy or, at the least, of a strong tendency toward convulsive disorder.

"The distinctions which the electroencephalogram makes between different types of seizures are of great practical importance. It has been found that the drugs which are now used against epileptic seizures tend to be effective against specific types of seizure. For example, the new drug, Tridione, is almost specifically effective against the 3-per-second dome and dart discharge of petit mal epilepsy, and is quite ineffective against other types of seizure.

"In addition to diagnosing and classifying abnormality the electroencephalogram aids in localizing an area of injury. For example, in Jacksonian epilepsy the abnormal waves begin in or are limited to the region surrounding the damaged cortex. Thus, tumors, particularly those causing epileptic attacks, can be better diagnosed and more accurately localized."

Value of EEG in Differential Diagnosis

Recently two patients were referred because of spells. One was a child of six who would "go blank" and sometimes faint. Her spells occurred once or twice a week and were attributed to excitement. The spells were short and were associated with an upward turning of the eyes, and transitory pallor. Petit mal was suspected, yet there was some doubt until the brain wave studies showed the characteristic 3-per-second dart and dome pattern. Tridoine was administered and has been remarkably effective. This child has been almost completely free of spells since this drug was prescribed in January, 1946.

Another patient had spells of fainting, also under excitement. Her history was charged with nervous upsets and emotional instability. A psychogenic basis for the spells was suspected – the brain waves proved to be perfectly normal. This finding did not rule out epilepsy (for as stated in Dr. Gibbs' discussion, on routine examination about 15 per cent of patients with seizures have normal electroencephalograms) but in this case is created a presumption that the condition was not epilepsy. We employed psychotherapy, not medication against attacks. The patient gained relief when she obtained clear insight into the nature of her symptoms and learned how to cope with a serious family problem.

Trauma and Epilepsy

Trauma to the brain is one of the important causes of epilepsy. Indeed, there are some writers who are of the opinion that many cases of so-called idiopathic epilepsy are the result of trauma during birth. As regards the direct effect of a brain injury in adult life as a cause of epilepsy, there is complete agreement. A skull fracture with hemorrhage in the underlying brain, or tearing of the brain substance by a bullet or other foreign body produces a scar tissue reaction. Such scar tissue, with adhesions of the pia and the dura, may interfere with the circulation of the cerebrospinal fluid and can cause "pulling" on the brain. Thus, Penfield and Foerster, who have studied this subject in great detail, have described a shifting of the ventricles, under the interesting title of "Wandering Ventricle." Penfield has furthermore shown how reactive changes proceed slowly and persistently over a period of years at the site of such a scar. The destroyed tissue replaced by a scar and particularly the area of slow healing and repair serve as a trigger mechanism to induce attacks. Brain wave studies will reveal that such a lesion is a center from which abnormal focal waves start.

Traumatic epilepsy sets in months or years after the injury has been sustained. In a study which I carried out some years ago (Mode of Onset of Epilepsy), I reported some eight cases in whom the epilepsy was distinctly traumatic in nature. The attacks began from months to eight years after the injury. The average was 18 months.

As an example, J. S., a young adolescent, had been accidentally shot in the head while hunting. A fragment of bullet had lodged in the brain and a hemiplegia resulted. Some 18 months after the injury the first Jacksonian attack appeared. These seizures recurred at intervals of approximately once a month for a matter of years.

The epileptic attacks that occur following injury are likely to be Jacksonian in character. The focal lesion in the brain sets off an attack which begins in a region of the body that corresponds to the injured area. This rule, however, is not universal, and there are some patients who have psychomotor attacks or generalized seizures. There will be a further discussion on the relationship of epilepsy and trauma in the next chapter.

Treatment

The aims of treatment are several: to prevent attacks, to build self-confidence of the patient, to assist the patient to maintain his social and industrial position.

A. Prevention of Attacks

The first duty is to discover if there is a specific cause for the attacks. If patient has syphilis of the brain or a brain tumor, this requires appropriate medical and surgical action. Traumatic epilepsy may be caused by a focal scar and, in certain instances, surgical removal of that scar may be advisable. The work of Penfield promised considerable benefit to those who have traumatic epilepsy. Thus far the results have not been quite as good as expected.

Patients who have a specific cause of epilepsy and those who are troubled by the idiopathic variety can be benefited by the use of anticonvulsant medication.

Sodium bromide had been the remedy of choice from about 1850 until 1912 when phenobarbital was introduced. Phenobarbital proved to be more effective and was less likely to produce skin eruptions and clouding of consciousness. It was prescribed in dosages beginning with gr. ½ (0.03 gm.) t.i.d. to gr. 1½ (0.1 gm.) two to four times daily. In adequate dosage phenobarbital was quite effective in reducing the frequency and intensity of grand mal convulsions but had only a moderate, if any, effect on petit mal spells. Then too, large doses of phenobarbital tended to make some patients dull and lethargic.

The introduction by Putnam and Merritt in 1938 of dilantin sodium was a remarkable advance in the therapy of epilepsy. This new drug was superior to phenobarbital in its anticonvulsant qualities. My experience with dilantin sodium may be summarized with the statement that it gave remarkable freedom from seizures to one-third of the patients, a substantial to moderate benefit to a third, and only doubtful help to the remainder. However, dilantin sodium produced several undesirable side actions: Swelling of the gums was common; tremors, incoordination and irritability occurred when the dosage was high; and occasionally more serious digestive or mental symptoms developed. Furthermore, dilantin sodium was of little value for petit mal spells.

To obtain the maximum therapeutic benefit with the minimum of side actions, it has been my custom to prescribe the dilantin sodium in graduated doses. For instance, the patient is given one capsule, gr. 1½ (0.1 gm.) daily, for the first week. A second capsule is then added for the second week. If the patient is still troubled by attacks, then we may increase the dose of dilantin sodium to a third capsule daily. If the spells still recur, it is my custom at this point to prescribe phenobarbital along with dilantin sodium. Here again we begin with 1½ gr. (0.1 gm.) and increase as is necessary. Many of my patients have not obtained substantial freedom from attacks until the dosage has reached 4½ gr. (0.3 gm.) of dilantin sodium daily plus 4½ gr. (0.3) of phenobarbital per day. When these drugs are combined, they tend to augment each other's anticonvulsant qualities while they offset the side actions.

Recently a new drug has been introduced for grand mal attacks, namely mesantoin (Sandoz Chemical Works). This new preparation, which is closely related to dilantin chemically, has proved to be effective as a substitute for dilantin. It is also administered in graduated doses, beginning with one or two tablets and increasing up to six, eight, or in rare instances even ten tablets daily. The combination of mesantoin with dilantin is highly satisfactory.

Kozol, who has had the most extensive experience with this drug, has found that it was effective in many patients in whom dilantin sodium had failed or had been of slight benefit. Furthermore it could be added to dilantin sodium and the two drugs combined exerted a stronger anticonvulsant effect than dilantin alone. The side actions of mesantoin were relatively mild, namely a rash in a small percentage of cases and some drowsiness when the dosage was increased to the larger amounts.

I have had experience with this preparation for a period of about two years. The patients who have received this preparation were either those who had not benefited to any great degree from dilantin sodium or had received no previous therapy. The substantial majority have reported considerable relief from attacks. Indeed, at this stage mesantoin gives promise of being an outstanding remedy.

The three most useful drugs, phenobarbital, dilantin sodium, and mesantoin, have failed to control petit mal. Another preparation, tridione, was first used by Lennox several years ago. Lennox has reported splendid results from tridione in the relief of all forms of petit mal attacks. My own experience has not been quite so favorable. However, in those patients who have petit mal spells without evidence of organic brain changes and in whose encephalogram there are clear-cut spike and dome waves, excellent results have been secured. There are several patients who formerly suffered from many minor attacks per day and who are now entirely free. Tridione comes in five gr. (0.3 gm.) capsules and is prescribed as follows: One capsule three times a day at the outset and the dosage may be increased to four, six, or even ten capsules if necessary.

Unfortunately tridione exhibits unfavorable side actions. Many patients mention a disturbance in vision in which all objects present a sparkling glare like fresh snow glittering in the winter sunlight. Although this hypersensitivity can be relieved by dark glasses, it is unpleasant for many patients. Less commonly a rash may occur. More serious, however, is the reported occurrence of severe anemia with destruction of the granulocyte cells from tridione. Because of these side actions I have limited the use of tridione to those cases of petit mal where the attacks are numerous and in whom there is no organic brain disorder. Furthermore, it is advisable to do blood studies at monthly intervals so that any change in the blood picture may be detected at a stage where the condition may yet be reversible.

The following general guides will help the physician in the medicinal treatment of epilepsy:

1. The dosage should be individualized and adjusted to the type of disease and the needs of the patient. It is best to start with a small amount of the drug and to increase gradually in accordance with the patient's requirements. Such a program of graduated dosage will reduce the tendency to toxic reactions.

2. The dosage should be adequate. The aim of therapy is not any specific number of pills but rather substantial relief from seizures. In the past physicians have tended to use insufficient amounts of anticonvulsant drugs.

3. Combinations of medication often have a superior anticonvulsant action to one drug alone. For instance, we can combine dilantin sodium and phenobarbital and thus secure an added anti-

convulsant protection, yet each drug offsets the side actions of the other.

4. Continuity of Treatment: The patient and his family should understand that epilepsy is a long-term illness and that the treatment with medication requires long-term care. Putnam has offered the interesting analogy that epileptic patients should receive drugs as diabetic individuals take insulin. Patients should therefore see the doctor frequently until the dosage is stabilized and optimum benefit obtained. Thereafter, the patient should be seen at intervals of once in two to three months as is required. The family must be warned against the tendency to stop drugs—a tendency that arises from two alternatives: The patient is better or he is unimproved. Instead of stopping the drugs, the former demands the continuation of therapy and the latter should be a demand for more medication.

If a patient develops status epilepticus, this is best treated by an injection of sodium phenobarbital, gr. two to gr. four intramuscularly. Should the attacks continue, then sodium amytal, gr. 7½ intravenously is helpful. If the above measures fail to stop the attacks, then large doses of paraldehyde intravenously or the use of ether as an anesthetic may be resorted to.

A minor item of some value is an identification card. It sometimes happens that an epileptic will have an attack in a street car or in some public place when he is alone. Then the emergency or ambulance is called and he is rushed to a hospital where he is subjected to many procedures before the nature of his malady is understood. After all, a patient who is unconscious or stuporous is a diagnostic challenge that requires prompt attention. Usually the patient awakens before the tests are completed and can explain. An identification card similar to that which certain diabetics carry would make the nature of the attack clear and would spare the patient unnecessary tests, expensive treatments, or even mishandling. I recall the case of one patient who, during the prohibition era, was found wandering in an ataxic, "drunken" manner. He was picked up by the police, who used forceful methods to try to find out his source of liquor supply. After about an hour, he was able to explain that he was an epileptic patient.

B. Psychotherapy for the Epileptic

In addition to the anticonvulsant medication, the epileptic

often is in need of an understanding of his illness and a removal of certain fears that have developed. Frequently the patient or his family dread the use of the term, epileptic.

One should offer hope to the epileptic and his family. There is always the possibility that the attacks may cease spontaneously or from medication. This rare occurrence, except in childhood, represents such good fortune that every epileptic may live in the hope that he too might enjoy such a blessing. Furthermore there is the hope that new therapies may prove superior to the medication now available. The epileptic patient should be encouraged with the confidence that his attacks will be reduced in frequency that he will be able to obtain a job and keep it, and that, with few restrictions, he may lead a normal life. Many of my patients are married and getting along well, and their children are free of epilepsy.

One may call upon figures from history such as Caesar, Mohamet, and Napoleon, geniuses who also had epilepsy. I frequently refer to the brilliant Russian writer, Dostoevski, who, at the age of 24, wrote a best seller, *Poor People*. Dostoevski had epileptic attacks throughout his life, yet at the age of sixty he was still capable of another masterpiece, *Brothers Karamazov*. Epilepsy obviously need not lead to deterioration.

Educational and Employment Problems of the Epileptic

If a child suffers from frequent attacks of grand mal type and these have not been adequately relieved by drugs, he will probably have trouble in school. Many an epileptic has been dismissed from class with instructions to the family that he will not be accepted again. In one city, Detroit, there is a special school for epileptic children. It is important that the boards of education appreciate their responsibility to provide sufficient education for the epileptic child as well as for any other handicapped pupil. Such children should be educated with a view towards a possibly restricted career. It is my custom to encourage the parents of an epileptic boy to cultivate interests in horticulture, nursery work, farming, as against railroad engineering or mechanical work that might expose the person to moving, dangerous machinery. Likewise, a girl student could be encouraged in lines such as crocheting and dressmaking, work that she could do on her own, as against let us say singing in public. There are certain situations in which an attack is rather embarrassing or hazardous.

It has been my experience also to confer with the school nurse and explain the nature of the child's difficulty. It may be necessary for the nurse to explain to fellow students the possibility of an attack. Life cannot be made shock-proof and it is better that children be exposed to the occurrence of such an attack without alarming, hysterical disturbance. It is part of education for the school nurse or school physician to give a brief talk to the class, in the absence of the epileptic student. His or her fellow classmates should be made to understand that anyone of us may have a fainting spell or become witnesses to a fit. They should be instructed on how to protect the person during his unconscious period and how later to assist him to a dispensary or to his home. One student might be selected or asked to volunteer as a "buddy" to keep an observing eye on the epileptic when he is going up and down stairs and when he is en route to and from school. Under such a regime, the classmates are active participants, not passive spectators whose emotions recoil unhealthily within themselves.

Epileptics who have attacks at work as a rule have been dismissed from employment. This was the practice before the war. As a result of such unemployment, I found many epileptic persons idle, self-conscious, worrisome, and impoverished. The search for another job was futile and heartbreaking. To meet this need, we established in the City of Cleveland a protected work-shop known as the Auracraft Shop. Here, under supervision and with emphasis upon aiding the person, practically every epileptic desirous of work was given a chance for training and employment. The work was of a routine character and relatively safe. Miss Bell Greve of the Association for the Crippled and Disabled was instrumental in helping to set up this shop.

During the war years, industry, hungry for manpower, was less critical in its employee selection. Many an epileptic who had been trained in the Auracraft Shop as well as others in private life were able to secure employment. In general, the work of the epileptic was satisfactory. There was no increased accident rate because epileptics, like other handicapped individuals, are so grateful for the opportunity to work and so conscientious that they did not have more accidents than the average. Furthermore, such epileptics had been receiving adequate anticonvulsant medication so that the attacks were few and far between.

In placement of the epileptic, one should be cautious about such hazards as sharp cutting instruments, open flames, driving automobiles, working around railroads, working on scaffolds, and other hazardous situations. Properly placed, the epileptic who has average intelligence and good personality, will prove to be a loyal and helpful workman.

REFERENCES

Lennox, W. G.: *Science and Seizures.* Harper & Bros., New York, 1941.

Fetterman, J. L., and Barnes, M. R.: Serial Studies of the Intelligence of Patients with Epilepsy. *Arch. Neurol. & Psychiat.*, 32:797, 1934.

Barnes, M. R., and Fetterman, J. L.: Mentality of Dispensary Epileptic Patients. *Arch. Neurol. & Psychiat.*, 40:903, 1938.

Paskind, H. A.: Extramural Patients with Epilepsy, with Special Reference to Frequent Absence of Deterioration, *Arch. Neurol. & Psychiat.*, 28:370, 1932.

Cobb, S.: Causes of Epilepsy. *Arch. Neurol. & Psychiat.*, 27: 1245, 1932.

Penfield, W., and Erickson, T. C.: *Epilepsy and Cerebral Localization.* Thomas, Springfield, 1941.

Gibbs, F. A., and Gibbs, E. L.: *Atlas of Electroencephalography.* Cummings Co., Cambridge, Mass., 1941.

Foerster, O., and Penfield, W.: Structural Basis of Traumatic Epilepsy and Results of Radical Operation. *Brain*, 53:99, 1930.

Fetterman, J. L., and Hall, V. R.: Mode of Onset of Epilepsy. *Arch. Neurol. & Psychiat.*, 38:744, 1937.

Merritt, H. H., and Putnam, T. J.: Sodium Diphenyl Hydantoinate in the Treatment of Convulsive Disorders. *J. A. M. A.*, 111:1068, 1938.

Fetterman, J. L.: Dilantin Sodium Therapy in Epilepsy. *J. A. M. A.*, 114:396, 1940.

Lennox, W. G.: The Petit Mal Epilepsies; Their Treatment with Tridione, *J. A. M. A.*, 129:1069, 1945.

Fetterman, J. L., and Greve, B.: The Auracraft Shop—A Work Project for Unemployable Epileptics. *Occupational Therapy and Rehabilitation*, 21:283, 1942.

Lennox, W. G., and Cobb, S.: Employment of Epileptics. *Industrial Medicine*, 11:571, 1942.

Gibbs, F. A., Gibbs, E. L., and Lennox, W. G.: Electroencephalographic Classification of Epileptic Patients and Control Subjects. *Arch. Neurol. & Psychiat.*, 50:111, 1943.

Merritt, H. H.: Treatment of Epilepsy, *J. Med.* 27:279, 1946.

Kozol, H. L.: Epilepsy. Treatment with New Drug. *Am. J. Psychiat.*, 103:154, 1946.

Putnam, T. J.: *Convulsive Seizures—How to Deal with Them.* J. B. Lippincott Co., 1943.

Chapter XI

THE PHYSICAL AND MENTAL SEQUELAE OF HEAD TRAUMA

INJURY abounds everywhere. Man is exposed to jars, to falls, to missiles, to all forms of violence. Such injury or trauma, when damaging the nervous system structurally or in its function, can set in motion a succession of emotional reactions of varying degree. The symptoms and defects which ensue from the structural loss, the admixture of organic loss and psychic reaction, or the psychoneurotic attachment to the event of the trauma constitute an interesting chapter in medicine.

The Physical and Clinical Changes Induced By Injury

When a passenger of a vehicle is hurled out onto the pavement, or when one is struck by the fist or hit in the head by a brick, what takes place inside the skull? The force of the blow is transmitted through the tissues of the brain and, if it is violent, there will be a temporary arrest in function of the ganglion cells, resulting in loss of consciousness. This is the simplest explanation of concussion. The effect of the jar disrupts function, chemically or electrically. This disruption may occur from the radiation of the blow and also from the temporary alteration in the circulation of the blood and in the cerebrospinal fluid. Courville, Hassin and others have demonstrated that injury produces dilation of capillaries, slowing of circulation or stasis. Likewise there occurs edema or swelling, within the brain cells as well as in the surrounding extracellular spaces.

Concussion is the clinical manifestation of a series of changes, including edema, slowing of circulation and stasis, which lead to brief unconsciousness, dazing, headache and stupor. Single instances of mild or moderate concussion rarely leave disabling handicaps. However, a potential neurotic unhappy in his assignment or tense and uneasy in a combat zone, clings to the symptoms of head injury. The fear about external danger is now displaced upon the painful area in his head: "I wonder if my skull is cracked. Will I be the same, or will I go insane?" His need of dependence is satisfied by the care he receives. His tendency to self-inspection finds in his many discomforts a fertile field. The conflict which has been going on between danger and duty, self-preservation and group loyalty, is resolved in favor of safety (with honor). Hence we find that after head injury neuroses are fairly common, especially if the milieu favors their development. An officer in Guadalcanal found such neuroses frequent among soldiers in the hospital after bomb explosion. The evidence for brain damage was slight, yet the patients' symptoms grew worse rather than cleared up. These patients became extremely sensitive to noises. The distant sound of a plane, friendly or otherwise, started them crying; an explosion, however far away, made them shake. The mild concussion had opened the door to a marked anxiety state.

If the violence be more severe, then the brain is shifted in its position within the skull. Such shift, as shown by Denny-Brown and Rowbotham, consists of suction of the brain from one side of the skull and pushing or compression against the opposite side. It involves also a certain degree of twisting or torsion at the brain stem. In this sudden movement of the brain in relation to the more or less fixed structures to which it is moored, physical damage takes place. Not only are there the stasis and edema of simple concussion, but there may be a contusion of the surface of the brain against a bony abutment, or a laceration against an unyielding shelf of dura or hemmorrhage within the substance of the brain.

Such trauma, which we may label as contusion or laceration of the brain, produces unconsciousness for hours or days and is followed by a train of more serious symptoms: prolonged and severe headache, dizziness, nausea, weakness, restlessness—even delirium. When the patient recovers from the immediate effects of the earlier days, he is likely to manifest nervous symptoms for a considerable period of time.

The hemorrhages which occur with trauma are of many types and degrees. Certainly in almost any severe head injury there will be some bleeding. *Courville says that unconsciousness lasting more than three hours following cranial trauma means hemorrhage.* There are several classical forms, each of which has some clinical or even surgical significance.

(a) PETECHIAL HEMORRHAGES: Spots of bleeding, often microscopic sleeves of red cells encircling tiny blood vessels, are found after injury. One may assume a few such small hemorrhages to be present in many instances, but they are widespread and numerous in fatal cases. For example, when a prize fighter is struck on the point of the chin and rendered unconscious for several hours and then recovers, it is probable that there were some small petechial hemorrhages. If he is "knocked out" in several subsequent bouts, then he may develop a form of encephalopathy from the accumulated damage of many such injuries. This is known on the sport pages as "punch drunk." If a fighter is struck a more severe blow to the chin, so that he becomes unconscious and remains unconscious until he dies 24 hours later, then it is probable that the autopsy will reveal multiple petechial hemorrhages.

(b) GROSS HEMORRHAGE: When the brain has been violently jarred, the inner movement leads to compression or laceration. In such instances, a gross hemorrhage develops at one area of the trauma in addition to possible diffuse damage. Such focal hemorrhage may be located at the tips of the frontal or temporal poles of the brain. For example, some years ago a man was driving his automobile and paid more attention to his sweetheart than to a parked automobile. In the collision he sustained a severe head injury which rendered him unconscious. There was bleeding from the nose and ears. He remained unconscious until he died some 48 hours later. The autopsy revealed a laceration and a large hemorrhage which destroyed a part of the left temporal lobe.

In the less severe cases, the hemorrhage may be absorbed and replaced by a glial scar, or in some instances the space left by the hemorrhage is filled in by fluid, forming a cyst. The damaged area may be near the surface or deeper within the substance of the brain.

The symptoms of a brain contusion and laceration are both general and focal, immediate and lasting.

The immediate general symptoms include unconsciousness, followed by confusion, and a gradual return to clarity. When the patient becomes conscious, he will usually complain of headaches, sensitivity to noise and to lights, and movements will induce dizziness, nausea and vomiting. For days this patient will be acutely ill, feverish, perspiring, and have a slow (or rapid) pulse.

Mentally he will pass through several stages, from deep coma to clarity. During this transition he may become delirious, disoriented as to time and place, hearing voices, fearful of danger, trying to get away from harm, or he may be eager to resume his work.

C. D. had been thrown from a coal truck and was brought to University Hospitals, unconscious. When he awoke, he thought he was still on the truck and demanded to be allowed to deliver the load. He did not understand that he was in a hospital and would not believe that the doctors and nurses were there to help him. Instead he was positive they were hold-up men who were going to hijack his truck. He cried for help when the attendants came near him. He "heard" his wife outside in the hall and pleaded for her to come to his rescue. On another occasion he believed that he must join the Army to rid the world of Hitler. For several days of his delirium he was completely unaware of headaches or painful bruises and could not recall any accident.

Subsequently, tests showed that he could not remember recent experiences, had a poor fund of information, was careless about his appearance, and could not continue any sustained activity. Likewise, he had emotional outbursts, sometimes gay (rarely), but more frequently quarrelsome. X-rays, using air injection, showed some brain atrophy and neurologic tests revealed damaged nerve pathways.

An example of severe head trauma showing both focal signs and mental symptoms is the case of corporal C. S., who was a passenger in a jeep traveling along the road when there was a violent collision. He was picked up - bruised, bleeding and unconscious. At the hospital he was critically ill, his pulse slow, the right side of his body weak. For several days he remained in a coma. The symptoms grew worse, so that there was reason to suspect a clot on the brain (subdural hematoma). The neurosurgeon explored the surface of the brain, but instead of a single clot pressing on the brain, he found numerous tiny, discolored areas. As the corporal recovered from his coma, he was confused and bewildered ("How did I get here? I am home; yes, this is home .... Who is this lady (wife)? It is someone I knew. She is a beaut ... I just came home from school ... Yesterday I was boating.") The corporal did not recall any accident and did not know where he was. When introduced to his wife, he finally recognized her, but an hour later could not remember her visit. One day he became delirious, smelled burning odors in the room and insisted that the mattress was on fire. He was fearful about food, suspecting poisoning. For the most part he was apathetic and paid no heed to the activities on the ward. He ignored a newspaper; he was unable to read it and unable to comprehend words. He had trouble with vision and could not tell time. His speech was affected, so that he would repeat the same phrase again and again. "Who is the lady who visited you?" he was asked. His answer was, "She is a killer-diller, a killer-diller, killer-diller" (a pet name for his wife). He would relate experiences that he had just completed (confabulations), made up of past events, wishes and imagination, such as "I just came back from fishing in a beautiful yacht – just got in." (He had been in bed three weeks.)

In this instance there were several stages, each merging into the other. First was the critical stage of coma. In this stage the patient's survival was uncertain. All consciousness was blotted out; even pulse, temperature and the blood pressure were affected by the diffuse injury. The patient then emerged from coma into a delirium-like condition. He was only partly in touch with reality. His words and thoughts were influenced by unchecked ideas from within; memory was poor and past events seemed to be happening now. Gradually, in a period of two months, the patient acquired a better grasp of contacts and became more alert, but was seriously handicapped by defects of motor control and thinking. Such residual handicaps represent diffuse and extensive islands of damaged brain tissue (traumatic encephalopathy). *Permanent defects are likely*.

An example of a *focal loss* is the man who receives a depressed fracture of the skull, with pressure upon a small area of the cortex, or the soldier with a bullet wound in the brain.

L. B. was shot through the left side of the head and he fell unconscious. He awoke 12 hours later, unable to remember what had happened, his head throbbing, his mind confused, and his right arm and leg paralyzed. He tried to speak but could utter only a few sounds and no words. X-rays of the skull and special tests revealed that a bullet had penetrated the skull, damaging the left lower frontal convolutions of the brain.

Two months had elapsed before I saw this man. He had improved considerably. He had regained power in the paralyzed arm and leg, so that he walked quite well, except for a slight limp, and there was still a moderate loss of skill in his right hand. He possessed power in the arm and forearm, but had not regained the finer, precise movements of his fingers. A more serious handicap was the loss of speech. He was unable to express what he wanted to say. Again and again he would struggle to find a word and would become red in the face when words failed to express his thoughts. He would start to talk, repeat the same word, remain blank, mispronounce a common word, repeat it and then give up, exasperated. He could understand what was said to him and could read and write, yet the faculty of expressing his ideas clearly in well pronounced words was severely damaged (*motor aphasia*). This defect was little improved in the two months which had elapsed and might persist as a chronic loss.

The immediate focal signs will be determined by the specific functions which have been damaged. One patient may exhibit tremors, weakness, or loss of sensation in one region of the body; another may show deafness, blindness, or even have hallucinations; some will be troubled by disturbances in speech. For example, a young man had been struck by a baseball. The blow was in the left parietal region. He was stunned but not unconscious. He was troubled by headaches for several days and by a specific defect in language. He talked freely but the words were inappropriate . . . *so-called sensory aphasia*. There was relative fluidity of speech but the words were ill chosen and did not make sense.

We will briefly touch upon the *hemorrhages which involve the lining membranes of the brain*, postponing a consideration of the sequelae until later in this chapter.

(c) SUBARACHNOID HEMORRHAGE: In some patients, head injury produces bleeding which is confined to the subarchnoid space. Of course, there may be subarchnoid bleeding in connection with laceration and gross hemorrhage in the substance of the brain.

In traumatic subarachnoid bleeding the injury may be slight in the milder forms and severe in the more grave or fatal types. My personal experience, fortunately, has been with the less severe, recoverable types. For example, a high school girl, playing basketball, ran into the wall, striking her head a glancing blow. She was dazed but not unconscious. Later she suffered intense headaches and became stuporous. She was taken to the University Hospitals for observation. At the initial examination she was drowsy and showed marked neck rigidity and total loss of reflexes. A lumbar puncture revealed pinkish spinal fluid under a high pressure (700 mm. H_2O). The removal of the spinal fluid resulted in a temporary improvement of the headache and of the stupor. This procedure was repeated several times, the patient's condition and the spinal fluid gradually returning to normal. Within two weeks she had become alert, the reflexes responded, and the spinal fluid was again clear and under a pressure of 150 mm. H_2O. This young woman remained well during a period of subsequent observation.

Another example is that of a star football player on a college team, who was stunned by a hard tackle. That afternoon he seemed dazed and could not remember details of the day's activity. He complained of headache and nausea, and had no appetite. For the remainder of the week he attended classes in a listless sort of way and even played football. However, his headache grew worse, so that he was sent to the hospital for observation. The neurological examination was essentially negative except for a minor difference in reflexes. The skull films were negative. The spinal fluid, however, was of a light yellow color and under increased pressure (300 mm. H_2O). This indicated a subarachnoid hemorrhage in the stage of resolution. This patient was kept in bed for two weeks and then allowed to resume activities gradually. He made a satisfactory recovery. Six months later he was seen again and was entirely symptom-free.

(d) SUBDURAL HEMATOMA: In some patients a relatively minor head injury is followed by gradually increasing symptoms of headaches, stupor and weakness on one side of the body. At operation a clot of blood is found under the dura, compressing the brain. In a typical instance, the patient may have sustained a blow to the head, perhaps the brow, which caused transitory unconsciousness. Indeed, he may not be able to recall the injury because the blow seemed trivial or because the dazed state obliterated his memory. The individual may go about his usual program of activity, troubled only by a headache. Then the headache grows worse and other symptoms develop. For example, C. J. had a blow on the head in an automobile accident. The headache troubled him moderately, so that an x-ray of the skull was taken. As this showed no fracture, he continued up and about, trying to do his usual work. Within two weeks he developed weakness in the left arm. Then the headache became intense and he was hospitalized at St. Alexis Hospital.

I saw this patient at the hospital with his physician, Dr. Rinaldi, some four weeks following the injury. He was lying in a deep stupor. He could be roused by strong stimula and gave coherent answers to questions and executed commands. The examination revealed a moderate paralysis of the entire left half of the body. There was also diminished sensation on this side. Dr. W. J. Gardner, who was called in consultation, performed an exploratory craniotomy and found and removed a large clot on the right hemisphere of the brain. C. J. made an excellent recovery.

A similar case was seen at the University Hospitals and successfully operated by Dr. Claude Beck.

There are other forms of such hematomata. Some are slow and chronic, consisting of fluid or clot within the lining of membranes; others are acute. The symptoms also vary, some patients exhibiting all forms of psychotic behavior.

(e) EXTRADURAL BLEEDING: A serious form of bleeding which occurs from a rupture of the middle meningeal artery leads to a clot outside the dura. In the classical instance, the patient has sustained a fairly severe blow on the side of the head, which has caused temporary unconsciousness. The x-rays commonly reveal a linear fracture of the temporal bone. The patient usually regains consciousness and remains lucid for hours or days. Then a series of symptoms occurs: headache, more marked on one side, and weakness of the opposite side of the body, due to the rapid accumulation of blood compressing the brain. *Immediate surgery is needed to save the patient's life.*

Other Immediate Effects of Trauma

We will merely mention in passing such injuries as depressed fractures of the skull, penetrating wounds of the brain, and injuries to cranial nerves. These and other lesions are caused by trauma. We will leave these subjects to the many excellent neurosurgical texts and take up *the sequelae of head injury*, such as:)1 Post-traumatic encephalopathy;)2 neuroses associated with trauma; 3) psychoses; 4) personality disorders; and 5) epilepsy.

Post-Traumatic Encephalopathy and the Post-Concussional State

When the brain has been injured, edema, anemia, hemorrhage and other lesions have taken place. Some of these, such as the edema, are reversible; others will be permanent. Destroyed ganglion cells and damaged nerve fibers are absorbed and replaced by glial scar tissue; gross hemorrhages may leave cysts which become filled with fluid. Processes of degeneration and repair may go on long after the injury. The sum total of these changes may be called post-traumatic encephalopathy.

Brief periods of unconsciousness with moderate symptoms may represent the clinical condition of concussion. In such instances many of the changes are reversible, but symptoms vary as to duration, in part due to the encephalopathy and in part to psychoneurotic admixture. *The most common symptoms*, representing a post-concussional state, according to Rowbotham, are headache, nervousness, change in disposition, unsteady gait, insomnia and dizziness.

Lynn and co-workers gave a series of *psychological tests* to patients who had suffered concussion and found a common group of defects: The rate of new learning and of forming new associations is slow; arithmetic problems and tasks involving numbers are likely to be somewhat difficult; the patient may be moderately productive in creative thinking but he is more trite and lacks the individuality of the normal.

Although such symptoms may represent actual brain lesions, it is difficult to appraise the part played by the inherent factors of the patient. Says Denny-Brown, "The problem of head injury is to a great extent one of the individual's reactions to trauma . . . and is conditioned by his original endowment." This same concept is expressed by Ruesch et al.: "The post-traumatic personality is more dependent on the pre-traumatic personality than on factors of the injury."

In concussion the changes are to a large extent transitory and tend towards recovery. In more serious cases the symptoms of post-traumatic encephalopathy depend upon the location, the extent of the pathology and the age and personality of the patient. The common symptoms are in the nature of headache, dizziness, irritability, loss of ability to concentrate and fatigability. The particular symptoms are correlated with the specific areas of destruction. *These constitute the so-called defect syndromes.*

For example, in the case of C. S. mentioned above, there was a disturbance in vision arising from a lesion in the brain stem. There was a moderate hemiparesis and there were, in addition, an impairment in memory and inability to concentrate. Months after the injury this patient could not recall the subjects recently discussed. He could not concentrate for any length of time on any one procedure. When he was given a mental test, he got tired after looking at a few cards and insisted on quitting. When he talked on any subject, he repeated the same phrase again and again. His walking was clumsy. He was troubled by headache and dizziness.

The symptoms were correlated with extensive pathology in the brain, for this man had been a very intelligent, pleasant person, of high attainment in his field. Their presence months after the injury pointed to the more or less permanent nature of the sequelae.

Another patient, N. A., had been brought to the University Hospitals in a delirious state, 24 hours after an automobile accident. She had no recollection of the injury and was disoriented as to time and place; she was noisy, talking in a loud, laughing voice, and was pleased with herself. For a time she was hallucinated, stating: "Christ appeared before me. He reached out to me and I knew that He wanted me to join Him. I reached for Him and He seemed to disappear." This patient remained delirious for about a week, during which time she had involuntary urination and defecation.

Gradually the mental state cleared and she became oriented. She took an interest in her environment and resumed some of her activities. She complained of headaches, could not remember well, and her gait was clumsy. Several months later, she was more alert and could manage some of her household tasks. However, she could not adjust very well to her duties. "I try to do my work but I forget my recipe. My mind seems dull, I burn my food, forgetting it is on the stove." When she spoke, she would repeat words and phrases: "My head feels as though there were a weight on it, a press, a pressure, a pressure on top of it." When this patient was seen a few months later she showed fair improvement. "My head feels clear and I can remember better." However, she continued to exhibit a religiosity unusual for her normal self, connected with the delusional experience which had taken place during the delirious period." I read the Scriptures and feel His presence when I do so. I now live according to the Scriptures." She had given up card parties, movies and drinking. Neurologically this patient had shown unequal pupils, positive Babinski in one foot, and some incoordination in walking.

After about 18 months the abnormalities of gait and minor reflexes were still present. She complained of occasional headache; her efficiency was decreased. The absorption in religious matters had declined, yet she was quite different from the well adjusted, capable person she had been prior to the accident. Here also we are dealing with sequelae resulting from structural damage to the brain.

Neuroses

The most common sequel of head injury is a psychoneurosis. It may be in pure form, represent a continuation of, or be merged with, encephalopathy. The occurrence of injury is a crucial event in the life of a psychoneurotic who has been making a relatively satisfactory adjustment to life, without disability. Quite suddenly he has been struck, jarred by an exploding bomb, thrown out of a vehicle. He was overwhelmed by an irresistible force, rendered unconscious, and awoke dazed, trembling, dizzy and aching. He finds himself away from the job he disliked or the front line danger which he dreaded and in the comforting arms of his wife or receiving the care of a nurse. He is the center of attention, the object of sympathy. An inner sense of guilt is satisfied; the tendency to blame others (projection) finds a ready target as he accuses the driver of the other car or the enemy sniper. Symptoms initiated by the trauma, such as headache and dizziness, grow in the culture medium of psychoneurotic mechanisms. The original symptoms flourish and new ones are added. In such patients the headache may be unusual, compressing, tightening, splitting. The vision is apt to be blurred, hearing sensitive or dull, appetite poor. Dizziness with the least movement, loss of memory, inability to concentrate, sleeplessness, and fear of losing one's mind are common symptoms. Then as the patient gets out of bed and attempts activity, he may complain of such additional symptoms as lightheadedness, staggering, weakness, tiredness, and or course inability to work. These and other specific symptoms such as were listed in Chapter II persist with tenacity.

In some cases where the injury was trivial, as in a patient who was struck in the head by a falling cardboard sign and who had no loss of consciousness, the symptoms are clearly functional. In others, where there was a concussion or more severe organic disturbance, *the psychologic features are superimposed.* For trauma tends to crystallize free floating anxiety . . . the contused and aching head draws attention upon itself . . . The organic symptoms are extended by the neurotic mechanisms.

The symptoms center chiefly upon the head, yet may extend to many other regions and functions. Furthermore, there is a tendency for the symptoms to grow worse in time, whereas the usual course of organic brain change is toward recovery.

The symptoms and course of psychoneurosis may become clearer by considering *the differential diagnosis between encephalopathy and neurosis,* taken from a paper published by Colonel W. C. Porter and myself. We listed a series of criteria in which there may be differences, acknowledging of course the confluence of symptoms from combined causes. These criteria are:

1. THE PRE-TRAUMATIC PERSONALITY: It is uncommon for neuroses to make their debut in adult life. More frequently the individual has, in his earlier days, revealed traits and habits of illness which stamp him as neurotic. Gillespie has outlined a series of traits of childhood which are fairly common precursors of adult neuroses. Gillespie's list includes pronounced morbid fears, timidity and lack of aggressiveness, habitual anxiety, inferiority feelings, and physiological instability in the form of habitual restless sleep, stammering, nail biting, bed wetting, fainting at the sight of blood, and excessive visceral reaction to emotion.

The above list of traits does not apply to the early life of every neurotic, nor is the normal person entirely free of them. However, the history of a majority of such characteristics and of previous illnesses suggestive of neurosis or hysteria is weighty evidence for functional illness. The examiner should make every effort to obtain a complete history. Though it seems time-consuming, such a history will actually abbreviate the examination and accelerate the recovery. Symonds makes the point that the discovery of psychopathic traits in the patient's personality will tell much more than an air encephalogram or other special procedures. "What's past is prologue," reads an inscription on the Archives Building in Washington. This is equally true for individuals as for nations.

2. THE TYPE AND SEVERITY OF THE TRAUMA: Although a minor accident might lead to serious consequences (subdural

hematoma), yet, all things being equal, the severity of the injury will usually determine the seriousness of the symptoms. A man hurled from a jeep and striking his head against a rock will suffer far more seriously than one whose head is bumped by a carton. Yet recently a soldier who sustained a minor bruise complained much more than the patient in the adjoining bed whose injury was a laceration of the brain.

3. ALERTNESS VERSUS AMNESIA AT THE TIME OF THE ACCIDENT: Loss of memory for the experience prior to the injury (retrograde amnesia) is the rule in a concussion of any severity. Indeed a patient may not be able to recall his activities for several hours, or even days, before the trauma. In neuroses there may be no amnesia. On the contrary, the neurotic patient may describe vividly how frightened he was, how he worried that the careless driver of the car would get him into danger. His worrisome awareness of all the details surrounding the episode may be remarkable. Pre-traumatic alertness and apprehension suggest a neurosis; pre-traumatic amnesia points emphatically to organic pathology. A striking exception is the retention of memory and consciousness in some penetrating injuries of the skull by a bayonet and the shearing of part of the skull and brain by a swiftly moving propeller blade (Rowbotham). Goldstein mentions instances in which a bullet of swift velocity penetrated the skull without causing a loss of consciousness.

4. UNCONSCIOUSNESS AND DELIRIUM: Loss of consciousness characterizes concussion. The disturbance in ganglion cell function from edema and vascular change consequent upon stretching and compressing of the brain blots out consciousness. *The duration of this loss of consciousness is a useful index of the severity of the injury* (Pilcher and Angelucci).

After a severe injury the patient goes through a clouded state and a stage of confusion and delirium before he becomes fully conscious. Memory for this phase is usually blotted out. Cairns uses the duration of this phase of post-traumatic amnesia as a prognostic timetable. According to Cairns, if the unconsciousness lasted five minutes to one hour, recovery can be expected in some six weeks; if the amnesia extends several days, the recovery period will last up to four months. When the amnesia extends over seven days, then the prognosis is poorer and improvement may take four to eight months. It is obvious that loss of consciousness reflects organic change, whereas a momentary dazing or no loss of consciousness is the rule in the neurotic reaction.

5. Neurologic Signs, Physical Findings and Laboratory Data: If a record of the initial examination at the time of the injury is available, it may furnish positive evidence. We will learn not only about unconsciousness and delirium, but about bleeding from the ears and nose, the presence of unequal pupils, twitchings and paresis, and the findings in the spinal fluid. Later we may obtain significant information from skull films, residual neurologic abnormalities and other tests. Sometimes a pneumoencephalogram will reveal the positive evidence of organic damage, but its use must be limited to definite indications (suspicion of subdural hematoma, epilepsy, and severe headache). Such evidence, of course, reflects more serious cerebral damage than has occurred in the usual post-concussion state and represents a contusion or laceration of the brain.

The study of the brain waves by *electroencephalography* promises to be remarkably helpful in ascertaining the site and severity of brain damage by trauma. Williams has demonstrated by serial brain wave studies the changes which are revealed in the early post-traumatic period and the improvement in the rhythm of such waves which runs parallel to recovery. Ultimately this procedure may simplify our problems, affording pictures of comparative value.

Other procedures may be utilized to establish a diagnosis. Goldstein's recent book outlines several tests which reveal defects of attention and memory. The Rorschach Ink Blot test may also be used because there are responses considered characteristic of organic damage. Psychological tests which reveal loss of previous capacities can be employed to reveal impairment in brain function.

6. Special Symptoms: Following a concussion the symptoms of headache, dizziness, weakness, and vasomotor instability have certain features. For example, they are made worse by movement, by heat and by drinking. On the other hand, a psychoneurotic may say that his head bothers him more when sitting idly, exercise in the warm sunshine makes him feel good and a few drinks make him happy. Several of the most severe head injury cases had no headache but marked loss of interest, undue cheer-

fulness, profound memory loss. Loud complaints of headache were common in the neuroses.

Other symptoms of the psychoneuroses include conversion disabilities; for example, paralysis and loss of sensation, altogether out of line with the organic pathology. The psychoneurotic may complain of loss of vision or loss of sensation in the entire half of his body where he was struck (conversion hysteria). His hearing, vision, and gait may be peculiar. The specific and the general symptoms do not conform to a characteristic organic syndrome.

7. THE MENTAL ATTITUDE AND THOUGHT CONTENT IN THE LATER PERIOD: The average person who has sustained head trauma is obviously distressed by his symptoms, yet he seeks help hopefully—he makes the best of his condition, tries to do as much as he can, even in a restricted manner. He looks forward toward hope of recovery, he directs his energy toward effort. Not so the psychoneurotic patient. Attention is concentrated upon the area injured. There is abnormal concern about sanity, paralysis or other dire consequences. The patient's major interest is now his head; the future looks dark; he shows undue dependence and attachment. The injury occupies the foreground of consciousness and reactions to the injury reappear frequently in dreams (Kardiner). Terror dreams featuring violence recur.

The preoccupation with the injury, the pessimistic mood, the tendency to blame others – these attitudes are more or less pronounced in psychoneuroses. The normal individual who has sustained concussion will also be concerned about it and will show some of the above reactions. The intensity, persistence and preoccupation characterize the psychoneurotic.

8. GAIN: ADVANTAGE OF THE SYMPTOMS TO THE INDIVIDUAL: Injury concerns the individual in his relation to his environment. The disability prevents the normal response to work and rest, disrupts plans and purposes, directs attention from outside problems to inner pathology. In civilian life, someone may be responsible for the injury and there is an instinctive effort to obtain redress. A claim for compensation may become a motivating force in the life of the injured person. During war time an injured soldier is taken from the dangers of the combat area, is withdrawn from the usual pressure of training, marching and fighting. He is placed in a relatively safe environment and receives sympathy, warmth and attention. Whether the gain be monetary in civilian

life or safety during war time, *it is a factor which tends to prolong the symptoms*. In the history of psychoneurotic illness, the element of gain looms large. The tendency to place the blame upon others, and the tenacious clinging to symptoms may serve an inner need. However, there is often a material advantage to the illness. The item of gain is an incentive in another group of cases. We refer to the sociopathic (the constitutional psychopathic) individual. Such a person uses the injury as an excuse for the further practice of his philosophy of life, namely, that society owes him a livelihood, and that any reason for his failure or non-desire to fulfill his obligations to society is sufficient and should be utilized to the greatest possible extent. This is an important consideration in those accident cases where the compensation may become an issue. There is a mixture of conscious simulation and wishful thinking. This mechanism should be differentiated from that present in the psychoneurotic individual where motives are largely unconscious.

9. SEQUENCE OF EVENTS: As a rule symptoms of a concussion are more intense at first and in the course of time they lessen. In the moderate case there is likely to be considerable relief and tendency toward further recovery. Cairns speaks of the common cycle which begins with unconsciousness, passes through a stage of confusion, a period of headaches and finally reaches the point of more or less total recovery. Such a curve of recovery is not smooth and steadily upward, but there are fluctuations from time to time. These variations, brought on by inner factors or external events, do not alter the trend of progress from ill health to wellbeing. Not so in neuroses. *The symptoms are markedly influenced by outside forces. They are responsive to situations.* For the average person, time is a therapist; in psychoneurosis it may be an opportunity for growth of symptoms.

The symptoms of the neuroses then are determined by inherent factors, reinforced often by the incentive of gain. The trauma is an incident seized upon by the psyche to provide defense for the ego or an attack upon society. Ruesch, Harris and Bowman compared a series of patients with acute symptoms and those who had prolonged chronic disabilities months or years after injury. Some of their comments are appropriate here: "Among these cases (chronic) the high incidence of mild injuries, requiring only brief or no hospitalization, was striking ... Many of these patients showed neurotic tendencies which often antedated the injury, as evidenced by the high incidence of neuropathic traits in childhood. Whereas social maladjustment seems to be associated with proneness for accidents, neurotic tendencies seem to predispose for prolongation of symptoms after injury. These individuals seem to be unable to cope with their minor problems and make the injury the 'cause' of the inability."

Psychoses

In the days immediately following head trauma, psychotic reactions are common. These are types of delirium, acute states of confusion and disorientation. Cerebral edema or hemorrhage, disrupting the normal functions, permits the release of inner fears and drives that take the form of a psychosis. The patient is confused as to time and place, has no recollection for the injury, "hears" voices or misinterprets a natural sound for the voice of friend or foe, believes that he has to execute some important duties. N. A. believed she was in heaven and that Christ had appeared and reached His hand out to her. Another patient insisted he leave "this place" (he failed to recognize the hospital) to destroy Hitler, as he was commanded by divine order. A man who had been in a hospital for several days insisted he had just come in from farming. "I brought in a wonderful crop – my fruit trees are doing well." When he was told that he had not left the bed for days, he smiled, but resumed, "You may be right, but I am sure I was plowing behind my team and that I brought in a large crop. Prices are high" – (Confabulation). Another patient, C. S., reported activities connected with boyhood loves—sailing and fishing. "I was in a sailboat outside Boston harbor. The wind was blowing – it was great fun. We have been out for several hours. I am going again tomorrow." Not only confabulation but confusion, fears, wild efforts to break away are manifestations of such traumatic psychosis.

Such psychotic disturbances are likely to be *brief*, lasting several days to some weeks. The tendency is toward recovery, as in most toxic psychoses, unless the damage to the brain be overwhelming and lead to death.

Psychoses of a persistent, chronic nature, resulting from injury, are uncommon. The usual psychoses, schizophrenias and manic-depressive states are not caused by injury, although *head trauma is so frequent in the lives of most of us that a clinical history may show some time connection between injury and mental illness.* The relatively minor role of injury in the causation of mental illness may be inferred from the fact that severing of brain fibers in the frontal area, *frontal lobotomy*, is used as a therapeutic measure for certain types of psychosis.

There are instances of persistent mental illness following trauma, largely in the form of failing attention, defective memory with gradual loss of interest in reality, and the appearance of amnesia and confabulation. Such examples usually represent the addition of alcoholism, arteriosclerosis, along with trauma. Denny-Brown agrees with the observations of an early impairment of intelligence and a ready fatigability due to injury. But there is a progressive improvement in functions in most cases, and residuals of intellectual defect occur in those whose posttraumatic disorientation and amnesia lasted many days (19 days or longer). Says this author: "It has long been known that traumatic dementia occurs mostly in old age and occurs much more frequently after falls than after penetrating cranial injuries. In cases admitted to the Boston City Hospital advanced age and alcoholism are prominent factors ... It is remarkable that no cases of persistent dementia have yet occurred in 119 cases of all types of head injury in healthy non-alcoholics between the ages of 15 and 55 followed up for six months or longer, without evidence of pre-traumatic impairment."

Palmer lists *the sequence of events in acute traumatic psychoses* as coma, stupor, semi-stupor, dazed bewilderment. Korsakoff phase, residual euphoria and recovery. Post-traumatic psychoneuroses and psychoses are usually psychogenic.

In a small number of patients the manifestations of an encephalopathy are in the form of a personality disorder. There are no gross intellectual defects and no obvious psychosis. *Yet the behavior pattern is changed toward impulsiveness, lack of control and overactivity.* Such was the case in a patient who sustained a head injury simultaneous with the passage of an electric current through his body. The case history is briefly as follows:

> C. S. had a normal birth and splendid early development. He grew physically and mentally; his school work was excellent and he appeared to be a well adjusted, healthy youngster.

PHYSICAL AND MENTAL SEQUELAE 319

The family history is essentially negative as far as neuropathic ancestry is concerned.

In May of 1934, at the age of 12, on a dare from his companions, he grasped a high tension wire and was thrown to the ground. (It was reported that he had received a shock of 4,000 volts.) He was taken to the hospital unconscious, his left palm burned and with burns across the buttocks, shoulders and head. In the hospital muscular twitchings and later generalized convulsions developed.

For about two weeks the youngster was critically ill and delirious. In his delirious state he was troubled by hallucinations, rarely auditory, frequently visual. The hallucinations had a zooscopic content; he saw pelicans marching, then fighting, being chased by large snakes. At times he would see sheep running and jumping. Occasionally he saw people swimming in a pool.

During this period he had extensive surgical treatment to the deep burns of the palms and fingers. Two of the fingers were amputated and several tendons sloughed. There were large burns of the scalp, with necrosis down to the bone.

Early in June there was improvement, though he still had occasional hallucinations and muscular twitchings. Toward the end of July the sloughing areas of the skull bone were improving and a plastic repair of the hand was undertaken. In August there were further operative procedures on the scalp, with an attempt to cover the denuded areas. By the middle of August the youth was improving and was discharged from the hospital.

Progress: From 1934 to 1936 the patient had shown considerable progress from the physical standpoint. The hand was healed, though with a residual deformity of the palm and fingers.

The chief difficulty was a gradually developing behavior problem, which will be presented in detail.

Present Status: According to the mother, he has been a changed boy since the accident. At first he was sick, weak and tired and was treated as an invalid. When he improved, however, and was asked to go back to school, it was found that he could not attend to his studies. Every report card showed deficiency. When corrected, he would become rebellious. "He is different. He now uses awful, vile language. He condemns me and his dad. If things don't suit him, he is like a perfect maniac. I must hold him or he will kill us. Once he knocked his father down. He used to be an affectionate boy, but now he punches me. He cries out, 'I want to hurt somebody. I would give anything to hurt someone.'

He seems like two different people. At times he will come into the room cheerfully, but if I happen to correct him, he will shriek and swear at me.

"His behavior is very restless. He is always into things. He may walk back and forth continuously. He will pick on things. He started to pick on the lamp shade and picked it to pieces. At school he does not study. He promises that he will do good work but never fulfills his promise. He seems full of mischief. One day he brought a pigeon into the classroom."

The patient himself says that he cannot concentrate, but at times his story is contradictory. He may even claim that he is a model boy, working very hard from morning to night.\"I have decided to become a doctor. I know I will be a good doctor. You see, I have suffered through it all and I am on the road to success. I like to try something different every day."

Examination: General: The youth is now a tall, well developed, healthy looking youngster of 14, who impresses one by his energetic, enthusiastic activity. He greeted the examiner with a broad smile and warm handshake and spoke cheerfully of his interest in our new hospital and of his own ambition to become a doctor. He seemed to ignore the scarred, deformed hand and was not introspective about the denuded area on the scalp.

Mental Status: There is restless overactivity. For a moment he would be sitting comfortably in a chair; then he would spring into his bed. A few minutes later he might curl up on the window sill and gaze out into space. He showed a fleeting interest in a large variety of subjects. He would observe the doctor's stethescope, his tie, the furniture, would make a comment on the demeanor of the nurse, refer to the psychologist as a "four-eyed wench." He seemed to show no respect for authority and position. His stories were frequently contradictory, with a tendency to confabulate. Most of the time he was animated, energetic and self-assertive, although with little insight into his own status.

Mrs. Barnes, a psychologist, made the following observations: "C. S. cooperated quite well on the Babcock test, apparently because in this test there is something new being presented continually. He got restless during the vocabulary test and fumed about the number of words there were in the list. He came the second time readily enough, but he repeatedly said that he was afraid he would be too late to return to the x-ray department before it closed, although he was assured that this was not the case. He refused to do the reading test after he first looked at it, saying that it was too easy, but he began working on it after it was explained that it became progressively harder. He started to work on the arithmetic without waiting for directions and was annoyed when stopped for directions.

"The Babcock test rated him as having barely normal average intelligence, but he showed no signs of general mental deterioration on it. However, when new learning is contrasted with old knowledge, there is a definite difference, about four and one-half years, showing that he acquires new learning with difficulty and not with anything like the facility normal to a boy of his intelligence."

A routine neurologic examination was essentially negative. The pupils were equal and regular and reacted to light and in accommodation. The discs show no changes. Visual fields were complete. Hearing and speech were normal. Muscular tone in the arms and legs was good. The reflexes were hypoactive; knee jerks were obtained only on reenforcement. The Babinski reaction was negative.

Summary: As a result of an electric shock and a fall on the head, a previously normal, well adjusted boy of 12 developed severe nervous symptoms. In the initial phase there was unconsciousness, followed by a period of convulsions, and then delirium. After recovery from this acute mental illness, the youth presented a tendency to overactivity, with psychomotor restlessness, resulting in difficulties at home and in school – a condition that may be called *a hyperkinetic behavior syndrome.*

Epilepsy and Trauma

One of the most serious sequels of head injury is epilepsy. The attacks may occur shortly after the trauma, during convalescence, or may develop months and even years later. Seizures which begin within two weeks of injury may come from a temporary disturbance (hemorrhage) and may cease spontaneously. Those which first appear months or years later are more likely to persist in chronic form.

The incidence of traumatic epilepsy is variable, as may be judged from the contradictory figures in the literature: from 2.5 per cent (Rowbotham) to 34 per cent (Ascroft; Cairns). This apparent discrepancy may be cleared up in part by a consideration of the nature of the injury, the time of the attacks and their type. In simple concussion, the incidence is low ... Penfield found that in 193 cases of scalp wound without fracture, one patient only developed epilepsy (0.5 per cent) and that among forty patients diagnosed as concussion, none had developed seizures. However, the figures for patients who had more severe injury were 5.1 per cent in cases of fractured skull without proven tear of the dura and 7.9 per cent in fractured skull cases with dural tear. The highest percentage of epilepsy occurs in penetrating head injury (Ascroft's figures – 45 per cent). Penfield's study shows a much lower percentage because he excluded the fits which developed within two weeks of the trauma, a symptom of surface hemorrhage and not necessarily an indication of later chronic epilepsy.

Another explanation for the apparent difference in figures is *the time when patients are studied*. The incidence rises with the number of years of follow-up.

Because of the potential danger of this complication, I advocated (1938) the use of anticonvulsant medication in severe head injuries in advance of the development of attacks.

The symptoms also vary and may account for the difference in figures. Some patients show only Jacksonian attacks; others exhibit petit and grand mal spells; then there are cases of psychomotor manifestations. Says Goldstein, "When only grand mal and petit mal attacks are considered, 15 per cent to 20 per cent of all patients with penetrating wounds suffer from epilepsy, but the incidence is higher if we count other forms of epilepsy."

Injury to the sensory-motor area of the brain is more likely to lead to epilepsy than injuries in the occipital lobe and in the cerebellum.

Traumatic epilepsy is an important subject as regards the health of veterans. Many soldiers have sustained brain injuries, particularly penetrating wounds of the skull. Epilepsy is a frequent complication of such an injury. Anticonvulsant therapy is recommended for such head cases even prior to the appearance of epilepsy. Such therapy may postpone or even prevent the occurrence of spells. In instances where attacks do occur, surgery may prove to be of benefit, as is being demonstrated by Walker et al.

Veterans who are troubled by epileptic spells deserve the utmost consideration along various lines. They are entitled to adequate compensation because of the potentiality of attacks. They require frequent attention of a physician with the use of the most modern anticonvulsant drugs available. Finally, vocational guidance and vocational opportunity should be made available to them in the hope that adequate treatment, a relatively safe and interesting job and proper compensation will enable such a veteran to make a satisfactory adjustment to life.

Treatment of Head Injuries

The immediate aim of treatment of any injured person is to save his life. Finer adjustments come later. The life-saving steps are to help control shock, check bleeding and prevent infection. A live patient beats a precise diagnosis.

Rest, warmth and blood plasma are useful in controlling shock. The sulfa drugs given orally and (according to some surgeons) dusted into the wound serve to reduce the possibility of infection, as does the intramuscular use of penicillin.

Once the patient has survived the collapse of the injury, the pallor, rapid pulse, falling blood pressure, then it is time to appraise the extent of the brain injury, the regions affected, and to plan effective measures to help. This appraisal includes a careful study of the patient: the state of consciousness, the pulse, color, blood pressure, the size of the pupils, the symmetry of the face, the voluntary and passive movements of the arms and legs, the reflexes and tests of sensation. These tests reveal to the examiner whether or not there is pressure upon the brain, what regions have been injured. A spinal puncture is valuable. It should be done whether the patient is co-operative or in a state of stupor. The color and pressure of the spinal fluid are clues to the type of injury; the removal of a certain amount of the fluid will temporarily reduce the pressure.

During the period between coma and complete consciousness is a phase of delirium. The patient is confused, does not know that he was hurt or that he is in a hospital. He is determined to get out of bed to attend to pressing duties; he tries to run away from enemies who lurk outside. *During this period, careful nursing observation is important.* Sedatives, such as paraldehyde or sodium amytal, may calm this restlessness. To relieve the edema many procedures have been in vogue, but their effect is temporary and sometimes doubtful. For the first 72 hours, if there are signs of increased pressure, then the intravenous injection of fifty cc. of twenty per cent sucrose will, for a short time, reduce the pressure and permit better metabolism of brain cells. Operations should be postponed except for such indications as extradural hemorrhage, subdural clots, and depressed skull fractures.

When the patient has become cooperative, x-rays of the skull may be taken. *These show the status of the bone, not the brain.* Hence x-ray examination (except in suspected depressed fractures) should be postponed until the condition of the injured person permits it. The electroencephalogram is a useful procedure which reveals the electrical status of the brain. There are diffuse, slow waves of high potential in coma and focal disturbances in other areas in which there are traumatic lesions. Such tests, especially if taken weeks apart (serially), provide a picture of progress and give early evidence of epilepsy.

Succeeding the earlier stages of coma and confusion is the stage of returning consciousness. The injured person makes his first efforts to observe, to act, to plan. For the distressing symptoms he requires medication, such as codeine, aspirin, phenobarbital, a liberal diet, and controlled activity. The old rule about an extended period of rest in bed has been discarded. *It is the practice in many clinics to permit the patient to get out of bed and to move about whenever he is able to do so.* Most patients who have received mild or moderate concussions are up and about within one week, not "imprisoned" in bed for six weeks. The prolonged period in bed did not necessarily assist the brain recovery but did cultivate worry and neurosis. *This new attitude not only is better for general well-being but apparently accelerates recovery.* Above all, it gives the patient a more hopeful outlook. Such progress tends to minimize neurosis and it should be backed up with hopeful remarks by physicians. At least, the doctor should refrain from encouraging anxiety by gloomy expression or pessimistic statements. (Of course, the family, and in necessary instances the patient himself, is told the facts of the brain injury.)

The period in bed then is primarily for rest until tissues resume healing and until freedom from distress enables the injured person to become active. It is a period for diagnosis, so that surgical measures may be carried out in proper cases. *Yet this period should be utilized to promote a return to activity.* Massage for unused muscles will prevent flabbiness, and active movement early will aid muscle tone. The patient should be kept interested, to the extent of his capacity, in radio, books, games and people. When he is able to walk, he should be permitted, indeed encouraged, to be outdoors, to do things for himself, and to become useful. Graduated activity, helping in the ward, exercise, occupation - all should be cultivated. The atmosphere on the ward should be RECOVERY. A hospital, military or civilian, should serve as a restorative to, not a retreat from, duty.

Special Measures of Treatment of Head-Injured Patients and For Readjustment

The most common symptom that incapacitates the patient is headache. The headache may be restricted to one spot or may be extensive. Heat and sunshine, excitement, rapid change in posture, and alcohol make it worse. The headache bears no direct ratio to the severity of the injury. P. C. was struck in the head by a large cardboard box while loading a truck for the Quartermaster Corps. Although the initial injury was slight, his complaint of headache was loud ... and persistent. B. I. was injured in an automobile collision, rendered unconscious for several days. After some months, he seemed dull, forgetful, took no interest in the news events of the day, although prior to the injury he was an avid reader of current events. At no time did he mention headache. Thus it is likely that the sensitivity of the person is more decisive than the site or size of the lesion.

For relief of the headache, we rely upon sedatives, time, and avoidance of the factors which increase it. When he returns to work, a person whose headaches are a disturbing factor after an injury should be given a light job, with the minimum exposure to heat, rapid moving and intense excitement. Medication, such as phenobarbital, aspirin and other analgesics, is beneficial. Injecting air into the spinal canal, replacing a like quantity of cerebrospinal fluid, *may* help. In certain instances of localized headache, section of the middle meningeal artery or an attempt at section of dural adhesions may be tried (Beck).

PARALYSIS: Head injury, especially when due to bullet wounds, may be followed by a partial or complete paralysis. The degree of recovery depends upon the tissue injury; the extent of usefulness depends upon the man and his treatment. Such a person should be treated as early as it is safe, in the hope of relieving the damage and improving the use of the non-affected parts of his body.

The paralyzed part should be massaged and kept active. The patient should try voluntarily to exercise the fingers and hand, or if no control is present, he should move the fingers with the good hand. Then he must start on a gross object—a ball which he clasps and throws. When this is mastered, he tries grasping smaller articles and using his fingers in writing or in handling tools, such as screw drivers. If there is a promise of progress, such exercises for the affected portion of the body should be continued. At the same time, the patient will instinctively use the good limb for everyday tasks. The left hand may require special training if the right side is paralyzed and the return to function is slow and imperfect. I have seen the futile effort to restore function to a paralyzed limb end in disappointment. The patient had a paralysis of the right arm from a bullet wound in the brain. Despite efforts at massage and movement, the arm became spastic and the fingers stiff and clenched in the palm. The man read a book on the *Power of the Will*. In it he read that one can achieve any goal, conquer any physical defect, if one has enough will power. Inspired by these words, he faced his paralyzed arm with set jaw and determined expression. He faced it as though it were detached from him, another person whom he must dominate: *I am going to make you do my bidding*. He glared, he talked firmly, he pleaded, he threatened. For days he concentrated on the paralyzed arm, set his mind on conquering the paralysis. He was doomed to failure; the nervous apparatus for voluntary motion had been destroyed, never to be restored. A sense of utter failure overcame this patient.

It is better, if serial examinations show that a paralyzed part will be improved little if any, to start training *the unaffected limb*. If the patient is not too old he can be taught to write, to manipulate the left hand and fingers. For example, M. M., a switchboard operator, developed a paralysis of the right arm, as well as loss of sensation in it. Recovery was slight. She was started using her left hand, placing round wooden pegs of different diameters into holes. Later she tried writing and finally needlework. In time she could use the left hand expertly. Aided by the clumsy grasp of the right hand, whose loss of sensation she had to compensate for by constant watching, M. M. resumed her job and rendered efficient service to her employer. Such success is possible if there is a desire to return to usefulness and if the patient can utilize other parts of the body.

SPEECH DEFECTS: Language is all-important in man's relation to man and to the past. It is the quickest way for man to socialize with fellow man, to communicate with him, however far the distance or however much time has elapsed. The Ten Commandments of Moses are read today; a letter from an aviator in Calcutta warms the heart of his mother in Chicago. Language is a shortcut for exchange of ideas. Language – speaking, understanding, writing – is dependent upon brain centers and their communications. Thus we encounter frequent examples of partial or serious loss of language in head injury cases. Such loss is far more disabling than we are inclined to believe. The person who cannot speak because of a brain injury doubts the axiom: "Silence is golden."

As a rule, the initial loss is not permanent. Some improvement takes place. Then such a handicapped person needs re-education of speech. There is no simple technique. Time and patience in helping a patient connect sound with pictures or with touch may restore forgotten memories or start new ones. As an infant, he learns to talk; so such a patient must once again be started on the road to language.

ATTACKS: The type and frequency of epilepsy have already been discussed. The treatment of such a complication is both surgical and medical. If a definite focus of scar tissue is found, surgical excision may be tried. But if there be many particles of lead or steel in the brain and diffuse damage, surgery is of no avail. Medical care in the form of anticonvulsant medication is distinctly valuable. I would advise starting such drugs early, even before attacks set in.

In the later stages of rehabilitation, the approach depends largely upon the degree of organic defect. For those who have sustained brain lesions with destruction of tissue, a restricted program that makes fewer demands is indicated. The patient should be permitted tasks that he can successfully accomplish. Those who have speech defects need teaching and need jobs that depend upon manual effort. Those who are subject to dizziness should be protected from climbing ladders or working on roofs. Patients who are troubled by headaches when stooping and when exposed to heat should for a time be kept out of hot furnace rooms and away from jobs requiring bending and stooping. So too, a veteran who has sustained a bullet injury to the brain, which makes him liable to epilepsy, should be guided into a career of relative safety and success. Depending upon talents and interests, he would be happier working for himself rather than for others; he would do better in gardening or farming than as a truck driver or in a steel mill.

For the patient whose major symptoms represent a psychoneurosis, treatment should follow along the lines outlined in Chapter III. Particular consideration needs to be given to the relationship of the patient to those whom he feels are responsible, his employer, the government, the "other party." The patient may feel unjustly treated by those allegedly responsible for the accident. He may seek "justice," demand revenge in the form of compensation. Indeed, illness is not limited to the individual but involves interpersonal relationships – the milieu.

Among the important influences in the milieu is the matter of compensation. Disability payments are not entirely a blessing. Financial aid during a period of obvious disability is certainly helpful to the injured man. *Continued compensation for neurotic symptoms is a boomerang.* Aring and Bateman demonstrated that continued monthly pensions given to the veterans of the last war tended "to nurture a national neurosis." Continued monthly payments for neurotic symptoms after head injury may be compared to the use of morphine for pain. In the acute stage such a measure (money or morphine) is beneficial. Continued beyond the acute stage, it tends to weaken initiative, prolong symptoms and delay recovery. The patient needs adequate diagnostic facilities, the benefit of psychotherapy, training to improve his vocational aptitude and assistance in securing employment. He may crave compensation, but, though compensation may please the patient, ultimately it will weaken his resolve and prove his undoing. In the interest of his ultimate welfare as well as from the standpoint of the community, such compensation must be limited. In a recent article by Lewy the following policy is advocated: "no compensation for any war neuroses."

The matter of indemnity for organic after-effects from brain injury is different. Here the loss of function is serious and often irreparable. Persons thus handicapped are entitled to generous financial assistance, but this aid should be coupled with a program of rehabilitation. If possible, the patient should be helped to a job and a pay check, not a hospital and a pension. Toward this goal, compensation should be in the form of vocational training, placement in a business or job. Compensation should then be adjusted either as a credit in reserve, as a lump sum advanced or as a partial monthly sum supplementing earnings. In no instance should compensation replace work. Training and reeducation may be necessary, and the type of work must be adjusted to the restricted capacities of the man; but practically every handicapped person possesses some capacities for usefulness. One should utilize the capabilities, not emphasize the difficulties, of those injured.

REFERENCES

Courville, C. B.: *Pathology of the Central Nervous System: A Study Based upon a Survey of Lesions Found in a Series of Fifteen Thousand Autopsies.* Pacific Press Pub. Assoc., Mountain View, Calif., 1937.

Courville, C. B.: Trauma to the Central Nervous System and Its Envelopes. In Tice, *Practice of Medicine*, Vol. X, Prior, Hagerstown, 1937.

Hassin, G. B.: *Histopathology of the Peripheral and Central Nervous Systems.* Wood, Baltimore, 1933.

Hassin, G. B.: General Pathological Considerations in Brain Injury. Chapter II in *Injuries of Skull, Brain and Spinal Cord*, S. Brock, Williams & Wilkins, Baltimore, 1940.

Denny-Brown, D., and Russell, W. R.: Experimental Cerebral Concussion. *Brain*, 64:93, 1941.

Rowbotham, G. F.: *Acute Injuries of the Head.* Williams & Wilkins, Baltimore, 1942.

Lynn, J. G., Levine, K. N., and Hewson, L. R.: Psychologic Tests for the Clinical Evaluation of Late "Diffuse Organic," "Neurotic," and "Normal" Reactions After Closed Head Injury. Chapter XIII in *Trauma of the Central Nervous System*, A. Research Nerv. & Ment. Dis. Proc., 24:296, 1945.

Denny-Brown, D.: *The Sequelae of War Head Injuries in Rehabilitation of the War Injured*, p. 9 Philosophical Library, New York, 1943.

Ruesch, J., Harris, R. E., and Bowman, K. M.: Pre- and Post-Traumatic Personality in Head Injuries. Chapter XXI in *Trauma of the Central Nervous System*, A. Research Nerv. & Ment. Dis. Proc. 24:507, 1945. Williams & Wilkens, Baltimore, 1945.

Porter, W. C., and Fetterman, J. L.: Diagnostic Approach to Head Injury Cases. *Diseases of the Nervous System*, 5:166, June, 1944.

Gillespie, R. D.: *The Psychological Effects of War on Citizen and Soldier*, Norton, New York, 1942.

Symonds, C. P.: Concussion and Contusion of the Brain and Their Sequelae. Chapter IV in *Injuries of Skull, Brain and Spinal Cord*, S. Brock, Williams & Wilkins, Baltimore, 1940.

Walker, Maj. A. E., Quadfasel, Capt. F. A., Marshall, Capt. C., Netsky, Capt. M. G. Fisher, Capt. R. G,. and Kaufman, 1st Lt. I. C., Gebhardt, 1st Lt. J. W., with technical assistance of Beresvord, E. N. *J. Nerv. & Ment. Disease*, 105:673–678, June, 1947.

Goldstein, K.: *After Effects of Brain Injuries in War.* Grune and Stratton, New York, 1942.

Pilcher, C., and Angelucci, R.: Analysis of Three Hundred and Seventy-Three Cases of Acute Cranio-Cerebral Injury. *War Medicine,* 2:114, 1942.

Cairns, H.: Head Injuries in War, with Especial Reference to Gunshot Wounds. *War Medicine,* 2:772, 1942.

Cairns, H.: Discussion on Rehabilitation After Injuries to Central Nervous System. *Proc. Royal Soc. Med.,* 35:295, 1942.

Williams, D.: The Electro-encephalogram in Chronic Post-Traumatic States. *J. Neurol. & Psychiat.,* 4:131, 1941.

Kardiner, A.: *The Traumatic Neuroses in War,* Hoeber, New York, 1941.

Denny-Brown, D.: Intellectual Deterioration Resulting from Head Injury. Chapter XVIII in *Trauma of the Central Nervous System,* A. Research Nerv. & Ment. Dis., Williams & Wilkins, Baltimore, 1945.

Palmer, H. A.: The Mental Sequalae of Head Injury. *J. Ment. Sc.,* 87:370, 1941.

Ascroft, P. B.: Treatment of Head Wounds Due to Missiles. Analysis of 500 Cases. *Lancet,* 2:211, 1943.

Penfield, W., and Shaver, M.: The Incidence of Traumatic Epilepsy and Headache After Head Injury in Civil Practice. Chapter XXVI in *Trauma of the Central Nervous System,* p. 620. A. Research Nerv. & Ment. Dis., Williams & Wilkins, Baltimore, 1945.

Aring, C. D., and Bateman, J. F.: Nurturing a National Neurosis. *J. A. M. A.,* 109:1092, 1937.

Lewy, E.: Compensation for War Neuroses. *War Medicine,* 1:887, 1941.

Brock, S.: *Injuries of the Skull, Brain and Spinal Cord.* Williams & Wilkins, Baltimore, 1940.

Kennedy, F.: Head Injuries: Effects and Their Appraisal. IV. Evaluation of Evidence. *Arch. Neurol. & Psychiat.,* 27:811, 1932.

Bowman, K. M., and Blau, A.: Psychotic States Following Head and Brain Injury in Adults and Children. Chapter XIII in *Injuries of Skull, Brain and Spinal Cord,* S. Brock, p. 309. Williams & Wilkins, Baltimore, 1940.

INDEX

A

Accident (see Trauma)
Accident proneness, 209, 317
Activity
  in depression, 123
  in psychoneurosis, 70
Adams, R. D., 279
Addiction (see Drug), 239
Adler, A., 8, 20
Aggressiveness, overcompensation for, 26
Air hunger, 39
Alcohol, influence on mood and thought, 119
Alcoholics Anonymous, 238
Alcoholism, 12, 232
  alcoholic hallucinosis, 236
  chronic, 233
  convulsions in, 236
  defined, 232
  delirium tremens, 236, 248
  diet in, 253
  in depression, 104
  in schizophrenia, 237
  Korsakoff's syndrome, 237
  neurological disturbances in, 235
  neuropsychiatric conditions the result of, 233, 239
  personality changes in, 232, (Case MF) 234, 237
Alexander, F., viii, 44, 47, 56, 57, 96
Allergies (physical), 23
Almansi, R. J., 203
Ambulatory electrocoma therapy, 172
Amnesia, 35
  hysterical, 35
  in epilepsy, 282, 284
  in head trauma, 313
  in malingering, 228
  in wartime, 228
  retrograde, 228
Amputees, 5, 6
Anemia, pernicious with psychosis, 257
Angelucci, R., 313
Anorexia
  in depression, 125
  in neurosis, 47
Anoxemia (of the brain), 244
Anxiety
  free-floating, 50
  neurosis, 33, 38, (Case PV) 52
Aphasia, 306

Appel, J. W., 30, 57
Argyll-Robertson pupils, 261
Aring, C. D., 328, 330
Arsenic, in neurosyphilis, 273, 276
Arsenoxide (Mapharsen), 273, 276
Arteriosclerosis, 119, 254
Ascroft, P. V., 322, 330
Aspirin, 324
Asthenic body type, 6
Asthmatic breathing due to emotional tension, 39
Ataxia (see Gait disorders), 261, 262
Athletic body type, 6
Atrophy
  muscular, 236
  optic, 262, (Case SM) 276
  traumatic cerebral, 303
Attacks (see Epileptic spells), 327
Auditory hallucinations, 129
Auracraft Shop, 299
Automatic behavior, 265, 284
Autistic thinking, 128
Avitaminosis in alcoholism, 240
  mental symptoms in, 246, 248

B

Back disorders, psychogenic, 41, 45
Bak, R., 203
Balser, B. H., 203
Barbiturates, addiction to, (Case WB) 239
  use in delirium, 252
  use in depression, 122
  use in neurosis, 78, 79
Barnes, M. R., 287, 300
Barrera, S. E., 203
Bateman, J. F., 328, 330
Baur, A. K., 203
Beck, Claude S., viii, 325
Behavior
  antisocial, (Case TM) 206
  automatic, in paresis, 265
  hyperkinetic syndrome, 321
  in manic states, 108
  in psychopathic personality, 206
  in schizophrenia, 134
  influences in children, 26
  manifestations in depression, 104
Belladonna, 79
Bennett, A. E., 124, 126, 183, 203
Beres, D., 203
Betalin, 153
Bibliotherapy, 70

Binkley, George W., viii
Birth trauma, 20
Bismuth, 265
  subsalicylate, 274
Blau, A., 330
Bleuler, E., 157, 224, 225, 241, 255
Body types, 6
Bond, E. D., 154, 157
Bonhoeffer, K., 254
Boston City Hospital, 318
Bowman, K. M., 241, 316, 330
Brain
  arteriosclerosis of, 254
  bullet wound in, 305
  electrical injury of, 318
  hemorrhages (see Head trauma), 301
    extradural, 308
    petechial, 303
    subarachnoid, 306
    subdural, 307
  injury, 20, 301
    confabulations in, 304
    neurological signs in, 314
    physical signs of, 314
    sequellae of, 309
  syphilitic involvement of, 259
  trauma, 301
  tumor, fear of, 37
Brain wave test (Electroencephalogram), 389, 314
Brewer's yeast, use of in delirium, 253
Brief psychotherapy, 63
Bromides
  addiction to, 240
  use in delirium, 252
  use in psychoneurosis, 78
Bruner, A. B., 276
Bruner, W. E., 276
Brunstig, L. A., 279
Brussel, J. A., 227, 241
Buerger's disease, 15

C

Cairns, H., 313, 321, 330, 376
Caldwell, J. M., 242
Catatonia, 143
Catharsis, 59
Character deviation, 22
Charcot's joint, 263
Childhood experiences, 24
Chloral hydrate, 79, (Case WT) 239
  in delirium, 252
Chloride, sodium, 253
Chronokinetic approach, in syphilis, 258
Circulatory symptoms, 42
  disturbances in insulin therapy, 152

Cleckley, H., 157
Cleveland State Hospital, viii
Climate, a factor in environment, 17
Cobb, S., 21, 55, 287, 300
Codeine, 324
Colfer, H. F., 203
Colitis, 18
Coma (see Electrocoma), (see Insulin coma), 318
Combat neurosis, (Case FS) 29, 62, (Case NE) 60
  relieved by psychotherapy, 62
Compulsions, 34
Concussion, brain, 301, 309
  sequence of events in, 316
  treatment of, 324
Confabulations, 245, 317
Consciousness
  clouding of, in alcoholism, 237
  diminution of, in epilepsy, 282, 284
  loss, in epilepsy, 280
Conditioned reflex, 240
Confusion, in psychosis, 245
  syndrome in electrocoma therapy, 183
Compensation, in head trauma, 329
  in neurosis, 95
Constitution, basis of personality, 4
Constitutional inadequacy, (Case LL) 205
Conversion hysteria, (Case DF) 23, 44, 315
  illustrative case history, 26
Convulsions, 265
  drug induced (see Insulin coma therapy), 152
  electrical (see Electrocoma therapy)
  in epilepsy, 280, 281, 283
  in paresis, 266
Coramine, 169
Contusion, of brain, 303
Counsel
  in depression, 121
  in psychoneurosis, 64
Countryman, M. A., 202
Courville, C. B., 301, 329
Coyne, A. R. M., 203
Craine, Gertrude E., viii
Criminalism, (Case EM) 208
Curran, F. J., 242

D

Darwin, C., 54
Dayton, N. A., 108, 126
Deaconess Hospital, 253
Deafness, in psychoneurosis, 36
Death wish, 12
Defect syndromes, 5, 309

INDEX

Deformity, postural, (Case MM) 41
Déja Vu, 284
Delirium, 243
  appearance in, 247
  course and prognosis of, 253
  death in, 253
  disorientation, 245
  disturbances of special senses in, 244
  fear reactions in, 245
  from bromides, 248
  in alcoholism, 248
  in brain injury, 313
  in drug addiction, 250, 252
  in febrile illness, 247
  memory disturbances in, 244
  peripheral nerve disturbances in, 244
  treatment of, 251
  tremens, 249
  tube feeding in, 253
  types of, 247
Delirium tremens, 236, (Case GU) 249
  treatment of, 252, 253
Delusions
  cosmic, 128, 133
  of grandeur, 265
  of persecution, 236, 237
  of visceral nihilism, 117
  somatic, 128
Dementia praecox (see Schizophrenia)
Dementia paralytica (see Paresis), 264
Dementia, traumatic, 318
Denny-Brown, D., 302, 309, 318
Depersonalization, 101
Depression (see Manic depressive psychosis), 199
  alcohol in, 104
  behavior manifestations in, 104
    agitation, 104
    aggressiveness, 106
    self-depreciation, (Case MC) 99, 101
  causes of, 115
  clinical example of, 112
  course of, 106
    cyclic swing, 108
    downward "D's," 123
    spontaneous improvement, 107, 108
  differentiated from psychoneurosis, 116
  duration, 108
  in organic brain disease, 98
  in schizophrenia, 118
  manic states in, 108, (Case SA) 109
    mixed manic depressive states, (Case CB) 110
  nature of, 119
  suicide and, 105, 123
  symptoms, 98, 102, 104
    anorexia, 125
    fatigue, 100
    feelings of unreality, 101
    insomnia, 102, 122
    somatic, 103
  types, 115
    endogenous, 98, 119
    involutional, 115
    reactive, 98, 115, 116, (Case LS) 198
    postpartum, 108
    schizo-depressive, (Case CU) 162
    stupor, 104, 115
  treatment, 120
    activity, 123
    counsel, 121
    electrocoma therapy, 125, (Case LS) 198
    medicinal procedures, 112
    psychotherapy, 120
    sedatives, 104, 123
    self-therapy, 105
    stimulants, 123
Deterioration
  in alcoholism, 237
  in epilepsy, 298
  in schizophrenia, 127
Diabetes, 256
Diencephalon, 8, 38, 188
Diet
  in alcoholism, 253
  in depression, 125
  in head injury, 324
  in neurosis, 80, 125
Digestion, disorders of, in psychoneurosis, 39, 240
Disability
  compensation for, 328
  formula to determine, 14
  in head trauma, 305, 309, 314, 317, 321
Disease, 16, 19
  mental (see Psychosis)
  metabolic, with psychosis, 254
  psychosomatic, 54
  thyroid in organic reaction types, 258
Disorientation, 245
Dissociation, in schizophrenia, 127
Dizziness
  in head trauma, 309
  in psychoneurosis, 37
Dostoevski, 281, 298
Dreams, interpretation of, 92
  terror, in head injury, 315
Drugs
  delirium from, 250
  in treatment of delirium, 251

in treatment of depression, 122
in treatment of epilepsy, 294
in treatment of head trauma, 323
in treatment of syphilis, 251
psychological need for, 240
Drug addiction, (Case WB) 239
Dunbar, F., 7, 57

E

Ebaugh, F. G., 108, 224, 241
Education, 1, 4, 13, 14, 64
  a factor in personality, 13
  of epileptics, 298
Ego, 3
  in neurosis, 46
Electrocoma therapy (shock), 158
  action, mode of, 185
  ambulatory, 172
    advantages, 172
    disadvantages, 172
  clinical change during, 192
  complications, 180
    death, the possibility of, 184
    delirium states, acute toxic, 183
    epilepsy, 193
    injury, 182
    memory disturbance, 176, 180
    traumatic, 182
  course, 167
  family, instructions to, 174, 176
  indications for, (Case SM) 160, (Case ME) 161
  in delirium, 253
  in endogenous depression, 125, 126
  in involutional melancholia, 161
  in manic states, 161, 187
  in manic depressive psychosis, (Case EO) 199
  in psychoneurosis, 94
  in reactive depression, (Case LS) 198
  in schizo-effective disorders, (Case MB) 197
  in schizophrenia, 149, 188, (Case BC) 195, (Case WB), (Case RI) 196
  insulin shock combined with, 193
  Introduction by Foster Kennedy, 158
  medication during, 169
  post-treatment care, 171
  psychotherapy, as an adjunct, 188, 191
  results of, 177, (Case EO) 178
  technique, 164
    apparatus, 164
    dosage, 166
    time factors, 166
  treatment, 168, 169
    maintenance dose, 167
  treatment-resistant cases, 189
Electroencephalogram, viii, 324
  in epilepsy, 289
  in head trauma, 314
  in malingering, a test for blindness, 232
  types of waves, 290
Electroencephalography (Brain Wave Test), 314
Emotional instability, (Case TM) 206
Employment (see Rehabilitation)
  of epileptics, 286, 298
  of syphilitics, 277
Encephalitis, 20
  syphilitic meningo- (General paresis), 261
Encephalopathy, 256, 318
  alcoholic, 243
  arteriosclerotic, 254
  differential diagnosis, 312
  post-traumatic, 308
  traumatic, 305
Endowment, 24, 27
Environment, 11, 13, 17
  an evocative force, 211
  changing the, 74
Epilepsy
  attacks, prevention of, 294
  types of
    grand mal, 280
    Jacksonian, 283
    petit mal, 282
    psychomotor equivalent, (Case JS) 293
    status epilepticus, 297
    uncinate gyrus fits, 284
  causes of, 287
  drugs in, 294, 296
  electroencephalogram, use in, 289
  education and employment in, 298
  history-taking in, 288
  medication in, 294, 296
  psychotherapy in, 297
  symptoms
    primary, 280
    psychological, 286
    secondary, 285
  trauma and, 293
  treatment of, 294
  types of
    idiopathic, 288
    symptomatic, 288
    traumatic, 293, 321
Erickson, T. C., 300
Escape, 46
  drugs, a means of, 240

Euphoria, residual, 318
Evans, V. L., 202
Extravert, 3, (Case CB) 4

F

Family, and illness, 19
 cooperation in electrocoma therapy, 174
Farrell, M. J., 57
Fatigue, 33
Fear, 3, 12, 18, 22, 33
 in psychoneurosis, 49, 50
 reactions, in psychosis, 245
 of syphilis, 28
Feldman, F., 185, 203
Fever therapy, in paresis, 119
Finesinger, J. E., 55
Focal loss, in head trauma, 305
Foerster, O., 293, 300
Foulkes, S. H., 96
Free association, 92
Freeman, W., 157, 203
French, T. M., vii, 68, 93, 96
Freud, Sigmund, vii, 3, 12, 20, 24, 51, 57, 106
Freudenberg, R., 157
Friedman, E., 202
Friedman, M. D., 182
Froelich's syndrome, 11
Frosch, J., 203
Frustration, 10, 14
 sexual, 43

G

Gait, disorders, 41, 46, 80
 hysterical, 41, 46
 in alcoholism, 236
 in brain injury, 309
 in locomotor ataxia, 262
Ganglion cells, 301, 309, 313
Gastro-intestinal tract
 disorders, due to emotion, 39, 47
 symptoms in depression, 103
Gellhorn, E., 188, 203
Genito-urinary tract, disorders in neurosis, 42
Gibbs, F. A., viii, 289, 300
Gillespie, R. F., 216, 221, 241, 254, 312, 329
Glial scar tissue, 309
Glucose, in delirium, 252
Glueck, S., 204, 222, 224, 241
Goals, 3, 10, 15
Goldman, D., 202
Goldstein, K., 46, 57, 314, 330
Gordon, Maurice B., viii, 149

Greve, B., 300
Grinker, R. R., 41, 51, 96, 300
Grothe, Phyllis, viii
Group spirit, 18
Group psychotherapy, 87
Guilt, 22, 29, 88
 in depression, 99, 104
 mechanism, in neurosis, 27
 sense of, (Case JH) 29
 skin symptoms, 44
Gumma (see Neurosyphilis), 259, 262

H

Hadfield, J. A., 80, 96
Hall, V. R., 300
Hallucinations, 129
 auditory, 129
 gustatory, 131
 in delirium, 247
 olfactory, 130
 tactile, 130
 visual, 130
 zooscopic, (Case CS) 319
Harbin, M., 41
Harris, R. E., 316
Harrison D. K., 217, 241
Hassin, G. B., 301, 329
Head trauma, 45, 301
 amnesia in, 313
 clinical and physical changes induced by, 301
 contusions and lacerations, 303, (Case CD) 304
 delirium in, 313
 effects of, 308
 encephalopathy, post-traumatic, 308
 epilepsy and, 321
 hemiplegia in, 305
 hemorrhage in, 302
 loss of consciousness in, 313
 neurological signs in, 314
 neurosis and, 311, 315
 personality affected by, 312
 psychosis in, (Case DS) 317, 318
 speech defects in, 327
 symptoms, special, 314
  advantage of, 315
 treatment of, 323, 325
 type and severity of, 312
Headache, 40
 in brain injury, 307
 in head trauma, 45
 in neurosis, 36, 314, 325
Health resort, a form of treatment, 18
Hearing disorders, 36
Heart

and circulatory symptoms in neurosis, 37
disease, 38
murmurs, 38
Hemiplegia, 46
  acute syphilitic involvement of the brain, 260
  in head trauma, 306
Hemorrhage, 301
  in brain injury, 302
  extradural, 308
  gross, 303
  petechial, 303
  subarachnoid, 306
  subdural, 306
Henderson, D. K., 211, 241, 254
Heredity
  and depression, 117
  and psychoneurosis, 22
Herzberg, A., 70, 96
Hinsie, L. E., 3, 20, 96
Hitch, K. S., 227, 241
Hoch, P. H., 150, 157, 203
Holbrook, C. S., 185, 203
Home
  atmosphere, 13
  influences on personality, 3
  security, 11
Homosexuality, 212
  of biological origin, 215
  cultural pressure in, 215
  delusions of, 128, 146
  true, 215
Hormones, use of
  in depression, 120
  influence of, on mood, 120
Horney, K., 25, 92, 97
Hospital environment, 19
Hostility, 8, 28
Hydrotherapy, in treatment of delirium, 252
Hyoscine hydrobromide, 252
Hypnosis, 80
Hypertension, emotional, 47
Hysteria, (Case DJ) 31, (Case MM) 41, (Case AB) 42
  amnesia in, 35
  conversion, 315
  dramatic convulsions, a form of, 18
  gait disorders in, 41, 46
  hemiplegia in, 46
  industrial pattern of, 20
  paralysis in, 52, 81, 82
  treatment of, 81, 82
  scoliosis and pain in, 41

I

Id, 3

Identification, 46
Illness, 3
  man and, 16
  mental attitude and, 14
Impastato, D. J., 203
Impotence, 43, 46
  in alcoholism, 237
Imitation of symptoms, 18
Inadequacy, feelings of, 8
Inductotherm, 275
Industry
  psychopathy in, 218
  vertebral neurosis in, 46
Inferiority, organic and physical, 8
Influenza, delirium with febrile illness, 247
Inheritance (see Heredity), 22
Insanity (see Psychosis)
Insomnia
  in depression, 122
  in post-concussional states, 309
Instability, emotional (see Psychopathic personality), (Case TM) 206
  in psychosis, 254
  psychological, 312
Instinct, 14
  of death, 20
  of love, 20
  of self-preservation, 18
Insulin
  in psychoneurosis, 79
  in treatment of delirium, 252
Insulin coma therapy, 149
  administration, technique of, 150
    course, 152
    dosage, 150
    manifestations during coma, 151
    termination of coma, 151
  complications of, 152
    circulatory disturbance, 152
    coma prolonged, 153
    convulsive reaction, 152
    death, 153
    hunger excitement, 152
    respiratory difficulties, 152
  illustrative case histories, (RI), (GR), 154
  indications for use, 156
  results, 153
Intelligence, 9
  in epilepsy, 287
Intocostrin, 169, 183, 185
Injury (see Trauma)
  a factor in nervous symptoms, 50
  back (see)
  head, 301
  mental attitude and, 14
Introvert, (Case PA) 3

INDEX

Involuntary movements, 41
Involutional melancholia (see Depression), 103, 115, 117
   indications for electrocoma therapy, 161

J

Jackson, A. H., 203
Jackson, Hughlings, 185, 283
James, William, 205
Jealousy, 205
Jelliffe, S. E., 95, 96, 157
Jennings, H. S., 211
Jessner, L., 150, 157, 203
Jones, M., 97

K

Kalinowsky, L. B., 149, 157, 161, 185, 202, 203
Kamellin, S., 265
Kardiner, A., 315
Karpman, B., 242
Katz, E., vii
Katzenelbogen, S., 203
Kennedy, A., 157
Kennedy, Foster, vii, 158
Kerman, E. F., 203
Kessler, M., 203
Korsakoff's syndrome, 237, 378
Kozol, H. L., 295, 300
Kraepelin, E., 137
Kraines, S. H., 157
Kretschmer, E., 6, 20
Kubie, L., 64, 69, 91, 92

L

Lakeside Hospital, 41, 237
Lennox, W. G., vii, 282, 287, 300
Levine, M., 70
Lewy, E., 330
Liberson, W. T., 200
Libido, 51
Liefer, W., 274
Lipetz, B., 203
Lobeline, 152
Lobotomy, 187, 194, 318
   in schizophrenia, 156
Lumbago, 40
Love
   instinct, 51
   object, 12
Lying, pathological, 207
Lynn, J. G., 309

M

Madden, J. J., 202
Maladjustment (see Psychopathic personality), 317

Malamud, W., 212, 241
Malaria, 247
   in treatment of syphilis, 275
   induced, 264
Malingering, (Case RB) 228
   amnesia in, 228
   detection of, 237
   feigned psychoneurosis, 232
   in service, (Case BM) 226
   symptoms of, 228
   types of, 226
Malzberg, B., 157
Manic depressive psychosis (see Depression), (Case EO) 199
   mixed, (Case CB) 110, (Case AL) 200
   typical example of, 113
Manic states, 108, (Case SA) 109
   in paresis, 268
Marijuana, 207
Masochism, 25
Masturbation, 68
Melancholia (see Involutional), 103
Memory disturbance
   in alcoholism, 237
   in brain lesion, 209
   in electrocoma therapy, 180, 244
   in psychoneurosis, 34
   in psychosis, 254
Menninger, K. A., 20, 21, 96
Menigitis
   acute in syphilis, 259, 261
   fear of, (Case JH) 28
Meningoencephalitis, 277
Merritt, H. Houston, 294, 297, 300
Mesantoin, 295
Metrazol, 149
Meyer, Robert, 226
Minnesota Multiphasic Test, 232
Mira, E., 50, 57, 217, 241
Mohr, C. F., 276, 297
Moore, J. E., 275, 276, 278, 279
Moriarty, J. D., 160, 202
Morphine
   addiction to, 149
   in delirium, 252
Müller, M., 153, 157
Muscular disorders, 40
Myerson, A., 22, 24, 203, 205, 211, 215, 223, 224, 228, 232, 241, 242

N

Napoleon, 2, 226, 298
Narco-analysis, 84, (Case TE) 85
Narco-synthesis, 84
Nembutal
   addiction to, 240
Neoarsphenamine, 205

Nervous manifestations (see Psychoneurosis),
Neurasthenia, 52
Neuritis
  alcoholic, 237
  peripheral, 244
Neuropsychatric Institute of Cleveland, vii
Neuropathic traits, 317
Neurosis (see Psychoneurosis)
Neurosyphilis, 258
  asymptomatic, 261
  classifications of, 261
  common clinical syndromes, 262
    gumma, 259
    meningovascular types, 261, 269
    optic nerve atrophy, 263
    paresis (dementia paralytica) 264
    tabes dorsalis, (Case PS) 262, (Case SB) 263
    tabo-paresis, 261
  course of, 261
  depression with, 119
  diagnosis of, 271
  dormancy of, 259
  hemiplegia in, 260
  laboratory and physical findings, 271
  rehabilitation of the patient, 277
  symptoms, causes of, 270
  treatment of, 272
Neymann, C. A., 202
Nomadism, (Case TM) 206
Norris, D. C., 226, 241
Noyes, A. P., 117, 126, 157, 205, 206, 241

O

Obsessions, 34
Obsessional neurosis, (Case ND) 34, 52
Occupational therapy (see Rehabilitation)
Organic reaction types, 254
O'Leary, James, vii, 276
Overcompensation, 8, 19
Overprotectiveness, 19
Oxophenarsine hydrochloride, 274, 276
Ozzipov, V. P., 227, 232

P

Pain, 4
Palmer, H. A., 318, 330
Paraldehyde, 239, 297
  in delirium, 252
Paralysis
  post-traumatic, 325
Paranoid states
  in alcoholism, 237
  in schizophrenia, 143
  in toxic psychosis, 286

Paresis (see Neurosyphilis), 119, 264
  personality changes in, (Case DW) 265, (Case LI) 266, (Case CW) 267
Parran, T., 278
Paskind, H. A., 300
Pathology
  in epilepsy, 288
  in head trauma, 302
  in paresis, 260, 270
  in tabes dorsalis, 262
  organic, 262
Patry, F. L., 203
Penfield, W., 288, 293, 300, 321
Perlson, J., 202
Perseveration
  in delirium, (Case RS) 248
  in organic reaction types, 255
Personality (see Psychopathic)
  antisocial, 12, 204, 206
  defined, 3, 4
  factors which influence, 3
    energy, 8
    environment, 11, 13
    intelligence, 9
    parents, 3, 12
    personal appearance, 10
    religion, 13
    trauma, 312
  inadequate, 205
  importance in illness, (Case PA), (Case CB) 4, (Case AC) 9, 12
  subdivisions of, 3
  types of
    extravert, 3
    introvert, (Case PA) 3
    pre-psychotic, 117
    psychopathic, 3, 204
    rigid, 3
    schizoid, 3
Phenobarbital, 79, 152, 282, 294, 324
  in epilepsy, 297
  in psychoneurosis, 79
Phobias, 34
Physiological reaction, 14
Picrotoxin, 124
Pilcher, C., 313, 330
Pneumoencephalogram, 389, 314
Polyneuritis
  in alcoholism, 236
Polysurgery, 95
Porter, William C., 217, 241, 312, 329
Post-war period and the veteran, 19
Posture disorders, 35
Pratt, J. H., 89, 96
Premature ejaculation, 43
Projection, 311

Psychoanalysis, 90
  analyst, dual role of the, 93
  fundamental concepts of, 90
  modifications of, 93
  procedures, 92
    dream interpretation, 92
    explanation and discussion, 92
    free association, 92
    transference, 92
Psychoneurosis, 22
  alcoholism in, 233
  brain injury with, 313
  causes of, 22
  childhood experiences, effect of, 24
  classifications of, 52
  combat, (Case FS) 29
  definition of, 22
  differential diagnosis of, 312
  drug addiction in, 239
  effect of injury in, (Case DJ) 50
  head injury with, 311
  heredity and, 22
  symptomatology of, 44
  symptoms of, 33
    choice of, 44
    circulatory, 37
    disorders of
      gait, 41
      posture, 35
      special senses, 35
    effectiveness of, 46
    gastro-intestinal, 39, 47, 52
    general, 33, 44
    genito-urinary, 42
    head, 36
    heart, 37
    mental, 34
    muscular, 40
    phobias, 34
    reality, sense of, 22
    respiratory, 39
    sexual, 43
    skin, 44
    sleep disturbances, 50
    tremors, 45
    vertebral, 11, 15, (Case MM) 41, (Case AB) 42, 45
    weakness, 33
  treatment of, 58
    electrocoma therapy, indications for, 94, 163
    medicinal, 78
    psychotherapy, 58
    recreational, 70
    suggestion, 37
    work, 72
  types of, 45
    anxiety, 52
    cardiac, 52
    constitutional, 53
    hysterical, 33, 44, 52
    neurasthenic, 59
    obsessional, 34, 52
    situational, 53, (Case NE) 60
    traumatic, 45
Psychopathic personality, 204
  causes, 221
  detection of, 232
  in the German Army, 218
  in industry, 218 (Case VG) 219
  nature of, 220
  treatment of, (Case BF) 223, 224
    analysis, 225
    hypnosis, 225
    psychotherapy, 224
    rehabilitation, 225, 263
  types of
    antisocial, 206
    constitutional inadequacy, 205, 211
    criminalism, 208
    emotional instability, (Case TM) 206
    female psychopath, (Case VM) 210
    inadequate personality, 205
    nomadism, 206, 212
    paranoid personality, 205
    pathological lying, 207
    sexual, 212
Psychosomatic disorders, 39, 54, (Case AJ) 56
  digestive, 39
  genito-urinary tract, 42, 43
  head symptoms, 36
  heart and circulatory, 37
  muscular, 40
  special senses, 35
Psychosis, 199
  treatment of
    electrocoma therapy, 169
    insulin coma therapy, 149
    psychotherapy, 191
  types of
    alcoholic, 104, 232
    arteriosclerotic, 254
    depressive, 160, 199
    involutional, 115
    manic depressive, (Case NZ) 113, (Case AL) 200
    organic reaction, 243, 254
    paretic, 264
    schizophrenic, 127, 253
    senile, 163
    toxic, 243, 253
    traumatic, 317, 318

Psychotherapy, 58
  adjunct of electrocoma therapy, 191
  brief, (Case NE) 60, 62, (Case MC) 63
  drugs and, 78
  group, 87, 90
  in alcoholism, 238
  in depression, 120
  in epilepsy, 297
  in psychoneurosis, 58
  in syphilis, 272
  methods of
    education, 64
    environmental change, 76
    hospitalization, 77
    hypnosis, 80
    narco-analysis, 84
    narco-synthesis, 84
    narco-therapy, 84
    occupation, 72
    persuasion, 64
    psychoanalysis, 90
    reasoning, 64
    suggestion, (Case DJ) 80, (Case MR) 82
  work an aid in, 72
Punishment, 13
Putnam, T. J., 294, 297, 300
Pyknic body type, 6

R

Rashkis, H. A., 90
Reactions, psychological, 45
Reality, 27
  adjustment to, in alcoholism, 237
  feelings of unreality in depression, 101
Religion, influence on personality, 13
Rehabilitation, 19
  in head trauma, 325
  in neurosyphilis, 277
  of the epileptic, 298
  of the psychoneurotic, 70, 72, 74
  of the psychopath, 26
Ressell, W. R., 329
Reynolds, F. W., 279, 297
Rivers, T., 252
Rorschach Ink Blot Test, 314
Ross, J. R., 157
Rossett, J., 244
Rowbotham, G. F., 302, 309, 321
Ruesch, J., 309, 316, 329
Ryan, V. G., 157, 203

S

Sakel, M., 149, 157
Sargant, W., 125, 126
Schilder, Paul, 17, 25, 26, 58, 88, 224

Schizo-affective disorders, 119, 143, (Case MB) 197
Schizo-depressions, 127
Schizophrenia, 127
  acute schizophrenic reaction, 196
  affect in, 134
  alcoholism and, 237
  causes of, 145
  common symptoms, 128, 136
    behavior disturbances, 134
    delusions, 136
    emotional disturbances, 134
    hallucinations, 129
      auditory, 129
      gustatory, 131
      olfactory, 130
      tactile, 130
      visual, 130
    ideas of reference, 136
    language disorders, 135
  course, 137
  treatment, 147
    electrocoma therapy, 160
    insulin coma therapy, 149
    psychotherapy, 148
  types of, (Case PF) 127, 142
    catatonic, 143
    dementia praecox, 127
    hebephrenic, 143, 195
    paranoid, 143, (Case RI) 196
    schizo-affective, (Case MB) 197
    simplex, 142
Schizophrenic-like reactions, (Cases SN, PB) 140, 146
School of Military Neuropsychiatry, vii
Scoliosis, 41
Schwartz, L. A., 97
Secondary gain, in psychoneurosis, 50
Sedation
  in delirium, 251
  in depression, 122
Self-depreciation, 35, 101, 117
Sex act, 13, 43
  aversion for, 43
Sex hormone, 124
Sexual difficulties
  impotence, 43, 46
  premature ejaculation, 43
Sezary, A., 259, 278
Shatzky, J., 3, 20, 96
Shock therapy (see Electrocoma therapy), 94, (Insulin coma), 149
Shurley, J. T., 154, 157
Silverman, D., 221, 241
Singer, H. D., 157
Skin, 44
Skull, depressed fracture of, 324

INDEX

Slater, E., 126
Sleep disturbances
  in depression, 102
  in psychoneurosis, 44
Social service data on selectees, 224
Sodium amytal, 80, 231, 232, 297, 324
  use of in delirium, 252
  use in drug addiction, 240
  use in electrocoma therapy, 235
  use in malingering, 232
  use in narco-analysis, 84
Sodium dilantin, 349
Solomon, H. C., 241, 242, 279
Speech
  defects in head trauma, 327
  disturbances in, 237
  loss of, (Case LB) 306
Spiegel, J. P., 46, 56, 57, 96
Spinal cord, degeneration in alcoholism, 236
Spinal fluid
  alterations in circulation of, 301
  changes of, in trauma, 365
  "paretic formula," 261
Status epilepticus, 297
Steiger, H. P., 276, 279
Stephen, K., 26, 57, 96
Strophanthin, 152
Stokes, J. H., 279
Storch, A., 133, 157
Strauss, M. B., 241
Strecker, E. A., vii, 108, 126, 163, 242, 252
Subdural haematoma, 304, 307, 312
Sucrose, 324
Suggestibility, of neurotics, 37
Suggestion, (Case DJ) 80, (Case MR) 82
Suicide, 105, 123
  in depression, 105
  "partial," 95
  prevention of, 123
Sulfa drugs
  use in delirium, 251
  use in head injury, 323
Sulfadiazine, 248
Superego, 2, 13, 24, 104
Susselman, S., 203
Symonds, C. P., 312
Symptoms
  imitation of, 18
  prolongation of, 317
  unique meaning of, 17
Syphilis (see Neurosyphilis)

T

Tabes dorsalis, 261, 262, (Case RE) 264
Taboparesis, 261

Templeton, C. H., 157
Tests
  Babcock, 320
  electroencephalogram (brain wave), 314
  Minnesota Multiphasic, 232
  psychological, 309, 314
  Rorschach, 314
  serological, 271
Therapy, 58
  bibliotherapy, 70
  electrocoma therapy, 158
  group, 87
  insulin coma (see)
  malaria fever therapy, 276
  occupational, 95
  penicillin, 276
  psychoanalysis (see)
  psychotherapy (see)
  self-therapy (secondary symptom in depression), 105
  shock, (see Electrocoma therapy)
  work as, (see Rehabilitation)
Thiamine chloride, 252
Thomas, G. A., 96
Thompson, G. N., 203
Tietz, E. B., 203
Titley, W. B., 117, 126
Transference, 92
Trauma (see Head trauma; also Injury), 301, 308
Treatment (see Therapy)
Tremors
  in alcoholism, 235
  in paresis, 265
  in psychoneurosis, 41
Tridione, 292, 296
Tryparsamide, 119, 264, 265
  in neurosyphilis, 277
Tubular vision, 35
Tumor
  brain, 243
  with psychosis, 257
Typhoid, delirium with febrile illness, 247

U

Unemployment and the veteran, 19
University Hospitals, 240
Urinary symptoms, 42
Urse, V. G., 212

V

Van Harreveld, A., 203
Vigotsky, L. S., 157
Visual disturbances
  in brain trauma, (Case AS) 309
  in neurosyphilis, 263
  in psychoneurosis, 35

Vertebral neurosis (see Back disorders)
Veteran, handicapped, 18
  psychoneurotic, 33
Vitamins
  in alcoholism, (Case ME) 236
  in toxic psychosis, 252
Von Jauregg, W., 275

W

War neurosis (see Combat)
Watts, J. W., 157, 203
Weakness, a symptom of psychoneurosis, 33
Wechsler, D., 21
Wechsler, I., 57
Weil, A. A., vii, 97, 160, 202
Wender, L., 97
Wilbur, C. B., 126
Wilcox, P., 202
Williams, D., 330
Williams, Guy, 186, 314
Wilson, E. J., vii, 287
Work (see Rehabilitation)
  interest in, 74
  material reward, 73
  social aspects of, 73
Wortis, H., 242
Wortis, S. B., 203

X

X-ray, in brain injury, 324

Y

Yakolev, P. I., vii, 241, 242

Z

Zilboorg, G., 21